Global Applications of One Health Practice and Care

Sandul Yasobant
Center for Development Research (ZEF), Germany

Deepak Saxena
Indian Institute of Public Health Gandhinagar, India

A volume in the Advances in Medical Diagnosis, Treatment, and Care (AMDTC) Book Series

IGI Global
DISSEMINATOR OF KNOWLEDGE

Published in the United States of America by
IGI Global
Medical Information Science Reference (an imprint of IGI Global)
701 E. Chocolate Avenue
Hershey PA, USA 17033
Tel: 717-533-8845
Fax: 717-533-8661
E-mail: cust@igi-global.com
Web site: http://www.igi-global.com

Library of Congress Cataloging-in-Publication Data

Names: Yasobant, Sandul, 1988- editor. | Saxena, Deepak, 1972- editor.
Title: Global applications of one health practice and care / Sandul Yasobant and Deepak Saxena, editors.
Description: Hershey, PA : Medical Information Science Reference, [2019] | Includes bibliographical references.
Identifiers: LCCN 2018008105| ISBN 9781522563044 (hardcover) | ISBN 9781522563051 (ebook)
Subjects: | MESH: One Health | Communicable Disease Control | Global Health
Classification: LCC RA441 | NLM WA 30.7 | DDC 362.1--dc23 LC record available at https://lccn.loc.gov/2018008105

This book is published in the IGI Global book series Advances in Medical Diagnosis, Treatment, and Care (AMDTC) (ISSN: 2475-6628; eISSN: 2475-6636)

British Cataloguing in Publication Data
A Cataloguing in Publication record for this book is available from the British Library.

Advances in Medical Diagnosis, Treatment, and Care (AMDTC) Book Series

ISSN:2475-6628
EISSN:2475-6636

MISSION

Advancements in medicine have prolonged the life expectancy of individuals all over the world. Once life-threatening conditions have become significantly easier to treat and even cure in many cases. Continued research in the medical field will further improve the quality of life, longevity, and wellbeing of individuals.

The **Advances in Medical Diagnosis, Treatment, and Care (AMDTC)** book series seeks to highlight publications on innovative treatment methodologies, diagnosis tools and techniques, and best practices for patient care. Comprised of comprehensive resources aimed to assist professionals in the medical field apply the latest innovations in the identification and management of medical conditions as well as patient care and interaction, the books within the AMDTC series are relevant to the research and practical needs of medical practitioners, researchers, students, and hospital administrators.

COVERAGE

- Medical Procedures
- Alternative Medicine
- Disease Prevention
- Medical Testing
- Experimental Medicine
- Emergency Medicine
- Internal Medicine
- Disease Management
- Cancer Treatment
- Diagnostic Medicine

IGI Global is currently accepting manuscripts for publication within this series. To submit a proposal for a volume in this series, please contact our Acquisition Editors at Acquisitions@igi-global.com or visit: http://www.igi-global.com/publish/.

The Advances in Medical Diagnosis, Treatment, and Care (AMDTC) Book Series (ISSN 2475-6628) is published by IGI Global, 701 E. Chocolate Avenue, Hershey, PA 17033-1240, USA, www.igi-global.com. This series is composed of titles available for purchase individually; each title is edited to be contextually exclusive from any other title within the series. For pricing and ordering information please visit http://www.igi-global.com/book-series/advances-medical-diagnosis-treatment-care/129618. Postmaster: Send all address changes to above address.

Titles in this Series

For a list of additional titles in this series, please visit:
https://www.igi-global.com/book-series/advances-medical-diagnosis-treatment-care/129618

Pre-Screening Systems for Early Disease Prediction, Detection, and Prevention
Thierry Edoh (Technical University of Munich, Germany) Pravin Pawar (Philips Research, India) and Sagar Mohammad (Philips Researc, India)
Medical Information Science Reference • ©2019 • 395pp • H/C (ISBN: 9781522571315) • US $245.00

Advanced Methodologies and Technologies in Medicine and Healthcare
Mehdi Khosrow-Pour, D.B.A. (Information Resources Management Associaton, USA)
Medical Information Science Reference • ©2019 • 591pp • H/C (ISBN: 9781522574897) • US $325.00

Handbook of Research on Critical Examinations of Neurodegenerative Disorders
Md. Sahab Uddin (Southeast University, Bangladesh) and Md. Shah Amran (University of Dhaka, Bangladesh)
Medical Information Science Reference • ©2019 • 597pp • H/C (ISBN: 9781522552826) • US $345.00

Effective Techniques for Managing Trigeminal Neuralgia
Steven Chang (Stanford University, USA) and Allen Ho (Stanford University, USA)
Medical Information Science Reference • ©2018 • 331pp • H/C (ISBN: 9781522553496) • US $225.00

Handbook of Research on Geriatric Health, Treatment, and Care
Barre Vijaya Prasad (Dharwad Institute of Mental Health and Neurosciences (DIMHANS), India) and Shamsi Akbar (King George's Medical University, India)
Medical Information Science Reference • ©2018 • 604pp • H/C (ISBN: 9781522534808) • US $375.00

For an entire list of titles in this series, please visit:
https://www.igi-global.com/book-series/advances-medical-diagnosis-treatment-care/129618

IGI Global
DISSEMINATOR OF KNOWLEDGE

701 East Chocolate Avenue, Hershey, PA 17033, USA
Tel: 717-533-8845 x100 • Fax: 717-533-8661
E-Mail: cust@igi-global.com • www.igi-global.com

Editorial Advisory Board

Table of Contents

Foreword xv

Preface xvi

Section 1

Chapter 1
Emerging Global Health Approaches at the Human-Animal Interface: Conceptual and Historical Issues of One Health 1
Walter Bruchhausen, University of Bonn, Germany

Chapter 2
We Are Not Part of Nature; We Are Nature: An African View on One Health 33
Ike Iyioke, University of Michigan – Flint, USA

Chapter 3
One Health Study Design 59
Punit Jhandai, Lala Lajpat Rai University of Veterinary and Animal Sciences, India

Section 2

Chapter 4
One Health and Parasites 82
Said Sajjad Ali Shah, Veterinary Research Institute, Pakistan
Adnan Khan, Wildlife Department, Khyber Pakhtunkhwa, Pakistan

Chapter 5
Veterinary Public Health: The Planetary Path to One Health 113
Utpal Das, The Kolkata Municipal Corporation, India

Chapter 6
Antibiotic Resistance in the Veterinary Perspective: A Major Challenge in Achieving One Health 142
Sophia Inbaraj, Indian Veterinary Research Institute, India
Vamshi Krishna Sriram, College of Veterinary Science, India
Prasad Thomas, Indian Veterinary Research Institute, India
Abhishek Verma, Indian Veterinary Research Institute, India
Pallab Chaudhuri, Indian Veterinary Research Institute, India

Section 3

Chapter 7
Risk Management and Risk Communication in the Case of Vector-Borne Disease: Case of Macedonia – Risk Management in VBDs 159
Sekovska Blagica, University St. Kiril and Methodius, Macedonia
Stefanovska Jovana, University St. Kiril and Methodius, Macedonia

Chapter 8
A One Health Perspective on Q Fever: Part 1 174
Rita Cruz, Polytechnic Institute of Viseu, Portugal
Carmen Vasconcelos-Nobrega, Polytechnic Institute of Viseu, Portugal & University of Trás-os-Montes and Alto Douro, Portugal
Fernando Esteves, Polytechnic Institute of Viseu, Portugal
Catarina Coelho, Polytechnic Institute of Viseu, Portugal & University of Trás-os-Montes and Alto Douro, Portugal
Ana Sofia Ferreira, University of Oporto, Portugal
Carla Santos, Polytechnic Institute of Viseu, Portugal
Cristina Mega, Polytechnic Institute of Viseu, Portugal
Ana C. Coelho, University of Trás-os-Montes and Alto Douro, Portugal
Helena Vala, Polytechnic Institute of Viseu, Portugal & University of Trás-os-Montes and Alto Douro, Portugal
João R. Mesquita, University of Oporto, Portugal

Chapter 9
A One Health Perspective on Q Fever: Part 2 195
Rita Cruz, Polytechnic Institute of Viseu, Portugal
Carmen Vasconcelos-Nobrega, Polytechnic Institute of Viseu, Portugal & University of Trás-os-Montes and Alto Douro, Portugal
Fernando Esteves, Polytechnic Institute of Viseu, Portugal
Catarina Coelho, Polytechnic Institute of Viseu, Portugal & University of Trás-os-Montes and Alto Douro, Portugal
Ana Sofia Ferreira, University of Oporto, Portugal
Carla Santos, Polytechnic Institute of Viseu, Portugal
Cristina Mega, Polytechnic Institute of Viseu, Portugal
Ana C. Coelho, University of Trás-os-Montes and Alto Douro, Portugal
Helena Vala, Polytechnic Institute of Viseu, Portugal & University of Trás-os-Montes and Alto Douro, Portugal
João R. Mesquita, University of Oporto, Portugal

Compilation of References 217

Related References 266

About the Contributors 299

Index 305

Detailed Table of Contents

Foreword xv

Preface xvi

Section 1

Chapter 1
Emerging Global Health Approaches at the Human-Animal Interface:
Conceptual and Historical Issues of One Health 1
Walter Bruchhausen, University of Bonn, Germany

The vagueness of the term one health is the result of multiple developments that it has brought together. Therefore, a historical and conceptual analysis, divided in three sections, is performed for understanding these tensions and their backgrounds. First, an account of different and changing attitudes towards animals and their health is given, especially in religion, modern philosophy, and pre-modern dealing with disease supposedly caused by animals and plants. The second part reconstructs early bacteriology as a search for environmental disease factors and a struggle with zoonoses in a globalized research effort. The final and largest section analyses the development of international policies on zoonoses and one health from the 1950s until today, sketching the way from a veterinarian and medical national public health issue via socio-economic perspectives to the perception of a global threat by emerging diseases which fueled inter-agency cooperation in an unprecedented manner.

Chapter 2
We Are Not Part of Nature; We Are Nature: An African View on One
Health..33
Ike Iyioke, University of Michigan – Flint, USA

This chapter explores holism as it pertains to health in African thought. Specifically, it uses the philosophical notion of personhood to illustrate holism within the biomedical research context. In African philosophy, nature is an organic whole, and the creation and sustenance of ecological balance or interdependence between human and non-humans, the visible and the invisible are most desired. The individual is anchored in a mesh of relationships within the family, village, environment, all of whom are primordial sources of that person's physical, psychic, and spiritual existence and wellbeing. It is a fallacy, indeed absurd to think that humans can exist or act as though they are independent of the environment they live in while continually sensing it via sight, touch, hearing, smell, and taste. In a sense, humans are not just a part of nature; they are nature. It is a holistic perspective, as opposed to anthropocentrism. The continued neglect of this philosophical perspective in favor exclusively of anthropocentrism or individualism is the cause of much human crisis.

Chapter 3
One Health Study Design...59
Punit Jhandai, Lala Lajpat Rai University of Veterinary and Animal Sciences, India

One health is an integrated approach that considers human, animal, and environmental health components that can improve prediction. One health implies that data on man and animal health and environmental indicators are studied and interpreted together. This chapter focuses on population-based quantitative and qualitative one health study designs with an emphasis on field surveys to understand disease dynamics and how to control measures being tested. The aim is not on early diagnoses of emerging diseases but instead of that on endemic zoonosis. It first describes examples on joint monitoring and surveillance to control diseases and then practical information on planning of a field study design, and concludes on the advantages of one health study designs. Also discussed are possible constraints for their implementation. For the examples, single sector approach could not explain the main epidemiological considerations.

Section 2

Chapter 4
One Health and Parasites 82
Said Sajjad Ali Shah, Veterinary Research Institute, Pakistan
Adnan Khan, Wildlife Department, Khyber Pakhtunkhwa, Pakistan

One health is a collective term used to address human and animal health issues under one platform. More than half of the diseases of humans are directly or indirectly related to animal health and spread from animals to humans or vice versa. Etiological agents of zoonotic diseases may be bacterial, viral, or parasitic in origin. Among them, parasitic agents are very important because they are either directly involved as etiological agents or as vectors of other pathogenic organisms. Parasitic zoonoses are transmitted to humans through vectors, food, or drinking water, and thus categorized as vector borne, food borne, and water borne parasitic zoonoses. Food borne and water borne parasitic zoonoses include all those parasitic diseases which are transmitted to humans by consuming contaminated food and water. An extensive alliance is necessary amongst physicians, veterinarians, and public health workers for timely response and approach to guarantee the prevention and management of infections.

Chapter 5
Veterinary Public Health: The Planetary Path to One Health............................113
Utpal Das, The Kolkata Municipal Corporation, India

Health and disease have always co-existed with man and animal. One medicine concept was developed in ancient times as recorded in the writings of Greek and Roman scholars. In the ecological context, animal activities tend to influence welfare of man in a number of ways and vice versa. The veterinarians are the only healthcare professionals likely to see both people and their animals and aware of the potential threat of zoonotic infections to clients. History behind conceptualization of veterinary public health to one health is discussed thoroughly, and eventually, veterinary public health is referred to as the planetary route and path to one health.

Chapter 6
Antibiotic Resistance in the Veterinary Perspective: A Major Challenge in Achieving One Health...142
Sophia Inbaraj, Indian Veterinary Research Institute, India
Vamshi Krishna Sriram, College of Veterinary Science, India
Prasad Thomas, Indian Veterinary Research Institute, India
Abhishek Verma, Indian Veterinary Research Institute, India
Pallab Chaudhuri, Indian Veterinary Research Institute, India

Antibiotic resistance is an emerging threat to achieving one health all over the globe. The phenomenon leads to the emergence of drug-resistant microbes previously susceptible to an antibiotic. Drug-resistant microbes are the major reasons for medical complications like patient mortality and treatment failure. Unregulated use of antibiotics in animal husbandry is one of the major reasons for the emergence of antibiotic resistance. The resistance enters the human population mainly through the food chain. The genetic markers associated with drug resistance spread among different bacterial species by horizontal gene transfer mechanisms. Therefore, regulation of antibiotics use in animal husbandry and proper safety measures at farm level are necessary to check drug-resistant microbes entering the food chain. This chapter discusses the antibiotics, antibiotic resistance, genetic mechanisms involved, the spread of resistance, and also the available strategies to combat antimicrobial drug resistance.

Section 3

Chapter 7
Risk Management and Risk Communication in the Case of Vector-Borne Disease: Case of Macedonia – Risk Management in VBDs 159
Sekovska Blagica, University St. Kiril and Methodius, Macedonia
Stefanovska Jovana, University St. Kiril and Methodius, Macedonia

Change in environmental and socio-economic, emerging zoonotic diseases will be an increasing challenge for public health in Europe and in Macedonia also. The risks and consequences triggered by vector-borne diseases (VBD) for public health in Macedonia are just starting to emerge in public awareness. This is clearly shown by recent events such as spread of hemorrhagic fevers in Europe. The term "public health" in the scope of this chapter suggests re-conceptualization of public health by adapting the risk governance framework developed by the International Risk Governance Council (IRGC) for this purpose. The IRGC approach is distinguished from more classical risk governance approaches, inter alia, by an explicit inclusion of a systematic concern assessment. However, unfortunately, not all countries are adapted on this innovative public health model. This chapter shows results of a risk management study based on interview in depth with the officials regard public health risk, in frame of one health concept in the Republic of Macedonia.

Chapter 8
A One Health Perspective on Q Fever: Part 1 174
Rita Cruz, Polytechnic Institute of Viseu, Portugal
Carmen Vasconcelos-Nobrega, Polytechnic Institute of Viseu, Portugal & University of Trás-os-Montes and Alto Douro, Portugal
Fernando Esteves, Polytechnic Institute of Viseu, Portugal
Catarina Coelho, Polytechnic Institute of Viseu, Portugal & University of Trás-os-Montes and Alto Douro, Portugal
Ana Sofia Ferreira, University of Oporto, Portugal
Carla Santos, Polytechnic Institute of Viseu, Portugal
Cristina Mega, Polytechnic Institute of Viseu, Portugal
Ana C. Coelho, University of Trás-os-Montes and Alto Douro, Portugal
Helena Vala, Polytechnic Institute of Viseu, Portugal & University of Trás-os-Montes and Alto Douro, Portugal
João R. Mesquita, University of Oporto, Portugal

Q fever is a worldwide zoonotic infectious disease caused by Coxiella burnetii and ruminants, namely, cattle, sheep, and goats, are known to be the main reservoir for human infection. C. burnetii infection in animals can result in epizootic abortions which are often associated with vast bacteria shedding in birth fluids and placentas. Human infections mainly occur in persons handling infected animals and their products. Here the authors describe the history, bacteriology, biosafety, and epidemiology of Q fever, now known to be a serious threat to veterinary public health.

Chapter 9
A One Health Perspective on Q Fever: Part 2..195
Rita Cruz, Polytechnic Institute of Viseu, Portugal
Carmen Vasconcelos-Nobrega, Polytechnic Institute of Viseu, Portugal & University of Trás-os-Montes and Alto Douro, Portugal
Fernando Esteves, Polytechnic Institute of Viseu, Portugal
Catarina Coelho, Polytechnic Institute of Viseu, Portugal & University of Trás-os-Montes and Alto Douro, Portugal
Ana Sofia Ferreira, University of Oporto, Portugal
Carla Santos, Polytechnic Institute of Viseu, Portugal
Cristina Mega, Polytechnic Institute of Viseu, Portugal
Ana C. Coelho, University of Trás-os-Montes and Alto Douro, Portugal
Helena Vala, Polytechnic Institute of Viseu, Portugal & University of Trás-os-Montes and Alto Douro, Portugal
João R. Mesquita, University of Oporto, Portugal

Q fever, a widespread zoonotic disease caused by Coxiella burnetiid, produces a complex and polymorphic disease in humans. As a zoonotic disease, control in animals will influence the level of disease seen in humans, thus resulting in interesting one health perspectives for disease control. Here the authors describe the clinical manifestations in animals and humans, as well as the current diagnostic methods available and the strategies for disease control. A review on the published information regarding Q fever as a disease with impact for veterinary public health and public health is presented.

Compilation of References 217

Related References 266

About the Contributors 299

Index 305

Foreword

I am extremely honoured and delighted to write a foreword for this wonderful compilation on One Health, as I believe in the holistic concept of One Health and its value for the society and Public Health in the country. One health, which initially started as a concept, has now become an approach and is gaining shape of One Health movement world over. Global emergence of this movement among the researchers, academicians and policy makers has offered a ray of hope in solving major Public Health challenges viz. Anti-microbial resistance, preventing emerging/re-emerging zoonotic diseases or food security issues etc. The expanded One Health encompasses any issues related to the human, animal and environment. I must appreciate that One Health is such a trans-disciplinary area, which needs a sky like umbrella to hold all the imperative stakeholders and move towards a successful collaborative effort.

This book comprises a compilation of past- history and development of One Health to the present situations and discusses about future in the form of challenges and opportunities. A glance through the pages of this book will reveal that it not only dissects the differential glances of One Health but also provides a basic understanding about the subject. Looking at this book into the context of Global Health, I would say that topics covered in this book will not only be useful for the readers, but will also pave path for the future, where we should take One Health further.

As Head of Division for "Establishment & Strengthening of state NCDC branches" at National Centre of Disease Control, India I look forward to the coming generation of researchers, members of academia and program managers engaged in the disease control adopting One Health approach to make the planet worth living by making better quality of life of all homo-sapiens on the planet.

Jai Karan
National Centre for Disease Control, India

Preface

'One Health' is an approach to designing and implementing programmes, policies, legislation and research in which multiple sectors communicate and work together to achieve better public health outcomes. It is now a recognized fact that health for all cannot be achieved unless human health is integrated with health of animal and safe environment. One health approach converges all three domains, but it requires collaborative efforts of multiple disciplines-working locally, nationally, and globally- to achieve the health for all. Although, One Health is not a new concept, but has not been in practice since long; however, with recent change in interactions between human, animal and environment, it has attracted more interest. Many factors have emerged resulting in close interactions between people, animals, and our environment; these changes have led to the emergence of diseases such as swine flu, Ebola, etc. and reemergence of many diseases such as rabies, diphtheria, TB etc. Hence, the concept of One health has gained more importance in rapidly urbanizing world.

Global Applications of One Health Practice and Care is a unique compilation in its kind; it covers diverse area of One Health practices including case studies. It discusses the theory of One Health evolution to current practices and major challenge for future in achieving One Health approach. This hand book emphasizes on various aspects of one health from the historical aspects to designing a one health study, from the different perspectives of one health to case studies on One Health. Viewpoints, research, and practices from across the globe gathered in this book will be a pathway and guides in future research.

This reference book will be useful for all the One health professionals who are into practice or planning to start research in this domain, it will also be very helpful for young scholars to think and deliberate on something different from the usual research. The primary audience for this book are students from the school of public health, veterinary science, environmental science, medical schools and policy planners, program managers, public health practitioners, animal health specialists and environmentalists.

The first three chapters of this book provides an insight from the concepts, historical perspective (Ch. 1), dimensions touching on holism aspects taking example from African perspective (Ch. 2) and how to design a one health research study with its advantages (Ch. 3). The next two chapters emphasize two aspects: one on human health i.e. one health and parasites providing a brief overview of public health aspect (Ch. 4) and the other on veterinary science perspectives especially how veterinary public health specialists can act for One Health (Ch. 5). A special chapter on antibiotic resistance aspects i.e. challenge in achieving one health for the future is being discussed in the next chapter (Ch. 6). The last three chapters are focused on disease specific from the One Health lenses; one on risk management and communication in case of vector borne disease (Ch. 7) and rest two on one health aspects of Q-fever (Chs. 8-9).

It is immensely satisfying to have contributions from prominent scientists and researchers of global repute who agreed to join this endeavor and penned their learnings on One Health represented as chapter for this book. It is also satisfying to see the outcome in a way as we originally envisioned. We hope that this book will be a source of inspiration to the readers to explore research in One Health. We challenge students at graduate and post-graduate level to read this book in detail, learn from it and grasp the fundamental ideas behind the One Health history and global practices. For researchers working in many different fields we believe that this book will provide a representative state-of-the-art overview in the field of One Health.

We wish all readers a fruitful time reading this book, and wish they experience the same excitement as we did – and still do – for moving with One Health.

Sandul Yasobant
Center for Development Research (ZEF), Germany

Deepak Saxena
Indian Institute of Public Health Gandhinagar, India

Section 1

Chapter 1
Emerging Global Health Approaches at the Human-Animal Interface:
Conceptual and Historical Issues of One Health

Walter Bruchhausen
University of Bonn, Germany

ABSTRACT

The vagueness of the term one health is the result of multiple developments that it has brought together. Therefore, a historical and conceptual analysis, divided in three sections, is performed for understanding these tensions and their backgrounds. First, an account of different and changing attitudes towards animals and their health is given, especially in religion, modern philosophy, and pre-modern dealing with disease supposedly caused by animals and plants. The second part reconstructs early bacteriology as a search for environmental disease factors and a struggle with zoonoses in a globalized research effort. The final and largest section analyses the development of international policies on zoonoses and one health from the 1950s until today, sketching the way from a veterinarian and medical national public health issue via socio-economic perspectives to the perception of a global threat by emerging diseases which fueled inter-agency cooperation in an unprecedented manner.

DOI: 10.4018/978-1-5225-6304-4.ch001

INTRODUCTION

The fact that a scientific and political area like One Health has developed and now deserves a research handbook on its practice and care is the final result of a long series and an enormous variety of experiences and reactions, of challenges and responses, of practical and theoretical developments – and accordingly contested. Therefore the (pre)history and theory of One Health may serve as a suitable introduction into this area of studying the highly heterogeneous practice on relations between man, animal and natural environment with regard to health. Thus this chapter will expose some of the fundamental ideas on the relations between humans and animals that informed and shaped the ways to One Health approaches – by critically looking at some of the established narratives as well as by adding some new stories. From the beginning of modern research and control of infectious diseases, a global perspective was indispensable. This is visible in the case of the cholera epidemics as starting point for the first international sanitary conferences in the 19th century. This global dimension affects the concept and history of One Health, too. Therefore most of the conceptual and historical developments described here – attitudes to animals, bacteriology, health governance – will have to be also linked to globalization and the emerging area of Global Health.

BACKGROUND: CHALLENGES FOR A HISTORIOGRAPHY OF ONE HEALTH

In accordance with the complex development of the field, collected volumes (Atlas, 2013; Bresalier, Cassidy, & Woods, 2015) and lectures (Vandersmissen, 2010) on One Health usually start with a historical account. Such short historical accounts, as common in medical issues, are rather historiography of science or history of the veterinary profession, i.e. a history and especially also prehistory of the academic and professional approaches to the issues. But the history of the field itself and the related practice, i.e. the relations between human, animal and environment health and the routine attempts to influence them, is rarely touched. The reasons for this narrow focus of the retrospective are quite obvious. They touch more theoretical, even ideological arguments as well as rather pragmatic ones. A dominant professional reason is the common function of history in the sciences: Celebrating important founding and other leading figures is a successful way to assert the reputability of a discipline. Compared to this, looking at past daily practices, at routine activities in struggling with a continuous challenge seems to be less exciting and interesting than quoting great names. This is also true for One Health: Pointing to its development as a scientific approach including well known physicians and veterinarians appears more academic and supportive for professional politics (Bresalier, et al., 2015, p. 1) than raising its issues as practice and care to be researched.

Equally, the practice of historiographic research has good reasons to deal with One Health as an academic instead of a practical field. A history of changing ideas can easily evade the question what realities in today's sense these concepts were addressing. And access to the necessary sources for a history of science is usually rather easy if they consist of original publications and secondary literature available in many libraries and even in the internet. Contrary to this comparatively simple approach to One Health as a recent Western science, a comprehensive history of health issues related to humans, animals and plants faces several challenges of epistemology and research practice.

The first challenge concerns the identification of historical accounts with today's medical classifications. As there was no concept of One Health centuries ago putting various developments, events and persons under this umbrella is our narrative, not any strand of the past. Similarly, the retrospective diagnosis of past illnesses by recent disease categories has rightly come into disrepute (Elmer & Peter, 2004). The reasons for this disrepute are not the same in different professional groups. For a historian the central problem is that past knowledge is judged by present knowledge. Thus the past accounts are not understood and explained by the horizon of the time – and therefore necessarily misunderstood whereas the present perspective is privileged as the only true 'knowledge'. For medical scientists on the other site this argument seems to be irrelevant as in this case they do not want to assess the intellectual quality of past colleagues, but just reconstruct 'facts'. Yet without an understanding of the contemporary classifications of a past time many accounts are misinterpreted as theory always determines perception and description. This has been extensively demonstrated for leprosy where many different skin afflictions that today doctors would probably attribute to syphilis or other treponematoses, to cancer or to circulation disorders have been labelled the same way. Similar difficulties are known with plague or anthrax (Wilkinson, 1993). Genomic analysis of germ DNA in human remains, e.g. found in graves of plague victims, prehistorical man or corpses in permafrost, has become the only scientifically reliable proof of the presence of certain pathogens, though not a causality beyond doubt. Thus in most cases we cannot be sure that a historical account of an epidemic or an individual illness corresponds to any category in the International Classification of Diseases, ICD-10 or now ICD-11. Certainly, this unavoidable uncertainty does not render a historical inquiry useless. Reactions to perceived illnesses or epidemics can be highly interesting and telling regardless of the precise nature of the pathogen.

A more practical than epistemological challenge for research in past relations between human, animal and environmental health is that the necessary data are not found in easily accessible articles by already known authors, but are scattered in sources of very different kinds and would have to be collected in highly time-consuming research projects. For some of the major zoonoses and vector-borne diseases several great books of both science and humanities, such as on bubonic plague (Scott & Duncan, 2001), malaria (Packard, 2007), sleeping sickness (Lyons, 1992), or rabies (Pemberton & Worboys, 2007), historical chapters in collected volumes on the scientific state of the art, such as on rabies (Wilkinson, 1988), contributions to historical encyclopedias and dictionaries, again on rabies (Patterson, 2003), anthrax (Wilkinson, 1993), leptospirosis (Gsell, 1993), trichinosis (Gilbertson, 1993), bubonic plague (Carmichael, 1993), or sound journal articles, e.g. on glanders (Wilkinson, 1981), have been published. Lacking the required mid-scale research project on primary sources for the history of such diseases, here my own account is necessarily based on such secondary sources.

The epistemological challenge does not only consist in the question whether a certain historical account can be attributed to a certain disease in today's biomedical sense, but even more in the ambiguity whether such diseases that a modern understanding sees as a zoonosis or related to food production should be treated in a retrospective as One Health issue. For before the 19th century, the transmission of a disease from an animal to man and vice versa (and even between human beings) was not an academically accepted concept. Thus it can be just investigated how phenomena of a disease that is classified as zoonanthroponosis today were perceived and treated in previous times.

Another challenge for a historiography of One Health lays in the complete opposite to the difficulties described so far, not in our difficulties in understanding distant times, but precisely in our lack of distance to current discourses. Nobody is able to say which of the many strands of the One Health discourses will be decisive for the future and which will be merely an ephemeron. Thus the more we approach the present, it will be only possible to introduce some of the many political and scientific initiatives in the field of One Health without a substantial claim to their superior importance.

Due to all these restrictions, the chapter can only be based on relevant research literature and official documents and can only give an account and analysis for some of the most prominent and common developments in the human attitudes towards animals, in zoonotic diseases and few human diseases caused by plant diseases, and in One Health as an emerging international movement.

MORE DIFFERENT OR MORE IN COMMON? PERCEPTIONS OF HUMANS, ANIMALS AND PLANTS

The Value of Non-Human Life

Today the most dominating areas of One Health are infectious diseases: zoonoses, food security and – with regard to the treatment of humans and animals with the same medicines – antimicrobial resistances. But in the classical and influential concept of 'one medicine' by US veterinarian Calvin Schwabe (1984) and more recent approaches such as that of the Swiss group of Zinsstag, Waltner-Toews, and Tanner (2015), the far reaching commonalities between human and animal nature that are expressed in anatomy and physiology, pathology and therapy are equal reasons for a common perspective. One result of this perspective was the call for more protection and rights of animals. This moral dimension is rather absent in the present scientific, medical and political mainstream debates on One Health. It forms, however, an important historical and cultural background that explains similar as well as highly different treatment of humans and animals also with regard to health. Most of the different treatment of human and non-human life, both within and outside health care, is based on concepts of different value. These concepts changed considerably over time and exhibit an enormous cross-cultural variety.

When in segmental societies totem animals of clans were revered and protected from killing or in early stratified societies like in ancient Egypt zoomorphic gods had a priesthood of their own at least some animals enjoyed a very privileged position. This did not exclude, sometimes even demanded their sacrifice for religious rituals and the use of their viscera for prophecy. As in Egypt often the same priests were responsible for such ritual handling of animals and for the healing of man and animal they gathered – according to Schwalbe (1978, pp. 84-107) – a considerably competence in comparative anatomy and pathology. This Egyptian knowledge stood quite in contrast to Mesopotamia where the healers of humans and cattle had been separate groups since early times.

Highly (though never exclusively) anthropocentric world views, such as the Greek-Roman, the monotheistic (Foltz, 2005) and the Confucian (Tucker, 2005) traditions which influence half of the world population and also Western science tended to privilege human life compared to that of other living beings. This does not exclude that admiration of the cosmic order and the genuine love for other living beings as fellow creatures might become quite strong, as in the Christian tradition the examples of the Celtic church or Saint Francis of Assisi show (French, 2005). And, on the other end of the moral scope, it does not exclude that for some rich and powerful individuals the lives of precious animals, e.g. for hunting, sports, warfare or breeding, are occasionally esteemed higher than the lives of humans regarded as inferior, such as slaves or barbarians. But in general, the far higher value of every human life is a dominating feature in these and some other traditions. The reason for the superiority of humans to animals was expressed in a central story of the bible common to Judaism, Christianity and Islam: the creation of the first humans Adam and Eva as final and highest part ('crown') of the world and their mission of taking the lead over the other beings which can be interpreted as either stewardship and care (dominion) or rule and exploitation (domination). Combined with Greek, especially Aristotelian philosophy, the distinction between the living, 'animated' beings was later systematized by Saint Thomas Aquinas (2004): plants had a vegetative soul (Latin: *'anima'*) only, animals a sensitive soul in addition, and only humans a vegetative, sensitive and intellectual/rational soul. The more Platonic or rather neo-Platonic 'great chain of being' was another, also scientifically applied metaphor for both connection and hierarchy in nature.

Other religious traditions that – like several Asian doctrines – assume an eventual pre- or post-mortal migration of a soul from humans to animals and vice versa might lead to a different view of animals (Wilkinson, 1992, p. 4; Schmithausen, 2005, p. 233; Narayanan, 2005, pp. 768-769) – but also to a different treatment of other human beings. One extreme result could be refraining from harming any living being, including the accidental swallowing of small insects. Some European approaches correspond to such strict avoidance of killing animals such as the 'ethics of reverence for life' of the physician, Christian theologian and philosopher Albert Schweitzer (2004).

Modern Western philosophy is divided on the issue of valuing animal life. The idealistic, continental European Kantian tradition would stick to the concept that rationality, especially as expressed in reflexive self-determination ('autonomy') privileges man over animals and therefore demands higher protection of any human life (Kant, 2004). In contrast, British utilitarian philosophy (Mill, 2004), based on the greatest happiness principle, holds in some variations, such as the Australian Peter Singer's preferential utilitarianism, that higher animals having and expressing interests, e.g. in feelings of pleasure and displeasure, demand more protection than early, defective or final stages of human lives that do not exhibit such interests (Singer, 2004). The latter view is partly based on a wide-spread tendency to an increased protection of animals (Vermeulen, 2010). In Europe, legal protection started in late 19th century since a cruel treatment of animals was regarded as threatening human moral feelings, thus ultimately leading towards cruel behavior against humans, too. Doctors should not do animal experimentation as they would develop similar attitudes towards their human patients. This 'anthropocentric' protection of animals, i.e. for the sake of humans, was replaced by a 'pathocentric' approach in the 20th century: Animals should be saved from cruel treatment for their own sake, i.e. in order to avoid their suffering.

Animal and Human Disease

The present concept of a zoonosis presupposes germ theory or another doctrine of transmission of diseases between living beings outside heredity. Thus in Western science, the concept became only possible in the late 19th century when previous vague ideas of 'contagion' were proven by experimental science and thereby accepted by academic medicine. The idea, however, that animal health may affect human health in a negative way is much older. It can be traced back to taboos and religious rules in many, probably most societies in the world. Animals that are not in good health or impure were regarded as unsuitable for human consumption, either in general or at least for certain groups. Many of these prohibitions became classified as 'superstition' by later science, but for some a positive effect on human health could be assumed. Thus some Muslims argue that the avoidance of pork or carrion is not just a religious duty, but they point to the possible negative effects on human health discussed in nutritional science and food hygiene – an argument not applicable, however, to the equally prohibited consumption of meat from animals sacrificed to others than God. Vegetarianism for religious reasons is similarly sometimes justified by hints to risks from infected animals.

The affection of human health by animals is not only imagined in such material concepts of impurity, but also in many concepts of spirit possession. Spirits of wild animals like lions might cause human disease in several African possession cults (Bruchhausen, 2006, p. 293). When such religious or other 'supernatural' ideas of disease causation were dispensed in more naturalistic systems of thought, such as Indian Ayurveda, some strands of Chinese medicine or ancient Greek medicine, eating or otherwise contacting sick animals was regarded as poisoning, as a threat to the healthy, i.e. balanced composition of the human body. With increasing empirical attention several transmissions of diseases between animals and humans were recognized already long before the establishment of bacteriology, e.g. by Albertus of Cologne (ca. 1200-1280) (Wilkinson, 1992, p. 18).

Other Food-Borne Diseases: Contamination and Degradation of Plants

As nearly all diseases of living plants do not directly harm humans the major impact of plant pathology on human health is the loss in food production causing under- and malnutrition, i.e. an issue of what is called food security today. A further negative impact may be by such contamination which does not damage the plant, but human health and by the degradation of plant products during processing, storage, transport, and sale, the issues of what is now called food safety. But there are some important exceptions to the rule that plant pathology itself does not spill over to humans: fungi infesting crop and intoxicating humans.

The best known of these mycotoxins are Ergot and Aflatoxins. Ergotism, the effect of alkaloids of *claviceps purpurea* infesting rye, and similar mycotoxins caused epidemics with ten thousands of deaths, not only in European medieval times, but even in the Soviet Union. Referred to as Saint Anthony's fire which could also name other gangrenous affections, the number of the sick initiated the care by the religious order of the Antonites in more than 370 special hospitals all over Europe (Bauer, 1973; Chaumartin, 1946; Haller, 2003). Later research distinguished gangrenous from convulsive forms and related the latter – besides regional differences in the content of different alkaloids – to an additional lack of vitamin A caused by low consumption of dairy products (Barger, 1931, pp. 24-26). This observation should caution against monocausal explanations in relations between human and plant health.

Toxic effects of Aflatoxins, ranging from acute vomiting including fatal cases to liver cancer, are rather the result of food storage in tropical and subtropical climates than a disease of the plants that produce peanuts or corns (Ainsworth, 2003). Such impact of storing and processing food on human health has recently become part of One Health discourses, too. Yet mycotoxins are sometimes also treated as food-borne diseases from animals since the human consumption of internal organs, milk and milk products from animals like pigs, poultry and cattle that have eaten food infested with fungi can transmit Aflatoxin M and Ochratoxin A with their (nephron) toxic, carcinogenic, teratogenic or immunosuppressive properties (Krauss, 2004, p. 557). Therefore such issues of plant health have to be included in a One Health perspective.

Germs Transgressing Species Borders: Zoonoses in Modern Science

When medicine was deeply transformed by experimental, quantifying and microscopic sciences and by an increased political interest since the early modern period One Health practice and care were at the center of these changes. Some challenges were of a rather 'pure' veterinary kind such as rinderpest destroying the cattle herds of Europe in this time which led to new public institutions for teaching and research. In these institutions scientific interest in the impact of animal health on human health, especially the diseases possibly transmitted from animals, both pet and lifestock, to humans, developed further. But in order to develop a true precedent of One Health, equal interest would have to grow on the side of human medicine which had become more and more separated from animal health by the institutionalization of veterinary medicine.

Interest in Pathogenic Factors: Zoonosis as Environmental Risk (Virchow)

In the history of modern scientific medicine as it was developed since the early 19th century the first reason for research in relations between human and animal health was the renewed interest in pathogenic factors. When young German medical scientists, among them Rudolf Virchow (1821-1902), founded a 'Society for scientific medicine' ('Gesellschaft für wissenschaftliche Medicin') in 1844 and also a new medical journal, called 'Medicinische Reform', in 1848 they demanded – besides other innovations – a new understanding and explanation of disease (Winau, 1987, p. 272). They did no longer accept inherited teachings on disease causation if they were not scientifically proven which meant confirmed by the results of controlled observation and experiments.

Although his academic reputation was largely based on his monography on cellular pathology, Virchow's scientific interest was far from being confined to the level of cells, tissues, and organs (Wilkinson, 1992, p. 193). As many pathologists, he looked at the variety of processes leading to the final picture of a disease. Close contact to domestic animals, eating meat, and drinking milk were certainly cases in point. By choosing the word 'zoonoses' as subtitle in brackets to the chapter 'Infections by contagious animal poisons' in the handbook of special pathology and therapy he had re-edited in 1855, Virchow used the word no longer for any animal disease, but for those transmitted from animals to humans (Virchow, 1855, p. 337; Krauss et al., 2004, p XIX). Thus the often found information that the word 'zoonoses' in the modern sense first appears with Ernst Wagner in 1876 (Stein, 2008) is certainly wrong, even earlier versions of the handbook by Wagner (1868, p. 159, 1874, p. 177) had already contained the word with this definition. Virchow could refer to some previous literature on transmission of disease from domestic animals to humans, especially a treatise by young doctor Jakob Levin that had won the award of the medical faculty of Berlin University (Levin, 1839). By uniting the three diseases rabies, anthrax and glanders in this chapter on zoonoses Virchow left the common system of classification in handbooks which had previously attributed rabies to 'neuroses' and skin affections like anthrax or glanders to the surgical diseases (*Handbuch*, 1841, p. 889). Later, Virchow especially dealt with the transmission from animals to humans in his research and his booklet on trichina (Virchow, 1864). Here he combined insights from microscopy, epidemiology and experiments, mainly feeding experiments, as well as human and veterinary medicine while developing and advocating meat inspection.

Virchow who never wholeheartedly embraced bacteriology as the new exclusive lead science and only explanation of infectious disease (Engelhardt, 1984, pp. 34-39) can be a guiding figure for One Health beyond his decisive contribution to the concept of zoonosis. The role model that he offers is that his central approach to disease causation and prevention was to be neither too general nor too narrow. Soon after Virchow's death it became obvious, even to Koch himself, that 'pure' bacteriology, i.e. without the look at other necessary conditions for infection, must run into theoretical and practical pitfalls (Berger, 2009). Its monocausal model could not explain why some individuals without previous contact to a certain pathogenic germs would not become infected despite strong exposition while others did. Virchow who was also attentive to other factors determining health and disease like nutritional status or polluted air could more easily accept a broader conditionality. In East African practice, 'Koch's method' of eliminating malaria by diagnosing and treating all carriers of the malaria plasmodium failed. If the vector, Anopheles mosquitoes, was not controlled the plasmodium could be too easily reintroduced by uncontrollable individual humans. Thus too narrow a focus on the germ could overlook other factors for explaining and fighting a disease.

On the other side, Virchow's scientific rigor waived aside too general explanations. Despite his harsh criticism of social misery, in his early reports on the living conditions in Silesia and the Spessart as well as his later career as a social politician, for him it was not enough to point to poverty or poor nutrition, but he wanted to have the precise contributing factors to ill-health clear.

This open attitude of Virchow could be a permanent warning for One Health not to become on the one side completely absorbed in single, for a certain period fashionable laboratory technologies and 'biomedical' mechanisms, like AMR or emerging diseases today, and on the other too general in a societal and ecological perspective by declaring all issues of economic inequality, animal welfare and ecology an indispensable precondition for human health. The reputation of such a reformative approach as One Health depends on both, on rigorous laboratory science and on a broader, but at the same time not unconfined perspective and relevance.

Simultaneous Teaching and Research in Human and Veterinary Medicine (Osler and Bollinger)

One of the next figures in the official ancestors' gallery of One Health has been – also as a pupil of Virchow (Saunders, 2000, p. 202) – deeply influenced by this transformation of European academic medicine, but is a typical North American professional by his pragmatism at the same time. Not too much troubled by questions of disciplinary belonging William Osler (1849-1919) thought as a physician at the medical school of McGill University also students of at the Montreal Veterinary College and acknowledged the many commonalities between the two largely separated fields. Thus he also worked on hog cholera. While it remains debated whether he developed a 'one medicine' approach out of this combined interest it is uncontested that he continued the tradition of 'comparative medicine'.

Osler was, however, not the only physician with a career in both, human and veterinary medicine in this period. In Munich from 1874 until 1880, Otto (von) Bollinger (1843-1909) simultaneously taught as professor of pathology at both, the Royal Bavarian Central School of Veterinary Medicine and the Medical Faculty of Munich University before he became the chair for pathology and later rector of the university (Krauße & Zandhof, 1990, pp. 83-84). After a teaching collaboration with the founder of the world-wide first institute of hygiene, the sceptic of exclusive bacteriology Max von Pettenkofer, he pioneered in public food hygiene, developing some of the first scientific measures for examining meat. His interest in zoonoses lead him to assuming a connection between human and bovine tuberculosis (Mayr & Mahnel, 1990, p. 169) even before Robert Koch identified the pathogenic microorganism common to both. The 'Bollinger corpuscles' for identifying poultry pox are a further result of his intensive study of diseases that possibly might affect humans and animals.

Early Bacteriology: Germs in Food and Zoonoses (Pasteur and Koch)

It has not been sufficiently noted, but is very telling that the initial history of bacteriology depended on food hygiene and zoonoses. The founder of bacteriology, Louis Pasteur (1822-1895), was a chemist working on food and was thus in close contact with both veterinarians and physicians. His early studies demonstrated that milk and wine were spoiled by microorganisms. Later he devoted his development of a first artificial vaccine to the most dangerous zoonosis, rabies, using tissue from an infected dog.

When Robert Koch (1843-1910) developed the experimental foundations of medical bacteriology the first two diseases he was successful with in his experiments were zoonoses: anthrax and tuberculosis. This was not by chance, but resulted from the requirements of his experiments that should prove the causation of disease by microorganisms. According to the postulates set up by his academic teacher Jacob Henle and expanded by himself, a microorganism would have to be identified and gained from one organism and transferred to another where it caused the same clinical picture. As he could not do such experiments in humans he needed an animal model and thus diseases that existed in both. The similarities between human and certain animal organisms in being susceptible to some germs made animal models of infectious diseases possible and allowed the transfer of bacteria from humans to animals.

Bacteriology Going Global: Tropical Health as Challenge for Zoonotic Research

Global health issues were a pacemaker for the research and control of zoonotic diseases as can be clearly seen from the history of tropical medicine (Scott, 1942, pp. 113-844). One reason was the size of protozoa and helminths as important tropical pathogens which facilitated their investigation, another the vector as easily accessible medium of transmission. Thus in Egypt already in 1851, many years before European bacteriology was established, the young German physician Theodor Bilharz (1825-1862) described the eggs and larvae of Schistosoma. Such research on the two human helminth diseases bilharziosis (by Schistosoma haematobium) and hookworm disease (by Ancylostoma duodenale or Necator americanus) became important for the zoonotic diseases caused by Schistosoma japonicum and Ancylostoma braziliense. In Algeria in 1880, the French doctor Alphonse Laveran (1845-1922) described the malaria plasmodium, later he worked on the zoonotic diseases by trypanosoma and founded the 'Société de Pathologie Exotique' in 1908. When in India in 1897 the British physician Ronald Ross (1857-1932) confirmed the previous beliefs of many natives and researchers that malaria is transmitted by mosquitos (Scott, 1942, pp. 160-161) the door for path-breaking research and effective control of vector-borne zoonotic infections was opened.

Although bacteriology with its research and control of zoonoses had been a very national enterprise at its beginning when Pasteur in France and Koch in Germany got extraordinary support from their respective national government it soon developed into an extremely global science and practice. An early step of this expansion was research on a purely human disease, the race between research teams from the two nations for the discovery of the Cholera bacterium, performed in the two British colonial territories of first Egypt and then India where Koch was successful in 1884/1885. But Koch's next international research involved animal health, first rinderpest in South Africa in 1896 (Wilkinson, 1992, pp. 195-196; Gradmann, 2010), a year later plague in India and German East Africa (today Tanzania), 1898-1999 malaria in Italy, Java and New Guinee, 1905-1906 sleeping sickness again in German East Africa and the neighboring British territory Uganda. During the same years researchers from other nations were successful worldwide in their research on vector-borne and zoonotic diseases by much smaller germs: on mosquito-borne viral yellow fever the Cuban Carlos Juan Finlay (1833–1915) and the US-American Walter Reed (1851-1902) in Cuba, on lice-borne typhus fever by rickettsia the Russian Ossip Motschutkowski (1845–1903) in Odessa, the US-American Howard Taylor Ricketts (1871-1910) in Mexico in 1910, and – both at the Hamburg Institute of Naval and Tropical Diseases – the Czech-Austrian Stanislaus (von) Prowazek (1875-1915) in 1913 and the Brazilian Henrique da Rocha Lima (1879-1956) in 1916.

The major pandemic zoonosis of this time was plague which had started as rather bubonic plague in one of its endemic spots in the Western part of Yunnan Province, China, in 1855, killed ten million people in India and had its final high-tide in a more pneumonic form in Manchuria in 1910-1911. As the germ and the transmission were discovered in these years – by the French physicians Alexandre Yersin (1843-1873) and Paul-Louis Simond (1858–1947) – the hunt on rats and other rodent populations became a central tool in disease control besides the older means of quarantine and isolation. Animal welfare was certainly not a core value in this approach. If we assume an animal origin, the Spanish Influenza of 1918 can be regarded as the last zoonotic pandemic which transgressed the threshold of ten million deaths within a few years.

TRANSGRESSING BORDERS BETWEEN SPECIES AND CONTINENTS: GLOBALIZATION AND ONE HEALTH

WHO, FAO and Zoonoses

Zoonoses had been already a prominent international issue in the inter-war period. In 1924, a cattle transport from India to Brazil via the Belgian port Antwerp caused an outbreak of rinderpest in Belgium. This led the League of Nations to found an organization for such issues, the *Office International des Epizooties (OIE)*, later renamed World Organization for Animal Health while keeping its acronym. Zoonoses were also a major topic of the rural hygiene conferences organized by the League of Nations Health Organization in these decades (Far Eastern Rural Hygiene Conference, 1937; WHA, 1954).

After 1945, one of the most important steps for establishing international collaboration and research on zoonoses was the Joint WHO/FAO Expert Group on Zoonoses, already founded in the first years of these two UN organizations for health and for food and agriculture, but without the OIE. The group was formed because many national governments asked the two organizations for assistance in this field. The report on the first session of this group was submitted after a five days meeting in December 1950 (Joint WHO/FAO Expert Group on Zoonoses, 1951, p. 1). The authorship of the first report, under the chairmanship of the former UK Chief Veterinary Officer Sir Daniel Cabot and with the membership of his successor Professor Thomas Dalling, had a complete veterinary and a rather high Northern bias: out of the fourteen experts, all from animal health institutions, none from human medicine, only two came from South America (Brazil and Argentina), two from geographical Asia (Israel and Indonesia), none from Africa or Oceania. The group was, however, aware that its recommendations must be valid 'in economically advanced and in less developed countries' (Joint WHO/FAO Expert Group on Zoonoses, 1951, p.5) and that collaboration with medical doctors is important: for the fight against bovine tuberculosis it states that the 'backing of the medical profession will greatly assist in obtaining public support' (Joint WHO/FAO Expert Group on Zoonoses, 1951, p.6).

The report defined the responsibility of veterinary medicine as protection against health hazards from ‚(a) contact with diseased animals', (b) consumption of their tissues or products, and (c) consumption of animal products contaminated during processing and delivery (Joint WHO/FAO Expert Group on Zoonoses, 1951, p.4). The new term 'veterinary public health' was affirmed as adequate name for these tasks. The report contained chapters of their own on 'tuberculosis in cattle', anthrax, Q fever, psittacosis and hydatidosis while listing 80 zoonotic diseases in an annex. When the Executive Board (EB) of the WHO accepted the first report in early 1951 it explicitly mentioned 'bovine tuberculosis, hydatidosis, and anthrax' as issues where effective measures exist, but need to be extended to more countries whereas 'virus encephalitides, tularaemia and leptospirosis' were named as examples for more neglected areas requiring further studies (1951).

The second report of the group, now called a committee, was submitted after its five days meeting in Stockholm in 1958 (Joint WHO/FAO Expert Committee on Zoonoses, 1959). Membership had changed nearly completely. Just one member of the first group, the representative of the Argentinian Ministry for Agriculture and Animal Husbandry, remained, three experts were shifted from 'members' to the enlarged 'secretariat'. The now slightly smaller expert group, ten members only, contained new experts from Pakistan and New Zealand, while the members from Israel, Brazil and Indonesia of 1950 were not part any more. Thus the percentage of former colonial territories did not change considerably. Human medicine and Public Health were represented this time, by experts on Rural Occupational Medicine and Hygiene from Poland and Tropical Hygiene and Geographical Pathology from the Netherlands as well as the eminent Swiss-American researcher Karl Friedrich Meyer (1884-1974) as the new chairman who had taught as a veterinarian also public health in the medical school. He had already prepared the document 'The Zoonoses in their relation to rural health' for the technical discussions at the Seventh World Health Assembly (1954). The tendency away from pure veterinary and microbiological experts towards more general public health and hygiene, i.e. integration of human medicine and public health is obvious.

'Three more major zoonoses, rabies, plague, and brucellosis', were once more excluded from the report since other WHO/FAO expert groups already worked on them (Joint WHO/FAO Expert Committee on Zoonoses, 1959, p. 5). The structure of the report again follows disease or microbiological taxonomy, with this time not only five chapters, but nine chapters and seven sub-chapters on particular diseases.

Salmonelloses and influenza as well as – following the recommendation by the WHO Executive Board – leptospirosis and viral encephalitis had been added as separate chapters. Toxoplasmosis, listeriosis, larva migrans, dermatomycoses, trematode infections, tularemia and cat-scratch disease were subsumed under the chapter title 'Other Zoonoses'.

The last chapter of the report is devoted to 'Emerging Zoonoses', already expects their increase due to changed land use, 'development' and growing populations, deplores the lack of research and proposes freeze-dried specimens for later retrospective epidemiology (Joint WHO/FAO Expert Committee on Zoonoses, 1959, pp. 55-56). Thus this report stands at the turning point from a rather static taxonomic approach to zoonoses to the dynamic perspective of developmental issues.

Economic Considerations and Interest Regarding Zoonoses

When in the late 1960 general interest in the socio-economic impact of development increased the World Health Assembly (1969) demanded a new joint report by the zoonoses experts from WHO and FAO, this time on the 'Socio-economic Consequences of the Zoonoses' and their prevention. In the next year, expert groups planning pilot studies for 'preparing methodology and criteria to be used in carrying out surveillance of zoonoses and evaluation of control programmes' were identified (Executive Board, 1970). The whole endeavor seemed to be far more complicated and ambitious than expected (Executive Board, 1971). It became especially clear that such research outside already existing research facilities would be quite expensive, and therefore the EB of WHO preferred the support of already established research into zoonoses to initiating new research institutions (Executive Board, 1972). Obviously, the expected economic gains were not justifying too expensive research – or at least economically interested donors could not be sufficiently recruited for sponsoring these fields.

Since the late 1980s, the Pan-American Health Organization (PAHO) as the regional office or branch of WHO developed some interest in zoonotic diseases, resulting in three volumes of a handbook (Acha & Szyfres, 1987, 2003a, 2003b). It is divided according to microbiological classification which means that practical, political or economic aspects in the control of the diseases that had spurred WHO interest in the 1970s are less prominent.

'One World, One Health™': Global Issues at the Human-Animal-Ecosystem Interface

Whereas international cooperation until the late 1990s had regarded zoonoses as rather local, national or regional phenomena this perspective rapidly changed after 2000. With the general fear of a 'return of the infectious diseases' which was set against the too optimistic attitude of the 1970s and fueled by the HIV/AIDS pandemic, scientific and political attention turned to 'emerging' or 're-emerging' infectious diseases with pandemic potential. Going beyond particular infectious diseases, a more general perspective on epidemiology and surveillance, control and preparedness for health risks at the now so called animal-human-ecosystems interface was taken. Also the initially very confined inter-agency collaboration within the UN system on zoonosis, that between WHO and FAO, was extended in several directions: economy and financing by the World Bank, child welfare by cooperating with the UN Children's Fund UNICEF, influenza by creating the UN System Influenza Coordination UNSIC within the UN Development Group in 2005 (World Health Report 2007) – and also wild animals.

The latter additional perspective was a rather new move, brought to public awareness by a 2004 meeting of the Wildlife Conservation Society with representatives from several UN agencies, titled 'One World, One Health: Building Interdisciplinary Bridges to Health in a Globalized World' (http://www.oneworldonehealth.org). Members of this society formulated the 'Manhattan Principles' accepted at this meeting. Besides more general imperatives for including the animal-human interface – ecosystems issues like water and land use were rather regarded as conditions than as goals – these principles contained two rules specific for wildlife:

1. Include wildlife health science as an essential component of global disease prevention, surveillance, monitoring, control and mitigation.
2. Recognize that human health programs can greatly contribute to conservation efforts (Cook, Karesh & Osofsky, 2004).

This coining of the term One Health already went far beyond the agricultural settings where the international discussion of zoonoses had started. This was a significant extension of attention from the anthropocentric concerns about human health and food security that WHO and FAO embodied to the welfare of both domestic and wild animals as a precondition for sustainable global health and agriculture.

Inter-Agency Agreements: Transforming Avian Influenza Into a One Health Issue

Despite the official international tendency away from specific diseases towards system perspectives it was particular outbreaks and pandemics after 2000 that triggered more interest in the human-animal interface: Avian influenza, the corona viruses SARS and later MERS, and especially Ebola in West Africa. The first of a series in according international conferences, inspired by the long-standing global cooperation on HIV/

AIDS, was the Geneva meeting of senior officials in November 2005. It reacted to the H5N1 threat and started a collaboration that led to the 'Global Program for Avian Influenza Control and Human Pandemic Preparedness and Response'. When the ministers met two months later in Beijing for their conference on this issue they took up the idea of a rather decentralized approach instead of a new vertical fund. Obviously the view that an inter-sectoral, i.e. systemic or horizontal approach is required was convincing and also decisive for the whole international process in which avian influenza was 'reframed' as a One Health issue (Chien, 2013, p. 213). The Fifth 'International Ministerial Conference on Avian and Pandemic Influenza' (IMCAPI) in New Delhi in 2007 led to a 'vision' of 'One Health and One World', required by the fact that 'Rising demands for animal products (associated with poverty reduction) and changes in ecosystems (due to population growth and climate change) are increasing human susceptibility to infection with animal diseases', while the hosting Indian government already issued a comprehensive national road map (Press Information Bureau Government of India, 2007).

The next year, a 'Strategic Framework for Reducing Risks of Infectious Diseases at the Animal–Human–Ecosystems Interface' was agreed by FAO, OIE, WHO, UNSIC, UNICEF, and WB (2008) which again chose the slogan 'One World, One Health' from the Manhattan principles in its title. The following IMCAPI in Sharm El Sheikh in 2008 welcomed this One Health strategy. Two years later, the World Bank published its two volumes on *'a One Health Approach for Controlling Zoonotic Diseases'* and *'The Economics of One Health' (2010a und 2010b)* intended to broaden the perspective from mainly avian influenza to all One Health issues and from merely pandemic to also endemic issues (World Bank, 2010a, p. x). The next IMCAPI in Hanoi the same year urged the implementation of these One Health approaches (Jonas & Warford, 2014, p. 3). A Tripartite Concept Note for collaboration in One Health was published by FAO, OIE, and WHO (2010).

The next high level technical meeting of senior officials in Mexico City in 2011 became somewhat ambiguous regarding vertical and horizontal approaches: On the one side, it recommend in its emphasis on cross-sectoral collaboration 'investing in existing systems' (FAO, OIE, & WHO, 2012, p. 30), i.e. a rather horizontal strategy, on the other side, it used rabies, zoonotic influenza and antimicrobial resistance (AMR) as 'entry points' (not as 'One Health global priorities' as some accounts misleadingly state, e.g. Jonas & Warford, 2014, p. 3) which might lead to the impression new vertical programmes are needed (p. vi).

In a report for the World Bank of 2014 on the accomplishments ten years after the first meeting, the authors who complained about a national and international neglect of 'veterinary and human public health capacities' in 'developing countries' called the response of the international community 'an unprecedented effort that coordinated animal health and human health interventions' and judged it as 'highly cost-efficient and evidence-based' because of its 'focus on prevention and preparedness for control of contagion at its animal source' (Jonas & Warford, 2014, p. 1). This focus on very early prevention and on preparedness already distinguishes One Health from other international programmes in the MDG era when interventions such as availability of anti-retroviral and anti-malarial therapy or mother-and-child health services dominated. The other difference to the rather vertical design of MDGs is the high emphasis on inter-sectoral collaboration within national governments. The recent One Health framework by the World Bank makes clear that global health threats can be most efficiently encountered by functioning national governance systems: 'Establishing multi-sectoral programs within governments to manage endemic zoonoses can provide solid ground for response to emerging diseases and outbreaks of major importance' (World Bank Group, 2018, p. 2).

Academic Perspectives: 'Health of Nomads' and Expanded One Health Concepts

As usual in WHO, the earlier work on zoonoses had been prompted by the interest of national governments, which not always represented the priorities of all their social and ethnic groups, and the more recent interest is spurred by global threats like SARS and Ebola. Because of the locally blind spots in these rather national and international perspectives, advocacy by health experts for neglected groups became a further, in this case quite influential factor for establishing One Health. Such a more recent European-African contribution to the One Health concept is the joint programme 'Health of Nomads' of the Swiss Tropical (and Public Health) Institute and the *Centre de Support en Santé International* in Chad since 1998 (Montavon et al., 2013). In interdisciplinary research between human and veterinary medicine, epidemiology, geography and anthropology it studied the relationship between humans and their cattle, disease patterns including the nature of the germs, nutritional status, perceptions of health issues and resulting practices among pastoralist groups in Chad (Schelling, 2002; Krönke, 2001; Diguimbaye-Djaibé et al., 2006; Schelling et al., 2005). As one of the practical results it lead to vaccination campaigns targeting humans and cattle at the same time (Béchir et al., 2004).

One of the principal investigators in this programme, the veterinarian Jakob Zinsstag, preferred the term One Health for such joint research and promoted it in articles, editorials and collected volumes. Within this series of publications by Zinsstag and colleagues a certain conceptual variety and dynamics between broadening and focusing can be observed. For the establishment of One Health, the broadening of perspectives from medicine to health and well-being and from disciplines to systems is emphasized (Zinsstag, Schelling, Waltner-Toews, & Tanner, 2011). As an integrating and integrated approach, One Health takes into accout the 'complex patterns of global change, the inextricable interconnection of humans, pet animals, livestock and wildlife and their social and ecological environment.' When to be distinguished from EcoHealth „pure" One Health is characterized by the disciplinary majority of veterinarians and public health practitioners and the main focus on communicable disease, food safety, nutrition and antimicrobial resistance, i.e. the immediate nexus between human and animal health (Zinsstag et al., 2012). In this narrow focus, One Health could learn 'ecosystem approaches' from EcoHealth.

A third line of argument for establishing One Health, after describing the wide scope and the relations to other similar concepts, is the emphasis on utility for donors and policy-makers. This reference to an added value that has accompanied One Health from its very beginnings is elaborated in the preface to the collected volume of 2015: 'We understand One Health foremost as any added value in terms of better health and well-being for humans and animals, financial savings and improved environmental services achieved from closer cooperation between practitioners and scholars concerned with human health, animal health and related outcomes, beyond what can be achieved by working alone.' (Zinsstag, Schelling, Waltner-Toews, Whittaker, & Tanner, 2015, p. xv). The 'theoretical issues' raised in their contribution to this volume, however, go far beyond the question of added value with its strong economic connotations. They include new, broadening perspectives compared to the hitherto dominating scientific approaches. These new aspects that are explicitly mentioned (Zinsstag, Waltner-Toews, & Tanner, 2015, p. 23) are

- 'Normative aspects (values) of the human-animal relationship with emphasis on improving animal protection and welfare in an inter-cultural context' with awareness of 'the social, cultural and religious background',
- Engagement 'with the public' and 'considering all forms of academic and non-academic knowledge for practical problem solving'
- Expansion towards 'Health in Social-Ecological Systems' (HSES).

These three expansions – towards the normative and inter-cultural, the public and non-academic, and the social and ecological – clearly reflect experiences in the Chad project, but at the same time intensify connections to Global Health. This openness for ethics, culture and social-ecological systems is important for a discipline like veterinary medicine which tends towards even more biological reductionism than human medicine as its patients themselves are less influenced by socio-cultural variety. Integrating the perspective of ecological systems brings One Health even more in line with the debates that shaped the Sustainable Development Goals. Not by short lived interventions themselves, such as joint immunization campaigns for humans and animals, but only by developing a broader perspective for any problem-solving One Health realizes its full potential. Hereby it might even be allowed to lose its essentially practical orientation temporarily if it sensitizes and encourages more disciplines to transgress their confinements.

One Health Beyond Animals: Food Security, Food Safety and Environmental Protection

Such risks for human health that grow from the quality of food related to zoonoses and AMR had been part of One Healt discourses at a very early stage. Issues of sufficient quantity, called food security since the 1970s, and of non-zoonotic food hygiene, especially microbial or toxic contamination and spoilage, dealt with under the term of food safety today, entered the arena of One Health only recently. Again, this is not so much a question of activities primarily, but of labelling. Nevertheless, for experts from food or agriculture on the one side and health or medicine on the other, working under a common heading might facilitate inter-sectoral and inter-disciplinary cooperation in many regards.

From the very beginnings of international cooperation on zoonoses, FAO had been a more or less equal partner to WHO. Nevertheless it is telling that early official UN documents on food, even if WHO participated in the consultations, avoided the term 'health'. Thus the influential Report of the World Food Conference in Rome in 1974, coining the concept of food security, does not contain the word 'health' at all. Its 'Universal Declaration on the Eradication of Hunger and Malnutrition' only speaks of all human beings' 'inalienable right to be free from hunger and malnutrition in order to develop fully and maintain their physical and mental faculties' (United Nations, 1975). Only in 1984, the World Bank made the link to health explicit when it added the condition 'enough food for an active, healthy life' to the definition of food security (World Bank, 1984). On the other side already in 1978, WHO had had made 'promotion of food supply and proper nutrition' the second of the eight prioritized constituents of its new Primary Health Care (PHC) strategy (WHO & UNICEF, 1978). In addition, nutritional information received a prominent place in health education, the first constituent of PHC. Nutritionists were educated and employed for PHC projects, and feeding centers with fields, gardens and kitchens for demonstration were attached to many district hospitals in areas with frequent malnutrition.

This continuous, nevertheless tension-filled convergence of perspectives and strategies at the inter-agency level has not been accompanied by similar large-scale cooperation between academic work on health and on food. Formal ties between medical and agricultural faculties remained rare and mostly weak. It were broad integrative approaches, like first that of Global Health in some of its more academic versions and then of One health, that opened up new links between food and health (von Braun, Ruel, & Gillespie 2010). To claim the label One Health for this connection, however, remains rare. Again for veterinarians One Health is seen as a chance to remind of the importance of veterinary services, now for a global livestock sector 'growing at an unprecedented rate, driven by urbanisation and rising incomes' (Kelly, Ferguson, Galligan, Salman, & Osburn, 2013, p. 739). Contrary to this, the United Nations System Standing Committee on Nutrition (UNSCN), the food and nutrition policy harmonization forum of the United Nations, does not even mention the term One Health in its comprehensive publications on nutrition and health (UNSCN, 2010, 2014, 2017a, 2017b, 2017c). Even the Global Nutrition Report 2017 where WHO and FAO are among the leading contributors does not refer to One Health (http://globalnutritionreport.org/the-report/). It seems that food and nutrition without relations to animal health are not regarded as areas for One Health by UN agencies.

A different position is taken by the Global Risk Forum (GRF) Davos, Switzerland, which organized the Third One Health Summit in 2015. Its list of One Health elements contains 'food safety & security'. If we compare the English version (http://onehealth.grforum.org/about/about-one-health/) and the German version (http://onehealth.grforum.org/de/one-health/one-health-kurz-erklaert/) we find a remarkable difference: In the graphic on the page in English the circle of One Health is divided into the thirds human, animal and environmental health, the quartered version on the German page shows a forth symbol, an apple referring to 'Food Safety & Security' and part of 'Agriculture'.

Another hint that German-speaking scientific communities tend towards this extension is the International Congress One Health & Food Safety at the University of Bonn, Germany, in September 2018 (https://www.onehealth.uni-bonn.de/).

Before the more recent attempts to import the established areas of food security and non-zoonotic food safety into One Health agendas the environment had already been a long-standing candidate, even officially acknowledged member in this club.

Figure 1.

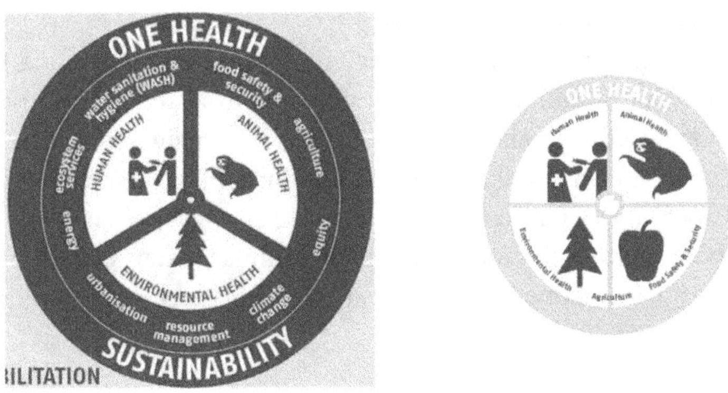

It is regularly mentioned in the titles of both political and academic publications on One Health. Yet even in 2018, it can not be regarded as an equal partner to human and animal health as a World Bank analysis clearly stated with regard to economic impact and donor motivation: 'While environment is one of three main sectors in the concept of One Health, in practice it is systematically underrepresented.' (World Bank, 2018, p. 57). Water which is not contaminated by pathogens or toxic chemicals is explicitly mentioned as the example where the integrity of the ecological system goes beyond merely intrinsic value and may have an enormous impact on human and animal health.

The main conceptual difficulty consists in the fact that the environment is not a living being in the same sense as humans or animals. Therefore it has not got a medicine of its own, and related to environment, the word 'health' is accordingly used in a rather peculiar way. In common use of language, the term 'environmental health' denotes a part of human public health, i.e. the impact of the environment on human health. 'Ecological Health' could mean either also a part of human medicine/public health or the condition of an ecosystem itself. Just in the new term 'EcoHealth' is the integrity of the system itself clearly addressed, but the use of 'health' is rather metaphorical. As an attribute to 'environment' so far the adjective 'healthy' means 'conducive to health', not 'being in good health'. There might be an ongoing semantic shift to the latter or from a metaphorical use to a technical term, but this is rather the result than the precondition of its inclusion in One Health or other more comprehensive health concepts. Certainly, the environment shares the ambiguity known from animals of having an intrinsic value itself on the one side and of being important, either useful or dangerous, for human health on the other. With those vectors, that are not diseased themselves, of diseases, that are not regularly included in lists of zoonoses therefore, the environment has in common that its own integrity might not be damaged by the pathogens it transmits to humans. The most enlightening debates in this field are those on differences between the 'three holistic approaches' EcoHealth, Planetary Health and One Health where the latter is characterized by a focus on 'safeguarding the health of vertebrates' (Lerner & Berg, 2017).

Thus some of the main reasons for including the environment and food issues in general into One Health are certainly different from those that initiated early concepts of One Medicine and One health. The main gains or at least potentials, however, such as enhancing inter-agency, inter-disciplinary, inter-ministerial and inter-professional cooperation by a more systematic and at the same time more problem-solving perspective, are remarkably similar, often even identical. The risk that such a broad notion of One Health prevents any conceptual clarity and operational practicability increases.

CONCLUSION: ZOONOSES – FROM GLOBAL OCCURRENCE AND INTEREST TO GLOBAL THREAT AND CHANCE

From the point of view of One Health practice and care, the history and theory of zoonoses is shaped by a broad, increasingly global variety of influences. One of the most prominent influences is certainly the professional interest of veterinarians who looked for more recognition of their discipline and work. The ubiquitous reference to the famous physicians Virchow and Osler mirrors this search for closer ties to the history of human medicine. The previous attempts to distance veterinary medicine from human medicine during the time of its academic establishment and professionalization are now reversed by an emphasis on commonalities.

Whereas for some time in the second half of the 20th century the overlapping area between human and animal health became to be regarded as a rather marginal field that would allegedly disappear with increasing urbanization and industrialization, it had enjoyed a very prominent position in medical research before. The fundamental scientific knowledge on which both human and veterinary medicine built on had been mainly gained at the interface between human and animal diseases, especially in the study of anthrax, tuberculosis and rabies. Insights at this interface stems from an intense academic interest in pathogenic factors in the middle of the 19th century and remains an important source for new perspectives in general questions of infectious diseases and immunology today. Without animal models that reproduce human diseases due to a certain degree of inter-specious transmissibility, much of current research in the life sciences would be impossible.

In the 19th century concepts of both pathogenic factors and bacteria, zoonoses were conceptualized as very local phenomena. Nearly only butchers and tanners with close contact to animals could attract anthrax. Trichinosis concerned eaters of the fresh meat only. And 'the colonial disease' sleeping sickness was confined to the environment of the cattle. The radius of its vector, the Tse-Tse fly, marked the precise borders as also in the case of malaria that of the Anopheles mosquitoes. But today, after more than a century of accelerated globalization, it is obvious that the major risks of zoonoses often concern far away events: New strains of the Influenza virus stemming from East Asian poultry threaten the rest of the world by pandemics, anti-microbial resistance caused by unrestricted use of antibiotics in animal husbandry in many countries is transferred by travelling patients or healthy carriers to patients at the other end of the world.

Although at least some zoonoses had been already part of the activities in rural hygiene in the inter-war period this group of diseases became a distinct part of international health in the 1950s only when the collaboration between WHO and FAO in this area started. Despite repeated inquiries into the economic consequences of these diseases it remained a rather invisible field, without a WHO programme or department of its own. This only changed with some alarming events after 2000: emerging diseases, some of them with pandemic potential, like avian influenza, SARS or Ebola, and the sharp increase in antimicrobial resistances. Since then, inspired by an initiative from wildlife conservation that promoted the term One Health internationally and especially supported by the World Bank, regular international meetings at minister level demand and monitor progress in some of these fields. Differing from the rather vertical and global programmes of the Millennium Development Goals on AIDS and malaria, mother and child health, the focus is on inter-sectoral cooperation at local, national and international level. Thus it has been recognized that functioning health systems, both for animals and humans, and their collaboration as well as health-in-all policies, including water, agriculture, trade, and education, are indispensable prerequisites for the early detection and the successful management of emerging diseases and thereby the protection of the global population. Whereas the environment has become an acknowledged part of One Health in the UN system, food security & safety still struggle to be recognized as other parts.

One Health was and still is an open learning process on all levels and in many sectors and disciplines. For this purpose, the often discussed vagueness of the term (Chien, 2013; Cassidy, 2016; Shresta, Acharya, & Shresta, 2018) is rather a chance and precondition than a disadvantage.

REFERENCES

Acha, P. N., & Szyfres, B. (2003). *Zoonoses and Communicable Diseases Common to Man and Animals* (Vol. 1-3). Washington, DC: Pan-American Health Organization.

Ainsworth, G. C. (2003). Fungus Poisoning. In K. F. Kiple (Ed.), *The Cambridge historical dictionary of disease* (pp. 132–134). Cambridge, UK: Cambridge University Press.

Atlas, R. M. (2013). One Health: Its Origins and Future. In J.S. Mackenzie, M. Jeggo, P. Daszak, & J.A. Richt (Eds.), The Concept and Examples of a One Health Approach = One Health: The Human-Animal-Environment Interfaces in Emerging Infectious Diseases, vol. 1 = Current Topics in Microbiology and Immunologie (pp. 1-13). Berlin, Germany: Springer. doi:10.1007/82_2012_223

Barger, G. (1931). *Ergot and Ergotism. A monograph based on the Dohme lectures delivered in Johns Hopkins University, Baltimore*. London, UK: Gurney & Jackson. Retrieved from http://ergotism.info/en/1931_barger_ergotism.htm

Bauer, V. H. (1973). *Das Antoniusfeuer in Kunst und Medizin*. Berlin: Springer Verlag. doi:10.1007/978-3-642-65768-9

Béchir, M., Schelling, E., Wyss, K., Daugla, D. M., Daoud, S., Tanner, M., & Zinsstag, J. (2004). Approche novatrice des vaccinations en santé publique et en médecine vétérinaire chez les pasteurs nomades au Tchad: Expériences et coûts. *Medecine Tropicale, 64*(5), 497–502. PMID:15771021

Berger, S. (2009). *Bakterien in Krieg und Frieden. Eine Geschichte der medizinischen Bakteriologie in Deutschland, 1890-1933.* Göttingen, Germany: Wallstein.

Bresalier, M., Cassidy, A., & Woods, A. (2015). One Health in History. In J. Zinsstag, E. Schelling, D. Waltner-Toews, M. Whittacker, & M. Tanner (Eds.), *One Health. The Theory and Practice of Integrated Health Approaches* (pp. 1–15). Wallingford, UK: CABI. doi:10.1079/9781780643410.0001

Bruchhausen, W. (2006). Medizin zwischen den Welten. Geschichte und Gegenwart des medizinischen Pluralismus im südöstlichen Tansania. Göttingen, Germany: v&r unipress/Bonn University Press.

Carmichael, A. (1993). Bubonic Plague. In K. F. Kiple (Ed.), *The Cambridge world history of human disease* (pp. 628–631). Cambridge, UK: Cambridge University Press. doi:10.1017/CHOL9780521332866.083

Cassidy, A. (2016). One Medicine? Advocating (Inter)disciplinarity at the Interfaces of Animal Health, Human Health, and the Environment. In S. Frickel, M. Albert, & B. Prainsack (Eds.), *Investigating Interdisciplinary Collaboration. Theory and Practice across Disciplines* (pp. 213–236). New Brunswick, NJ: Rutgers University Press.

Chaumartin, H. (1946). *Le mal des ardents et le feu Saint-Antoine. Etude historique médicale, hagiographique et légendaire.* Vienne, France: Imprimerie Ternet-Martin.

Chien, Y.-J. (2013). How did international agencies perceive the avian influenza problem? The adoption and manufacture of the 'One World, One Health' framework. *Sociology of Health & Illness, 35*(2), 213–226. doi:10.1111/j.1467-9566.2012.01534.x PMID:23095003

Cook, R. A., Karesh, W. B., & Osofsky, S. A. (Eds.). (2004). *The Manhattan Principles on 'One World One Health.* New York, NY: Wildlife Conservation Society.

Diguimbaye-Djaibé, C., Hilty, M., Ngandolo, R., Mahamat, H. H., Pfyffer, G. E., Baggi, F., … Zinsstag, J. (2006). Mycobacterium bovis isolates from tuberculous lesions in Chadian zebu carcasses. *Emerging Infectious Diseases, 12*(5), 769–771. Available at http://www.cdc.gov/ncidod/eid/vol12no05/pdfs/05-0691.pdf

Elmer, P. (2004). *The healing arts: Health, disease and society in Europe, 1500-1800.* Manchester, UK: Manchester University Press.

Executive Board. (1951). *EB7.R78 Joint WHO/FAO Expert Group on Zoonoses: Report on First Session*. Geneva, Switzerland: WHO.

Executive Board. (1970). *EB45.R4 Socio-economic Consequences of the Zoonoses*. Geneva, Switzerland: WHO.

Executive Board. (1971). *EB47.R44 Socio-economic Consequences of the Zoonoses*. Geneva, Switzerland: WHO.

Executive Board. (1972). *EB49.R11 Socio-economic Consequences of the Zoonoses*. Geneva, Switzerland: WHO.

FAO, OIE, WHO, UNSIC, UNICEF, & WB. (2008). *Contributing to One World, One Health: A Strategic Framework for Reducing Risks of Infectious Diseases at the Animal–Human–Ecosystems Interface*. Authors.

FAO, OIE, & WHO. (2010). *The FAO-OIE-WHO Collaboration: Sharing Responsibilities and Coordinating Global Activities at the Animal–Human–Ecosystems Interfaces. A Tripartite Concept Note*. Available from http://www.fao.org/docrep/012/ak736e/ak736e00.pdf

FAO, OIE, & WHO. (2012). High-Level Technical Meeting to Address Health Risks at the Human-Animal-Ecosystems Interfaces. Mexico City, Mexico 15-17 November 2011. Authors.

Far Eastern Rural Hygiene Conference. (1937). *Current Science, 6*(2), 70-72.

Foltz, R. C. (2005). Islam, Animals, and Vegetarianism. In *The Encyclopeadia of Religion and Nature* (pp. 873–875). London: Continuum.

French, W. (2005). Francis of Assisi. In *The Encyclopeadia of Religion and Nature* (pp. 670–672). London: Continuum.

Gibbs, S. E. J., & Gibbs, E. P. G. (2012). The Historical, Present, and Future Role of Veterinarians in One Health. In J.S. Mackenzie, M. Jeggo, P. Daszak, & J.A. Richt (Eds.), The Concept and Examples of a One Health Approach = One Health: The Human-Animal-Environment Interfaces in Emerging Infectious Diseases, vol. 1 = Current Topics in Microbiology and Immunologie (pp. 31-47). Berlin, Germany: Springer. doi:10.1007/82_2012_259

Gilbertson, D. (1993). Trichinosis. In K. F. Kiple (Ed.), *The Cambridge world history of human disease* (pp. 1055–1058). Cambridge, UK: Cambridge University Press. doi:10.1017/CHOL9780521332866.207

Gradmann, C. (2010). Robert Koch and the invention of the carrier state: Tropical medicine, veterinary infections and epidemiology around 1900. *Studies in History and Philosophy of Biological and Biomedical Sciences*, *41*(3), 232–240. doi:10.1016/j.shpsc.2010.04.012 PMID:20934644

Gsell, O. (1993). Leptospirosis. In K. F. Kiple (Ed.), *The Cambridge world history of human disease* (pp. 840–842). Cambridge, UK: Cambridge University Press. doi:10.1017/CHOL9780521332866.143

Haller, J. S. Jr. (2003). Ergotism. In K. F. Kiple (Ed.), *The Cambridge historical dictionary of disease* (pp. 120–121). Cambridge, UK: Cambridge University Press.

Handbuch der speciellen Pathologie und Therapie der chronischen Krankheiten nach den Erfahrungen der bewährtesten Ärzte unserer Zeit systematisch dargestellt. (1841). (Vol. 1-3). Berlin: Veit.

Joint WHO/FAO Expert Committee on Zoonoses. (1959). *Second Report = WHO Technical Report Series, 169, FAO agricultural studies, 47.* Author.

Joint WHO/FAO Expert Group on Zoonoses. (1951). *Report on the first session = WHO Technical Report Series, 40.* Author.

Jonas, O., & Warford, L. (2014). *Global Program for Avian Influenza Control and Human Pandemic Preparedness and Response. Project Accomplishments.* Washington, DC: The World Bank.

Kant, I. (2004). Animals may be Used. In A. Linzey & P. B. Clarke (Eds.), *Animal Rights: A Historical Anthology* (pp. 78–79). New York, NY: Columbia University Press.

Kant, I. (2004). Duties to Animals are Indirect. In A. Linzey & P. B. Clarke (Eds.), *Animal Rights: A Historical Anthology* (pp. 126–127). New York, NY: Columbia University Press.

Kelly, A. M., Ferguson, J. D., Galligan, D. T., Salman, M. Osburn, B. I. (2013), One health, food security, and veterinary medicine. *Journal of the American Veterinary Medical Association*, *242*(6), 739-743. doi:10.2460/javma.242.6.739

Krauss, H., Weber, A., Appel, M., Enders, B., Graevenitz, A. v., Isenberg, H. D., … Zahner, H. (2004). Zoonosen. Von Tier zu Mensch übertragbare Infektionskrankheiten (3rd ed.). Köln, Germany: Deutscher Ärzte-Verlag.

Krauße, G., & Zandhof, K. J. (1990). Institut für Hygiene und Technologie der Lebensmittel tierischen Ursprungs. In A. von den Driesch (Ed.), 200 Jahre tierärztliche Lehre und Forschung in München (pp. 83-96). Stuttgart, Germany: Schattauer.

Krönke, F. (2001). *Perception of Ill-health in a FulBe Pastoralist Community and Its Implications on Health Interventions in Chad* (Doctoral dissertation). Available from http://pages.unibas.ch/diss/2002/ DissB_6478.htm

Lerner, H., & Berg, C. (2017). A Comparison of Three Holistic Approaches to Health: One Health, EcoHealth, and Planetary Health. *Frontiers in Veterinary Science*, *4*(163). doi:10.3389/fvets.2017.00163 PMID:29085825

Levin, J. (1839). *Vergleichende Darstellung der von den Hausthieren auf Menschen übertragbaren Krankheiten*. Berlin: Schroeder.

Lyons, M. (1992). *The Colonial Disease: A Social History of Sleeping Sickness in Northern Zaire, 1900-1940*. Cambridge, UK: Cambridge University Press. doi:10.1017/CBO9780511583704

Mayr, A., & Mahnel, H. (1990). Institut für Medizinische Mikrobiologie, Infektions- und Seuchenmedizin. In A. von den Driesch (Ed.), 200 Jahre tierärztliche Lehre und Forschung in München (pp. 169-179). Stuttgart, Germany: Schattauer.

Mill, J. S. (2004). Duties to Animals are Direct. In A. Linzey & P. B. Clarke (Eds.), *Animal Rights: A Historical Anthology* (pp. 138–140). New York, NY: Columbia University Press.

Montavon, A., Jean-Richard, V., Bechir, M., Daugla, D. M., Abdoulaye, M., Bongo Naré, R. N., ... Zinsstag, J. (2013). Health of mobile pastoralists in the Sahel - assessment of 15 years of research and development. *Tropical Medicine & International Health*, *18*(9), 1044–1052. doi:10.1111/tmi.12147 PMID:23834073

Narayanan, V. (2005). Hinduism. In *The Encyclopeadia of Religion and Nature* (pp. 763–777). London: Continuum.

Packard, R. M. (2007). *The making of a tropical disease. A short history of malaria*. Baltimore, MD: Johns Hopkins University Press.

Patterson, D. (2003). Rabies. In K. F. Kiple (Ed.), *The Cambridge historical dictionary of disease* (pp. 270–275). Cambridge, UK: Cambridge University Press.

Pemberton, N., & Worboys, M. (2007). *Mad dogs and Englishmen. Rabies in Britain, 1830-2000*. Basingstoke, UK: Palgrave Macmillan.

Press Information Bureau Government of India. (2007). *'Vision and Road Map' released at the conclusion of the three-day International Ministerial Conference on Avian and Pandemic Influenza*. Retrieved on 14 August from https://www.cdc.gov/onehealth/pdf/delhi/vision_roadmap.pdf

Saunders, L. Z. (2000). Virchow's Contributions to Veterinary Medicine: Celebrated Then, Forgotten Now. *Veterinary Pathology*, *37*(3), 199–207. doi:10.1354/vp.37-3-199 PMID:10810984

Schelling, E. (2002). *Human and animal health in nomadic pastoralist of Chad: Zoonoses, morbidity and health services* (Doctoral dissertation). Available from https://edoc.unibas.ch/57/1/DissB_6478.pdf

Schelling, E., Daoud, S., Daugla, D. M., Diallo, P., Tanner, M., & Zinsstag, J. (2005). Morbidity and nutrition patterns of three nomadic pastoralist communities of Chad. *Acta Tropica*, *95*(1), 16–25. doi:10.1016/j.actatropica.2005.03.006 PMID:15866506

Schmithausen, L. (2005). Buddhism. In *The Encyclopeadia of Religion and Nature* (pp. 232–236). London: Continuum.

Schwabe, C. W. (1978). *Cattle, Priests, and Progress in Medicine*. Minneapolis, MN: University of Minnesota Press.

Schwabe, C. W. (1984). *Veterinary medicine and human health* (3rd ed.). Baltimore, MD: Williams and Wilkins.

Schweitzer, A. (2004). Duties to Life. In A. Linzey & P. B. Clarke (Eds.), *Animal Rights: A Historical Anthology* (pp. 152–153). New York, NY: Columbia University Press.

Scott, H. H. (1942). *A History of Tropical Medicine* (Vol. 1-2). London, UK: Arnold.

Scott, S., & Duncan, C. J. (2001). *Biology of Plagues. Evidence from Historical Populations*. Cambridge, UK: Cambridge University Press. doi:10.1017/CBO9780511542527

Shrestha, K., Acharya, K. P., & Shrestha, S. (2018). One health: The interface between veterinary and human health. *International Journal of One Health*, *4*, 8–14. doi:10.14202/IJOH.2018.8-14

Singer, P. (2004). All Animals are Equal. In A. Linzey & P. B. Clarke (Eds.), *Animal Rights: A Historical Anthology* (pp. 138–140). New York, NY: Columbia University Press.

St Aquinas, T. (2004). Animals are not Rational Creatures. In A. Linzey & P. B. Clarke (Eds.), *Animal Rights: A Historical Anthology* (pp. 7–11). New York, NY: Columbia University Press.

Stein, M. (2008), Zoonosen. Fragile Barriere zwischen den Arten. *Research*Eu. Magazin des europäischen Forschungsraums, Sonderausgabe Oktober ‚Mensch sein Tier sein'*, 34.

Tucker, M. E. (2005). Confucianism. In *The Encyclopeadia of Religion and Nature* (pp. 407–411). London: Continuum.

United Nations. (1975). *Report of the World Food Conference in Rome, 5-16 November 1974*. New York, NY: United Nations.

UNSCN. (2010). *Progress in Nutrition. 6th report on the world nutrition situation*. Geneva, Switzerland: UNSCN.

UNSCN. (2014). *Nutrition and the Post-2015 Sustainable Development Goals. A Technical Note*. Geneva, Switzerland: UNSCN.

UNSCN. (2017a). *Global Governance for Nutrition and the role of UNSCN*. Discussion Paper. Geneva, Switzerland: UNSCN.

UNSCN. (2017b). *By 2030, end all forms of malnutrition and leave no one behind*. Discussion Paper. Geneva, Switzerland: UNSCN.

UNSCN. (2017c). *Sustainable Diets for Healthy People and a Healthy Planet*. Discussion Paper. Geneva, Switzerland: UNSCN.

Vandersmissen, A. (2010). *'One Health': From a Classical Concept to a Modern Dynamics for Global Co-operation*. Paper presented at Operationalizing 'One Health': A Policy Perspective -Taking Stock and Shaping an Implementation Roadmap, Stone Mountain, GA. Retrieved 14 August 2018 from https://www.cdc.gov/onehealth/pdf/atlanta/alain_vandersmissen.pdf

Vermeulen, V. (2010). Forschung an Tieren. In *Forschungsethik. Eine Einführung* (pp. 82–97). Stuttgart: J. B. Metzler.

Virchow, R. (1855). Infectionen durch contagiöse Thiergifte. In *Intoxicationen, Zoonosen und Syphilis = Handbuch der speciellen Pathologie und Therapie, 2(1)*. Erlangen: Enke.

Virchow, R. (1864). *Darstellung der Lehre von den Trichinen mit Rücksicht auf die dadurch gebotenen Vorsichtsmaaßregeln für Laien und Ärzte*. Berlin, Germany: Reimer.

von Braun, J., Ruel, M. T., & Gillespie, S. (2010). Bridging the gap: Linking agriculture and health to achieve the Millenium Development Goals. In P. Pintrup-Andersen (Ed.), *The African Food System and its Interaction with Human Health and Nutrition* (pp. 279–303). Ithaca, NY: Cornell University Press.

von Engelhardt, D. (1984). Kausalität und Konditionalität in der modernen Medizin. In H. Schipperges (Ed.), *Pathogenese. Grundzüge und Perspektiven einer Theoretischen Pathologie*. Berlin, Germany: Springer.

Wagner, E. (Ed.). (1874). *Handbuch der allgemeinen Pathologie*. Leipzig, Germany: Otto Wigand.

Wilkinson, L. (1981). Glanders: Medicine and veterinary medicine in common pursuit of a contagious disease. *Medical History*, *25*(04), 363–384. doi:10.1017/S0025727300034876 PMID:7038356

Wilkinson, L. (1988). Understanding the Nature of Rabies: An Historical Perspective. In J. B. Campbell & K. M. Charlton (Eds.), *Rabies = Developments in Veterinary Virology, 7* (pp. 1–23). Boston, MA: Springer. doi:10.1007/978-1-4613-1755-5_1

Wilkinson, L. (1992). *Animals and Disease. An introduction to the history of comparative medicine*. Cambridge, UK: Cambridge University Press.

Wilkinson, L. (1993). Anthrax. In K. F. Kiple (Ed.), *The Cambridge world history of human disease* (pp. 582–584). Cambridge, UK: Cambridge University Press. doi:10.1017/CHOL9780521332866.070

Winau, R. (1887). *Medizin in Berlin*. Berlin, Germany: Walter de Gruyter.

World Bank. (1986). *Poverty and Hunger: Issues and Options for Food Security in Developing Countries*. Washington, DC: World Bank.

World Bank. (2010a). People, Pathogens, and Our Planet: Vol. 1. *Towards a One Health Approach for Controlling Zoonotic Diseases*. Washington, DC: The World Bank.

World Bank. (2010b). People, Pathogens and Our Planet: Vol. 2. *The Economics of One Health*. Washington, DC: The World Bank.

World Bank Group. (2018). *Operational Framework for strengthening human, animal and environmental public health systems at their interface = Report number 122980-GLB*. Washington, DC: World Bank.

World Health Assembly. (1954). *WHA7-TD-8 Report of technical discussions at the Seventh World Health Assembly*. Author.

World Health Assembly. (1969). *WHA22.35 Socio-economic Consequences of the Zoonoses*. Author.

World Health Organization. (2006). The Control of Neglected Zoonotic Diseases: A Route to Poverty Alleviation: Report of a Joint WHO/DFID-AHP. Meeting with the participation of FAO and OIE = WHO/SDE/FOS/2006.1, Geneva, Switzerland.

World Health Report. (2007). *A Safer Future: Global Public Health Security*. Geneva, Switzerland: WHO.

Wydra, K. (2012). The One Health Concept in a development context. In M. Kappas, U. Groß, & D. Kelleher (Eds.), *Global Health - A challenge for interdisciplinary research*. Göttingen, Germany: Universitätsverlag.

Zinsstag, J. (2012). Convergence of Ecohealth and One Health. *EcoHealth*, *9*(4), 371–373. doi:10.100710393-013-0812-z PMID:23392841

Zinsstag, J., Mackenzie, J. S., Jeggo, M., Heymann, D. L., Patz, J. A., & Daszak, P. (2012). Mainstreaming one health. *EcoHealth*, *9*(2), 107–110. doi:10.100710393-012-0772-8 PMID:22777051

Zinsstag, J., Schelling, E., Waltner-Toews, D., & Tanner, M. (2011, September 1). From "one medicine" to "one health" and systemic approaches to health and well-being. *Preventive Veterinary Medicine*, *101*(3-4), 148–156. doi:10.1016/j.prevetmed.2010.07.003 PMID:20832879

Zinsstag, J., Schelling, E., Waltner-Toews, D., & Tanner, M. (2011). From "one medicine" to "one health" and systemic approaches to health and well-being. *Preventive Veterinary Medicine*, *101*(3-4), 148–156. doi:10.1016/j.prevetmed.2010.07.003 PMID:20832879

Zinsstag, J., Schelling, E., Waltner-Toews, D., Whittaker, M., & Tanner, M. (2015). Preface. In J. Zinsstag, E. Schelling, D. Waltner-Toews, M. Whittacker, & M. Tanner (Eds.), *One Health. The Theory and Practice of Integrated Health Approaches* (pp. xv–xvi). Wallingford, UK: CABI. doi:10.1079/9781780643410.0000

Zinsstag, J., Waltner-Toews, D., & Tanner, M. (2015). Theoretical Issues of One Health. In J. Zinsstag, E. Schelling, D. Waltner-Toews, M. Whittacker, & M. Tanner (Eds.), *One Health. The Theory and Practice of Integrated Health Approaches* (pp. 16–25). Wallingford, UK: CABI. doi:10.1079/9781780643410.0016

Chapter 2
We Are Not Part of Nature; We Are Nature:
An African View on One Health

Ike Iyioke
University of Michigan – Flint, USA

ABSTRACT

This chapter explores holism as it pertains to health in African thought. Specifically, it uses the philosophical notion of personhood to illustrate holism within the biomedical research context. In African philosophy, nature is an organic whole, and the creation and sustenance of ecological balance or interdependence between human and non-humans, the visible and the invisible are most desired. The individual is anchored in a mesh of relationships within the family, village, environment, all of whom are primordial sources of that person's physical, psychic, and spiritual existence and wellbeing. It is a fallacy, indeed absurd to think that humans can exist or act as though they are independent of the environment they live in while continually sensing it via sight, touch, hearing, smell, and taste. In a sense, humans are not just a part of nature; they are nature. It is a holistic perspective, as opposed to anthropocentrism. The continued neglect of this philosophical perspective in favor exclusively of anthropocentrism or individualism is the cause of much human crisis.

DOI: 10.4018/978-1-5225-6304-4.ch002

INTRODUCTION

This chapter explores the notion of holism[1] in African thought as it relates to One Health. Specifically, the African perception of a person (e.g., a research participant) is used to illustrate the understanding of holism within the context of biomedical research or healthcare. Given that African philosophical considerations for the individual person are always in relation to his/her family, community and environment; it follows that individual persons ought to be understood holistically; not as detached entities.

Scant support for aspects of holism has been long in coming, including from philosopher-ecologist Aldo Leopold and environmental naturalist John Muir. Also, more contemporary support for the unanimity of environmental and human health has been noted by the likes of Potter (1971; 1988; 1990; 1995; 1998 and 1999) and Pierce and Jameton (2004). Such support gained strength in a 2014 WHO report. In *Guidance Framework for Testing of Genetically Modified Mosquitoes* (GMM),[2] the WHO doubles down and draws a parallel between environmental and human health.

These strands of support shall be ploughed in for illustration as they merely echo the centuries old African philosophical perspective which holds that every earthly element possesses respective intrinsic value while being intimately connected to everything else in ranked order of being. For instance, the GMM protocol seems to make an about face by breaking with Euro-American liberal tradition as if to recognize the African philosophical disposition to oneness; wholistic healing included.

By comparison, modern Euro-American realization of One Health is in its infancy. For instance, only recently, Craddock (2015) acknowledged it as a well-timed term that is gaining traction to capture and address the complex connection between human, animal and ecological health. Earlier, she had argued that "There is potentially much to be gained by incorporating the interrelations of animal and human ecosystems, as well as the expertise of veterinary, medical, and public health practitioners" (Craddock, 2014, p. 36). Likewise, the intricate patterns of global change and its connection with human, domestic and wildlife and their social and ecological environment, have forced a re-evaluation of integrated approaches to human and animal health and their respective social and environmental implication (Zinsstag, Schelling, Waltner-Toews & Tanner, 2011). With specific reference to challenges posed in recent decades by pandemic infectious diseases such as A(H1N1), HIV/AIDS, SARS and Influenza, need for new approaches and concepts have been urged "in order to understand how biological emergencies and health alerts deploy new scales of action" (Tirado, F., Gomez, A., & Rocamora, V., 2015).

In terms of diseases that are zoonoses, One Health approach creates a confluence for physicians and veterinarians to unify their efforts (Dantas-Torres, F., Chomel, B., & Otranto, D., 2012). An assortment of disease-producing microorganisms such as viruses, bacteria, protozoa and helminths, have life cycles that require passage through the vertebrate host. "Major tick-borne infections of humans are typically an infringement of a circulation between wildlife animal reservoirs and tick vectors" (Baneth, 2014, p. 591). Hence,

One World One Health' (OWOH), 'One Medicine' and 'One Health' are all injunctions to work across the domains of veterinary, human and environmental health. In large part they are institutional responses to growing concerns regarding shared health risks at the human, animal and environmental interfaces. (Hinchliffe, 2015, p. 28)

METHODOLOGY AND ANALYTIC APPROACH

To proceed, the chapter starts with a clinical trial example – the 1996 Trovan experimentation in Nigeria – and briefly examines its implications with respect to the African notion of personhood. Next, a major part of this chapter reviews the philosophical considerations that presaged the development of GMM for the fight against malaria and dengue fever-carrying mosquitoes. The highlighting of relevant parts of the GMM framework will show how they sharply differ from the Trovan clinical trial process in their considerations of study 'subjects' vis-à-vis the environment. Hence, the author will reference in detail the WHO inter-disciplinary report that was formulated to guide the GMM clinical trials process. While it is still early to determine the protocol's full merits nevertheless, its rich vein of form seem to make it a model for other clinical trial protocols, including those that use human subjects and those that potentially have both direct and indirect ecological implications. Next, the chapter examines tenets of environmental ethics and healthcare ethics with a view also to highlight the unity between environmental and human health. The analysis wraps up with a closer examination of holism in African philosophy. The take away message is that even as humans occupy a pivotal place in the web of life, because all reality is interrelated and interdependent, considerations for individual research subjects ought to be extended to everything in the physical, social and spiritual environments in ranking order.

AN AFRICAN TEST CASE

The American pharmaceutical giant, Pfizer, in 1996, administered Trovafloxacin (Trovan), an antibiotic, to many pediatric patients as part of its effort to determine the effectiveness of the experimental drug in treating meningitis during a concurrent epidemic of cerebro-spinal and bacterial meningitis, measles, and cholera in children in Kano, Nigeria. The drug had never been tested on children. All the children in the study were picked from among the long lines of people seeking care. That action was blamed for the death of 11 children; while scores more suffer permanent disabilities such as brain damage, paralysis, muteness/ slurred speech, and blindness (Stephens, 2006, p. A01). A series of lawsuits by the victims and the Nigerian government, filed under the U.S. Alien Tort Claims Act, commenced in 2001, but were withdrawn in the Supreme Court in September 2010. Pfizer had struck a $75-million out-of-court settlement for claims related to the fiasco. Also, later that same year, Pfizer offered to build a $25-million hospital in the city, a gesture aimed to further appease the people (Independent, 2009).

Pfizer claimed it followed all necessary protocols, but because the suits could not run their full course in court, numerous allegations remain unanswered, including that Pfizer took advantage of the chaos from the medical crisis as an opportunity to quickly conduct the study (a potentially dangerous treatment) on young children, something it had been unable to obtain permission to do elsewhere. Other allegations were that Pfizer obtained no assent from any of the children participating in the trial (or informed consent from their parents); and that Pfizer provided no explanation to the children or their parents that the treatment was experimental and that they were free to refuse it in favor of the known effective treatment available at the same hospital free of charge. Lastly, that Pfizer never received the necessary approvals (either from the Nigerian government or the hospital administration) to conduct the research, but when the FDA began to conduct an audit of Pfizer's Trovan records, suddenly a letter dated March 1996 surfaced stating that the hospital's ethics committee had approved the Trovan study (but the hospital had no ethics board).

The default assessment procedure for the Pfizer action would be to adhere to the yardstick established to regulate biomedical research, namely, the four principles of research ethics.[3] This set of principles arose in response to numerous historical acts of experimental callousness which debased human subjects as in the Nuremberg atrocities, among others. To help curtail future recurrence, the Nuremberg Code (and other similar codes) established human subject protection guidelines. However, these principles which are rooted in Western individualistic notions of personhood, are inadequate in for example Africa, which sees the person not as an isolated individual, but as part of the community who is embedded in kinship, community and the environment. The principlist approach is borne out of typical Euro-American thinking which emphasizes the individual and his rights. In the eyes of the experimentalists, the Trovan test subjects were just that – individuated test subjects. But, the African holistic worldview is its opposite and there is no better illustration of this than the understanding of the concept of personhood in African lore.

In African thought (a philosophical tradition that precedes all others) philosophy is about the search for the meaning of being, existence, life – all life in their order, interrelated as one continuum that finds fulfillment in the creator (God). At the fulcrum of that continuum is 'man,' the center of all earthly life, all creation and in whom creation is most made manifest. Put otherwise, the African 'man' is a living vital force who exists in a hierarchical relationship to other beings – his family, clan, descendants, ancestors and deity. Ontologically, he is in a similar relationship with his land; with all that the land contains or produces; with all that grows or lives on it; and all that dwells on it and in it (Tempels, 1959).

Under normal African custom, the individual does not exist alone except corporately. We are who we are because of our roots; hence the individual,

...owes his existence to other people, including those of past generations and his contemporaries. The individual can only say: 'I am because we are; and since we are, therefore I am'. This is a cardinal point in the understanding of the African view of man. (Mbiti, 1970, p.108)

By implication, the fulfillment of a person's life depends on and is enhanced by the support and enrichment of all other life forces (humans/spirits) around, as well as other elements in the environment (say, minerals). In concert, a person's life's worth can either collaterally be enhanced or diminished by other forces and elements around. So, beyond being a social being, the human person is suffused and suffuses in all creation. This relationship is so constitutive of the self that any impact on that oneness, can lead to concomitant impact on the person (and vice-a-versa). And in the view of De Craemer (1983), the far-reaching relationship is therefore believed to be supernaturally, as well as naturally threatening and potentially destructive to the family, the community, and the environment. This all-encompassing perspective has variously been referred to as group solidarity (Menkiti, 2004); communalistic character (Wiredu, 2004); communitarian view (Matolino, 2011); eco-communalism (Tangwa, 2004); cultural collectivism (Schwartz and Bilsky, 1987); communalism (Ikuenobe, 2006); or communalism thesis (Kaphagawani, 2004). Thus, communalism is the most distinguishing feature in understanding the human person in the African thinking. In this chapter, that perspective is called one-in-all relationship or bio-eco-communalism (BEC).[4]

It is against this backdrop; and owing to the intensified practice of transnational biomedical research (particularly the outsourcing of clinical trials from the Global North to the Global South); plus, the considerable controversy about the mainstream ethics of research which is narrowly constructed with individualistic philosophy, that the crafting of GMM framework could not have been better. Its thorough review now follows.

THE GMM MODEL

The GMM intervention is a preventionist precautionary strategy that is built on attacking mosquito vectors *ab initio* and viewed as the most effective way to reduce transmission of diseases in endemic areas. The mechanics of the technology works when lab-hatched genetically modified mosquitoes are,

... made sterile and thus unable to pass the genetic modification on to future generations through mating. In other cases, the GMM are meant to mate and introduce the effect briefly into the local mosquito population, but the modification will gradually be diluted out by crossing with local mosquitoes over a number of generations until it is lost. (WHO GMM, 2014, p. xi)

For a method this new, one main concern was that some unknown outcome could result outside of its intended purpose, potentially engendering grave ethical, environmental, social and other consequences. Considering this, the team of experts[5] devised implementation strategies for the testing of the modified vectors. The result was the following two-tenet agreements:

- *Field testing must begin with release of sterile or otherwise self-limiting modified male mosquitoes in order to gain experience with the technology under circumstances where its effects can be reversed by halting releases.*
- *Testing of modified mosquitoes incorporating gene drive must begin under physical confinement. No genetically-modified mosquitoes designed to replicate and spread the modification to wild-type mosquitoes [should be] tested outside of the laboratory.* (WHO GMM, 2014, p. xi)

This is a confidence-booster and fosters quality and consistency in the processes for testing and regulating new genetic technologies.

Intense calls for ethics and public engagement in public health research is a claim that is often made, and the GMM guideline underscores its importance to the hilt. So crucial and integral are ethics and engagement efforts that it was urged they be initiated early and at intervals throughout the study (and even after). Rightly noted, the role of ethics and engagement becomes clear in the way that tensions are doused between scientists who are absorbed in the quest to realize the envisioned results of their research, and some in the public who view them as lacking in moral sensibility or fellow-feeling. Primed to be a 4-phased trial, the GMM report recommends that engagement activities be introduced during Phases 1 and 2,[6] to ensure the goals and methods of the project are well defined and communicated to meet genuine stakeholder needs.

Field researchers stand to benefit when community engagement activities are expanded in Phase 3 specifically because they address ethical responsibilities beyond the formal permissions required at the individual level (informed consent/assent) and the governmental level (regulatory compliance). If it hasn't been made apparent already, meaningful engagement with the community, among other related actions, smoothens the path to obtaining authorization to conduct study.

The larger philosophical point that the GMM proposal precisely advocates is that ethics of engagement aims to identify and recognize the interests of stakeholders and their legitimate entitlements, rights, other types of claims and obligations, including what actions or activities that are necessary by the principle of respect for communities hosting the trials. (WHO GMM, 2014, p. 60).

The GMM ethics and community engagement approach follows a concentric relationship: from the core 'human research subjects' (residents), to their friends, families, and the larger community. The outer spectrum recognizes individuals who do not typically fall within the definition of human subjects but who might be affected by the conduct of research, either because they reside near the research project site, or that their daily activities and/or livelihood, including economic interests, could be affected by the research activities.

Ordinarily, these are not the sorts of engagement activities standard research budgets accommodate as far as most scientific studies are conceived and conducted. However, it would be conceded that many scientists often view their work as having value and a social purpose, and this may be especially so for those conducting research on public health and disease control. But the hint in the GMM guidelines is that scientists are often not very transparent. Also, scientists do not always articulate the purpose of their research explicitly or discuss its value with others. In contrast, the GMM guidelines sought to make explicit the value and social purpose of the scientific research project and initiate a broader reflection that serves several key functions and interests.

Ziman (1998) makes that ethical burden more explicit particularly as scientific outcomes become increasingly integrated into the social fabric. Hence, "scientists are having to perform new roles in which ethical considerations can no longer be swept aside" (p. 5396). This thinking is reflected in Elliot's (2011) discussion of "Ethics for Experts" or 'ethics of expertise,' EOE. There, he develops a set of guidelines to assist researchers in sharing their study plans and findings; a move that will in turn assist the citizens, activists and policy makers as well to enable them to understand better the ramifications of the research they do on the social environment.

One of the major shortcomings of principlism is the lack of recognition that all research, directly or otherwise, do affect the larger communities and not just the individual study subjects. Hence, the GMM guidelines have highlighted this apparent implication particularly that the effects of the trials will largely be at the community level as well as on the environment. Recognition of this factual rarity (particularly in a prominent literature representing the world body) that fuses human health and environmental health is delightful. But more importantly, it is a widely shared philosophical perspective, for instance, in Africa which recognizes the holism or interconnectedness and the intrinsic value of everything in nature in ranked order of being.

The point here is simply to give readers a picture of some of the reasons a research team on a clinical trials mission might find the prospect of considering the safety of the environment appealing and as an integral part of their work. In certain clinical trial cases (e.g., the GMM trial) the connection is obvious, in others (e.g., the Trovan trials), it might be subliminal. Here, the GMM guideline further gets at the point by way of *biosafety*. By biosafety, the guidelines highlight the connection and proffer plans to address the safe use of technologies "through the management of risks to the environment and to human health posed by the application of the new technology" (WHO GMM, 2014, p. 33).

The design of this public health intervention tool strongly considers the need to target the pathogens in a way that does not harm either environmental or human health (plus, health of non-human animals too). The key word here is risk, how to avoid it if possible, or limit it as much as possible, and manage it to acceptable levels, if a hazard results. This, according the GMM report, is done through 'risk analysis,' a phrase that incorporates, risk concern, risk assessment, risk management and risk communication. It explicates risk concern to mean alertness to and reason to worry about issues pertaining to both technology and social values, and in both cases supported evidence that a concern is valid. For risk assessment and management, the development of risk frameworks are necessary whereby qualitative, and where possible, quantitative pieces of evidence are used to assess the probability that an adverse event will occur and the consequences associated with the occurrence of that event. A risk analysis procedure accounts for the possibility of an event happening but which may or may not be harmful in particular circumstances. Ultimately, effective risk management can render many risks acceptable and manageable.

Per the WHO framework, biosafety risk assessment aims to determine,

(i) the potential hazards and the mechanisms of impact for GMM on wild populations of target and non-target organisms; (ii) the likelihood and magnitude of impact of the GMM on the receiving environment; (iii) the levels and consequences of uncertainty associated with the effects; and, (iv) appropriate risk management measures needed to mitigate any harm or uncertainty associated with changes to target organism populations or the wider receiving environments. Risk communication ensures that there is a well-documented explanation of what risks have been identified, how they have been assessed, what the acceptable level of risk is, and how risk management may be able to achieve acceptable levels of risk with implementation. (WHO GMM, 2014, p. 33)

Ostensibly, estimating the degree of ecological risk from the introduction of a new technology such as GMM, involves an admixture of ethics, culture, science, economics and health. Equally useful would be to apply lessons from other environmental health programs, which typically involve unavoidable risks and as such not amenable to ethical procedures that presume an opportunity to exit or opt out of the risk bearing situation.

In releasing transgenic mosquitoes into a designated site, it was hypothesized that some of the key consequences will likely be the alteration of ecosystem functions (such as role of mosquito larvae in the food chain for predators) and other impacts on target organisms through destabilization of local mosquito populations. The possibility of these unintended reality may pose a risk, according to the guideline, particularly to human health if the GMM vector control system fails after a release program is well advanced. "This might include assessing local mosquito populations for the evolution of resistance to the transgene function, the evolution of the disease pathogen to resist transgene function or changes in host range of targeted mosquito species" (pp. 49-50).

To itemize specifics, the ecological consequences that might occur, as identified by the GMM report, include, effects on biological diversity; persistence of the transgene in the ecosystem; evolutionary responses (especially in target mosquito vectors or pathogens); and, unintentional trans-boundary movement (including international borders).

Finally, the guidelines prescribe that biosafety measures ought to be buoyed further by independent constituencies or review boards. This appears to fit with its promise of maintaining transparency and permitting of objectivity and candor.

Such groups can provide oversight of the risk assessment and risk management within each phase of testing and provide independent scientific advice on the risks of GMM to human health and the environment. (WHO GMM, 2014, p. 51)

All in all, the foregoing marks a shift from considering ethics of research within the bare bones of principlism, to considering the ethics of research in a much broader sense. For instance, the GMM model for biosafety and ethics of engagement, reveal the need to improve the links between research and health care delivery and to promote the environmental, cultural, socio-political and economic processes that are involved, thus widening the understanding of the vicissitudes of the impacts of public health research – or any other research for that matter.

Couched within the philosophical commitment to evaluate clinical trials in terms of ecological and human health, the GMM project seems to have restored a healthy debate. It does so while pursuing efficacy, transparency, responsible sense of purpose, quality and consistency in the process of testing and regulating new genetic technologies. After several decades of regarding bioethics and environmental ethics as distinct disciplines, it appears that mankind's collective capacity to understand and discuss them jointly, is now revamped. Biomedical researchers, bioethicists and environmental philosophers should now take up the challenge to refocus on that discussion.

ENVIRONMETAL ETHICS AND HEALTHCARE ETHICS

Not many people are aware that environmental ethics used to be embedded in bioethics.[7] Pierce and Jameton's (2004) opening salvo lamented about the separation even as both fields remain hinged on a common philosophical substratum. But, the inspiration by the GMM framework already provides a renewed vigor in the direction of resolving that splinter. Properly considered, environmental and human matters should not be separated from each other; that includes ecological and human health issues.

One influential view that seemed to blaze an early trail in fusing human needs with nature was that of John Muir, a Scottish-American naturalist and an early advocate of wilderness preservation in the U.S. He believed in the intrinsic value and rights of all creatures and that a divine spirit flows in nature. But, he equally valued nature for the sake of scientific research, for recreation, aesthetic enjoyment and spiritual inspiration. It was an attribute that didn't quite distinguish him just like most of his 19th century preservationist peers in America (Highland, 2001). However, Aldo Leopold's was one distinctive 19th century perspective that hit the point well out of the ball park. In advocating a land ethic – the view that mankind's moral concern should cover the natural environment and its nonhuman contents – he inspired several thinkers to advance the idea for "moral obligations toward ecological wholes, such as species, communities, and ecosystems; not just their individual constituents," (Stanford Encyclopedia of Philosophy). At Leopold's urging the argument goes that individual interests and well-being should be subsumed under the holistic good of the earth's biotic community. Hence his famous line:

That land as a community is the basic concept of ecology, but that land is to be loved and respected is an extension of ethics... A thing is right when it tends to preserve the integrity, stability, and beauty of the biotic community. It is wrong when it tends otherwise. (Leopold, 1949, pp. 224-225)

In 1970, when Porter used the term *bioethics*, his concern went beyond the confines of medical ethics. He was troubled by the emerging global environmental crisis and the challenges of the earth's survival. That explains why, two decades later, he reframed it as *global bioethics*, to accurately capture his thinking and foster a re-conceptualization of an ethics of health care as it relates to Earth care and global survival. Porter, an oncologist, saw a constant thread of unity whether it was in his cancer research or any other aspect of life and concluded that much of mankind's problems were their inability to forge a synergy between the two broad cultures of science and the humanities.

Ethical values cannot be separated from biological facts. We are in great need of a Land Ethic, a Wildlife Ethic, a Population Ethic, a Consumption Ethic, an Urban Ethic, an International Ethic, a Geriatric Ethic, and so on. (Potter, 1971, p. 55)[8]

To the extent that this disconnect cannot be endured for too long presses the need for the immediate bridging of medical and ecological ethics recognizing them as one and their critical role in the future of health and environmental planning for all species, human and non-human. Whitehouse (1999) draws directly from Potter's original intuition to characterize the syndrome and to recommend a treatment plan. The bridging effort should be seen as the most expansive aspiration that contributes to the "development of viable programs of sustainable medicines in a sustainable environment" (p. 41). Similarly, the work of Pierce and Jameton (2004, p. vi) is primed exactly to achieve that aim. It maintains that high quality and ethically sound health care are guaranteed to be available, if and only if the larger environment is robustly viable enough to sustain good health.

It all seems intuitive and straight forward, yet mankind is reminded that they cannot, in their constant quest for specialization, continue to compartmentalize their daily lives, their health and wellbeing, from reality – essentially, the myriad elements in the ecosystem (human and non-human) that are interdependent on each other in the web of life. From microorganisms and tiny entomological species to large mammals, and the role each plays; to thinking about the safety of the water we drink and about the quality of air. To insist that there is a distinction between environmental implications of mankind's decisions and ethical judgments in health care policies, and to pay little attention to axiomatic philosophical action theory, seems a serious lapse in scholarly rigor. Genetic epidemiology has long proven that human diseases result from a combination of genetic inheritance and the environment and no other affirmation highlights the premise of that argument better (Khoury, M. 1997).

It is easy to discern why there is constant connection in everything. As an illustration, consider the long process in a drug or medical device production whereby biomedical scientists produce a medical device or a cancer drug; IRB committees determine which of them meet clinical trial protocols – federal and state laws; and FDA decides when to approve for market-wide use. What is less known is how often, if at all, any of the actors involved pauses to ponder possible ecological root cause or causes of the cancer disease that may be targeted. But findings such as the ones by a 2013 WHO study might have put paid to that disconnection just as Porter envisioned. Data for the WHO finding show that 223,000 deaths from lung cancer around the world were caused by air pollution in 2013.

The International Agency for Research on Cancer (branch of WHO) that did the study, now classifies air pollution in the same category as tobacco smoke, UV radiation and plutonium. And although air pollution had been known to cause heart and lung diseases, latest evidence provides additional data that it also was causing cancer. So, the next time there is a search for the cure of certain cancers, it should be noted that answers could be residing in plain sight right within the immediate environment. Curiously, the 21st Century Cures Act initiated by President Barak Obama with a $6.3 billion investment for Cancer Moonshot Force, does not do that (Korte, 2016).

Questions that Pierce and Jameton (2004) posed and the compelling answers they proffered to prove their point, are instructive. The questions include: What concepts from environmental ethics can be applied to health care and how can they be combined with more traditional health-care ethics concepts? What kinds of case studies in health care highlight both clinical and environmental principles? Ultimately, it is reasonable to conclude that environmental principles are the pivot of a responsible inclusive understanding of bioethics and conduct of healthcare.

A clarion call from Australia – another effort resembling the African holistic perspective – has aimed to re-interpret the definition of sustainable development with more ecocentric reorientation. If this call from 'Down Under' typifies similar calls that are anticipated from the Western bloc, it could be a sign indicating the shifting posture which adds impetus that holism could be catching on. Imran, Khorshed, and Beaumont (2014) have further exposed the limitations in the contemporary anthropocentric conceptualization of sustainable development with a utilitarian ethic; and strongly argue for a more ecocentric reinterpretation of its definition that is more inclusive of the socio-ecological values. That seems like a recourse to finding lasting global resolution and a framework for sustainable development based on a reinterpretation that recognizes the interdependence of humans with the rest of the ecosphere.

HOLISM AS HALLMARK OF AFRICAN PERSPECTIVE

The trending argument thus far represents strands of philosophical viewpoints that touch on the meaning of holism which itself is built on the simple thought that all reality is a unity. It is still the case that despite advanced technologies and sophisticated modern life; holism is undeniable. One simple action by some actor could have the potential to produce a ripple effect on the rest of reality. Hence, there is a moral burden to maintaining order or else; and how the status quo holds depends on the relationship between individuals, and between humans and the natural ecosystem. Nelson (2010) delineates environmental ethical holism as

...the position that moral significance attaches to wholes over and above the individuals they include, or the idea that environmental wholes can and do matter morally and directly, or that they possess intrinsic value ... We are exploring or desiring a system that allows us to directly morally include species, ecosystems, watersheds, biotic communities, or entities we typically consider collectives.

Following Marietta (1995), Verharen's (2006) three-pronged view of holism is enlightening as well. First, it is a claim that all reality constitutes a single being; then that it is a commitment to join together what has been split apart; and lastly, that it is a claim that a single principle binds all existence together. Earlier, Verharen (1995) explained, as did Diop (1974), that most ancient Egyptian cosmologies attributed the origins of the universe to a single principle such as *Nun*, through a process of becoming out of an original chaotic matter (water).[9] "Through that same creative process, *Khepera*, the basic physical elements come into being, and from those elements evolve the gods, humans, and the world as we know it" (p. 960). The ancient Egyptians joined spirit together with matter, in which case humans were not separate from animals and even gods. Hence, the ancient African progenitor inspired holistic philosophies that have exerted a powerful hold on the human imagination.

While Aldo Leopold is probably modern time's most prominent influence on proponents of holistic ethics, unfortunately very little (if any) credit has been attributed to the ancient African root of that philosophical orientation. As it has been made clear here, the African thinking sees nature (reality) as an organic whole. That African philosophical point of view about which Kelbessa (2011) illuminates is the belief that is further depicted by Oromo ecotheology which teaches a positive relationship between the environment, humanity and their deity.[10]

There is a positive relationship between God and the Earth, humans and the natural environment. All creatures are essentially effected and affected by the harmonious relationship between Waaqa and the Earth. Waqaa is the creator of various creatures and is responsible for their existence. He requires humans to responsibly cohabit the Earth with other creatures... (p. 55)

For the African, here exemplified by the Oromo, the land is not simply a property to be exploited by humans without due respect and care. It is intrinsically valuable and requires respect and protection on the part of its inhabitants. If humans continuously despoil the land by breaking traditional rules and the cosmic purpose, it may not support all creatures indefinitely. The Oromo believe that the present generation has responsibility to pass on natural resources in good order to a future generation. That is why the Oromo are concerned with the health and peace of the environment and its inhabitants. They depend on environmental resources to heal themselves (Kelbessa, 2011).

It follows that in African philosophy, nature (reality) is an organic whole, and the creation and sustenance of ecological balance or interdependence between human and non-humans, the visible and the invisible are most desired. The individual is integrally anchored in a mesh of relationships within the family, village, environment, and even the spiritual world; all of whom are primordial sources of his/her physical, psychic, and spiritual existence and wellbeing (Iyioke, 2016). It is a fallacy, indeed absurd to think that humans can exist or act as though they are independent of the environment they live in even as they ceaselessly rely on it and are unrelentingly sensing it via sight, touch, hearing, smell and taste. In a sense, humans are not just a part of nature, they *are* nature. It is a holistic perspective, as opposed to anthropocentrism (a social paradigm that values nature instrumentally and maintains the isolation of humans from nature and only sees its usefulness to humans). The African traditional belief is that everyone is perpetually incomplete and is eternally being added to others and is fully fulfilled after they are enmeshed with others and with their environment (Niehaus, 2002).

As a disposition that contrasts with much of the prevailing (Euro-American) intellectual stance, this approach strives to introduce the African view point by making explicit the import of the self in a re-contextualized health research arena. Viewed as such, biomedical research (and healthcare service at large) ought to go beyond autonomy-based considerations for the individual with absolute right to self-determination; and embrace a more holistic-based approach that embeds the individual in his/her family, community and the environment.

The point seems to be that the continued neglect of this philosophical axiom in favor exclusively of anthropocentrism or individualism, is the bane of much of human crisis (including health). For instance, Ingwe, R.; Ebegbulem, J.; & Ikeji, C. (2010) have blamed anthropocentric policies and crises in climate/environment, finance and economy (especially by advanced economies) to the complete neglect of ecocentric world view. Specifically, pursuing the objectives and interests of human beings without consideration for the "inter-relatedness of human and non-human natural systems is responsible for the climate-environmental crisis" (p. 03).

In inventing 'eco-bio-communitarianism,' Tangwa (2004) expresses the fear that humankind is living in an age of,

... myriad problems of global pollution (of air, water, and soil); global climate change; of massive risks to plants, animals, and humans from toxic industrial wastes and from sophisticated weapons (conventional, nuclear, chemical, and biological); risks of upsetting nature's ecological balance; risk of accidentally triggering the collapse of the very foundations of life via gene technology, etc. (p. 393)

Hence, a back-to-the-roots solution is recommended on all fronts to refocus and reinstitute various disciplines in the nexus of the development of both human and non-human natural environmental systems.

There is the claim that in the last few decades, environmental ethics has become an inherently holistic pursuit. Consequently, rapid calls for its adoption in both environmental and human health policies have assumed Doppler proportions whenever the issue came up for discussions in African thought (Iyioke, 2016).

By some unintended way, globalization might shed its negative image with the saving grace embedded in the ontological concept of African holism. For one, the immensely complex global economy, have within the last 20-odd years, surged to integrate at a vortex, thanks to globalization. By the same token, the ultimate reduction of complexity to simplicity which is found in the philosophy of holism might just be the solution. Hence, Verharen (2006) concludes that,

The roots of all humans, as the whole world, is finally beginning to discover are in Africa... Unlike the history of the universe [the Big Bang Theory], the history of thought has moved in the direction of simplicity, defined as the smallest number of symbols capable of describing the greatest range of experience. (p. 961)

Agreed.

Figure 1. Environmental/human health, GMM framework, and African holism – one health

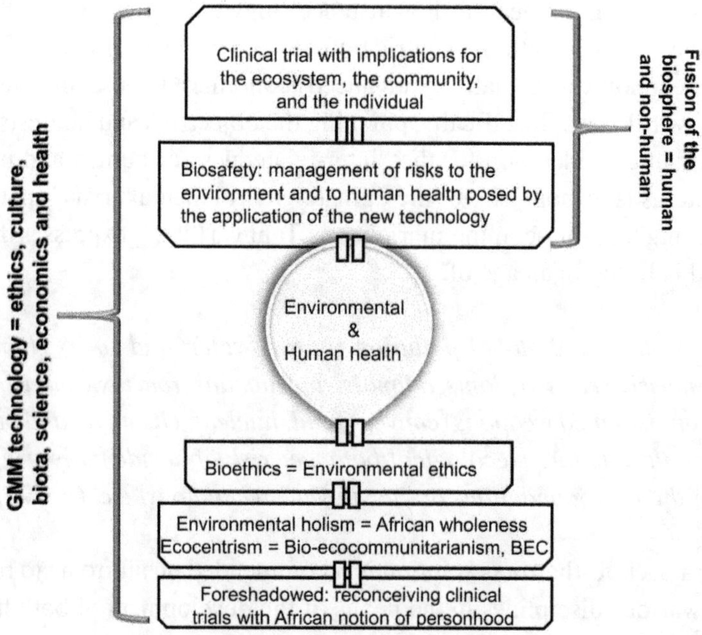

CONCLUSION

In an ideal bedside healthcare delivery, for example nursing care, holism regards the human being as composing of "mind, body and soul integrated into an inseparable whole that is greater than the sum of the parts, [and] is in constant interaction with the universe and all that it contains" (Erickson, 2007, p. 139). In the context of this chapter, holism is taken to a whole new level to represent the totality of reality, or the natural ordering of things which encompasses the natural relations of everything to everything else. The African philosophical tradition regards this interrelationship and interdependency of beings as sacrosanct, such that the preservation and sustenance of the natural order (nature/reality/environment), is a prerequisite to the preservation and sustenance of the elemental forces (humans and non-humans) that exist in it. To guarantee the physical and spiritual well-being of humans, mankind must in tandem ensure the well-being of the surrounding environment in which humans are encased.

When the holistic principle is applied to the health theme, the interconnectedness and interdependence of human persons with everything else in the society and in nature are easily discernible. As such, whatever happens to the individual happens to the community in which he belongs, and to the environment in which everything is contained. This principle rejects individualism and its cousin anthropocentrism.

The conventional biomedical research with human subjects represents anthropocentric/individualistic approach that often seeks to satisfy the needs of the individual person (though desirable as it is); but negates the needs of his/her community, and even exploits nature. When science fashions a project to serve such agendas, the avowed purpose of dominating nature can unwittingly turn into the domination of the human person.

This chapter is a rich constellation of literature touching on holism. A major source being the blaze-trailing GMM clinical trial protocol that fuses human and environmental health, which origin could be traced to ancient African tradition. As summarized in Figure 1, the GMM framework has rendered a catalogue of services that fits perfectly with the author's thesis. 1) The over-arching aim to reconceive responsibility in clinical trials with comprehensive considerations that include research subjects along with their family, community engagement, respect for culture, and the environment. 2) By headlining the intimate connection, namely the inseparability between environmental and human health, the GMM report hits at the heart of a long-nursed intuition that brings together bioethics (here via clinical trials) with environmental ethics. 3) The GMM's methodology further buoys the author's inclination for holism – a widely shared philosophical perspective in African thought; and the intrinsic value of nature in ranked order of being. 4) Even when the protocol does not directly deal with human study subjects, nonetheless its approach is yet another indictment of sorts on the four principles of research ethics. It marks a shift from considering ethics of research solely within the bare bones of principlism to considering the ethics of research in a much broader sense. It engages the transgenic project in the fight against malaria and dengue fever as an all-encompassing endeavor revealing the need to improve the links between environmental health research and human health; and promotes the cultural, socio-political and economic processes that are embedded.

The parallel emergence of such technologies as GMM and One Health approach is striking. Lezaun and Porter (2015) agree,

The development of the One World, One Health agenda coincides in time with the appearance of a different model for the management of human-animal relations: the genetic manipulation of animal species in order to curtail their ability as carriers of human pathogens. (p. 96)

Put together, this chapter benefits from relevant discourses to build a persuasive argument. As a clinical trial protocol with an exceptional merit, it is here argued that the steps GMM method recommends should be standard practice for *all* clinical trial protocols. And, for melding human and environmental health, the argument here bolsters the views of a section of the philosophy community who pine for the urgent reconciliation of healthcare and environmental ethics both of which share a fundamental basis for the pursuit of a common purpose. So fundamentally similar that they both share significant overlap on many issues – ethical approaches, concepts, and moral considerations. That, in and of itself, extends to the eco-centric philosophical view of holism and the intrinsic value of the biospheral elements in ranked order of being. This is best expressed in the communalism principle that is being espoused here, a.k.a., bio-eco-communalism, BEC.

As opposed to autonomy-based principlism, BEC is a communitarian perspective, and is here proposed as the preferred alternative model. This move draws further attention to the inadequacy of the principlist approach particularly in multicultural settings. A re-conceptualized clinical trials process transcends the bare bones of principlism to concentrically accommodate the interests of *all stakeholders* in biomedical studies: human subjects, family, host community, the physical environment, animals, and minerals. As a contribution authored from within the domain of bioethics via African philosophy, the emphasis here is the understanding that African philosophical concepts are never considered as individuated concepts; they are holistic. If therefore, mankind is concerned about their well-being, it must adequately cater for the well-being of every being – human and non-human – in nature. As the foregoing exposition has shown, the African philosophical default position is that everything in nature is ringed together in a web.

This fusion of elements (human and non-human) by implication makes a strong statement about the interrelatedness/interconnectedness of such factors as ethics, culture, the biota, science, technology, and economics. In so doing it has adequately positioned biosafety, namely the management of risks, as an integral point of consideration on issues relating to the environment and to human health.

The wider policy implications resulting from the trans-disciplinary approach in formulating the clinical trials process are many. They include that (the autonomy-based) research ethics principles can no longer be assumed to be universal everlasting ideas or transcendental truths (Rendtorff, 2002). Autonomy-based theoretical approach regards persons as autonomous, self-interested, accumulative and having independent agency which is measured in terms of control over others. By inference, the individual's interests are opposed to the interests of other individuals, his immediate community, the larger social whole, and the environment (Piot, 1990). However, individuals do not exist in a vacuum. So, while individualism and individual rights is the primary concern for research ethics in the mainstream practice; that consideration is here deemed insufficient. Holistic approach is a reminder to pivot to BEC – an understanding that results from re-conceptualizing personhood within the context of communitarianism. With the right awareness, bioethicists, biomedical researchers, medical practitioners, technocrats, scholars, policy makers, and students would benefit from this reformulated approach.

To circle back, the connection of holism in African thought as it pertains to One Health is simple. The ancient African thought adopted holism as conventional custom long before life became complicated. That simple but needful approach has become even more pertinent at current stage of development.

Today's era of globalization is characterized by intensified interspecies encounters, growing ecological concerns and the (re-)emergence of infectious diseases, manifesting themselves in the interplay of medical and biological, but also social, cultural and political processes. One health approaches – which combine multidisciplinary efforts to stimulate collaborations between different health professionals such as veterinarians, medical practitioners, biologists, and public health professionals – can be understood as a response to this complex interconnectedness. (Wolf, 2015, p. 5)

As it stands, the adoption of One World One Health is mankind's resolve to mobilize resources that had for too long existed in separate disciplinary silos and muster an arsenal like never before to address their myriad health and other needs (Mutsaers, 2015).

REFERENCES

Asante, M. (2000). *The Egyptian philosophers: Ancient African voices from Imhotep to Akhenaten*. Chicago, IL: African American Images.

Craddock, S. (2014). Precarious connections: Making therapeutic production happen for malaria and tuberculosis. *Social Science & Medicine*, *129*, 36–43. doi:10.1016/j.socscimed.2014.07.039 PMID:25142906

Craddock, S., & Hinchliffe, S. (2015). One world, one health? Social science engagements with the one health agenda. *Social Science & Medicine*, *129*, 1–4. doi:10.1016/j.socscimed.2014.11.016 PMID:25434985

Danta-Torres, F., Chomel, B., & Otranto, D. (2012). Ticks and tick-borne diseases: A One Health perspective. *Trends in Parasitology*, *28*(10), 437–446. doi:10.1016/j.pt.2012.07.003 PMID:22902521

De Craemer, W. (1983). A cross-cultural perspective on personhood. *The Milbank Memorial Fund Quarterly. Health and Society*, *61*(1), 19–34. doi:10.2307/3349814 PMID:6552386

Diop, C. (1974). *The African Origin of Civilization: Myth or Reality*. Chicago, IL: Lawrence Hill & Co.

Elliot, K. (2011). *Is a little pollution good for you?* New York, NY: Oxford University Press. doi:10.1093/acprof:oso/9780199755622.001.0001

Erickson, H. L. (2007). Philosophy and theory of holism. *The Nursing Clinics of North America*, *42*(2), 139–163. doi:10.1016/j.cnur.2007.03.001 PMID:17544676

Highland, C. (2001). *Meditations of John Muir*. Berkeley, CA: Wilderness Press.

Hinchliffe, S. (2015). More than one world, more than one health: Re-configuring interspecies health. *Social Science & Medicine*, *129*, 28–35. doi:10.1016/j.socscimed.2014.07.007 PMID:25022470

Ikuenobe, P. (2006). *Philosophical perspectives on communalism and morality in African traditions*. Oxford, UK: Lexington Books.

Imran, S., Alam, K., & Beaumont, N. (2014). Reinterpreting the definition of sustainable development for a more ecocentric reorientation. *Sustainable Development*, *22*(2), 134–144. doi:10.1002d.537

Ingwe, R., Ebegbulem, J. & Ikeji, C. (2010). Ecocentric and anthropocentric policies and crises in climate/environment, finance and economy: Implications of the emerging green policy of the Obama administration for Africa's sustainable development. *African Journal of Political Science and International Relations*, *4*(1), 1-12.

Iyioke, I. V. (2016). *Re-conceptualizing responsibility in clinical trials: An insight with the African notion of self* (Unpublished doctoral dissertation). Michigan State University, East Lansing, MI.

Kaphagawani, D. (2004). African conception of a person: A critical survey. In K. Wiredu (Ed.), *A Companion to African Philosophy* (pp. 332–342). Blackwell Publishing; doi:10.1002/9780470997154.ch26

Kelbessa, W. (2005). The utility of ethical dialogue for marginalized voices in Africa. In Proceedings of Sharpening policy tools for marginalized managers of natural resources. Addis Ababa University.

Kelbessa, W. (2011). Indigenous Environmental Philosophy. In J. Garfield & W. Edelglass (Eds.), *The Oxford Handbook of World Philosophy* (pp. 574–581). Oxford, UK: Oxford University Press. doi:10.1093/oxfordhb/9780195328998.003.004

Kelbessa, W. (2011). *Indigenous and Modern environmental ethics: A study of the indigenous Oromo environmental ethic and modern issues of environment and development*. Washington, DC: Cultural Heritage and Contemporary Change, Series II.

Korte, G. (2016, December 13). Obama signs $6.3 billion law for cancer research, drug treatment. *USA Today*.

Leopold, W. (1949). *A Sand County Almanac*. Oxford, UK: Oxford University Press.

Marietta, D. (1995). *For People and the Planet: Holism and Humanism in Environmental ethics*. Philadelphia, PA: Temple University Press.

Matolino, B. (2011). The (mal) function of "it" in Ifeanyi Menkiti's normative account of person. *African Studies Quarterly*, *12*(4), 23–37.

Mbiti, J. (1970). *African Religions and Philosophy*. New York, NY: Praeger Publishers.

Menkiti, I. (2004). On the normative conception of a person. In K. Wiredu (Ed.), *A companion to African philosophy* (pp. 324–331). New York, NY: Blackwell Publishing.

Mutsaers, I. (2015). One-health approach as counter-measure against "autoimmune" responses in biosecurity. *Social Science & Medicine*, *129*, 123–130. doi:10.1016/j.socscimed.2014.09.042 PMID:25446776

Nelson, M. (2010). *Teaching holism in environmental ethics* (Unpublished pedagogical paper). Michigan State University, East Lansing, MI.

Niehaus, I. (2002). Bodies, heat, and taboos: Conceptualizing modern personhood in the South African Lowveld. *Ethnology*, *41*(3), 189. doi:10.2307/4153025

Pierce, J., & Jameton, A. (2004). *The ethics of environmentally responsible health care*. Oxford, UK: Oxford University Press, Inc. doi:10.1016/j.scitotenv.2004.03.034

Piot, C. (1999). *Remotely global: Village modernity in West Africa*. Chicago, IL: The University of Chicago Press.

Porter, V. R. (1999). Fragmented ethics and 'Bridges Bioethics.'. *The Hastings Center Report*, *29*(1), 38–40. doi:10.2307/3528538 PMID:10052010

Porter, V. R., & Whitehouse, P. J. (1998). Deep and global bioethics for a livable world. *Scientist (Philadelphia, Pa.)*, *12*(1), 9.

Potter, V. R. (1971). *Bioethics: Bridge to the future*. Englewood Cliffs, NJ: Prentice-Hall, Inc.

Potter, V. R. (1988). *Global bioethics: Building on the Leopold legacy*. East Lansing, MI: Michigan State University Press.

Potter, V. R. (1990). Getting to the Year 3000: Can global bioethics overcome evolution's fatal flaw? *Perspectives in Biology and Medicine*, *8*(2), 185–186. doi:10.1080/10590509009373376 PMID:11642811

Potter, V. R., & Potter, L. (1995). Global bioethics: Converting sustainable development to global survival. *Medicine and Global Survival*, *2*(3), 9–17. PMID:14627015

Quigley, D. (2006). A review of improved ethical practices in environmental and public health research: Case examples from Native communities. *Ethical Practices in Environmental and Public Health*, *33*(2), 130-147. doi:. doi:10.1023/A:1021132602330

Schwartz, S. & Bilsky, W. (1987). Towards a universal psychological structure of human values. *Journal of Personality and Social Psychology*, (53), 550-562.

Tangwa, G. B. (2004). Some African Reflections on Biomedical and Environmental Ethics. In K. Wiredu (Ed.), *A Companion to African philosophy* (pp. 387–395). Oxford, UK: Blackwell Publishers.

Tempels, P., Rubbens, A., & King, C. (1959). *Bantu philosophy*. Paris: Présence Africaine.

The Internet Encyclopedia of Philosophy. (n.d.). *Bioethics*. Retrieved June 26, 2014, from http://www.iep.utm.edu/bioethic/#SH2a

Tirado, F., Gomez, A., & Rocamora, V. (2015). The global condition of epidemics: Panoramas in A (H1N1) influenza and their consequences for One World One Health program. *Social Science & Medicine*, *129*, 113–122. doi:10.1016/j.socscimed.2014.09.003 PMID:25218795

Verharen, C. C. (1995). Afrocentrism and Acentrism: A marriage of science and philosophy. *Journal of Black Studies*, *26*(1), 62–76. doi:10.1177/002193479502600105

Verharen, C. C. (2006). Philosophy against empire: An ancient Egyptian renaissance. *Journal of Black Studies*, *36*(6), 958–973. doi:10.1177/0021934705286128

Whitehouse, P. J. (1999). The ecomedical disconnection syndrome. *The Hastings Center Report, 29*(1), 41–44. doi:10.2307/3528539 PMID:10052011

Wiredu, K. (2004). Introduction: African philosophy in our time. In K. Wiredu (Ed.), *A Companion to African Philosophy* (pp. 1–28). Blackwell Publishing.

Wolf, M. (2015, March). Is there really such a thing as "one health"? Thinking about a more than human world from the perspective of cultural anthropology. *Social Science & Medicine, 129*, 5–11. doi:10.1016/j.socscimed.2014.06.018 PMID:24961737

World Health Organization, International Agency for Research on Cancer. (2013, October 17). *Press Release, No. 221*. WHO.

World Health Organization. (2014). Guidance framework for testing of genetically modified mosquitoes. A health information product by the WHO-executed UNICEF/UNDP/World Bank/World Health Organizations Special Program for Research and Training in Tropical Diseases. Geneva, Switzerland: WHO.

Ziman, J. (1998). Why must scientists become more ethically sensitive than they used to be? *Science, 282*(5395), 1813–1814. doi:10.1126cience.282.5395.1813 PMID:11645122

Zinsstag, J., Schelling, E., Waltner-Toews, D., & Tanner, M. (2011). *From "one medicine" to "one health" and systemic approaches to health and well-being*. Academic Press.

KEY TERMS AND DEFINITIONS

All-in-One (One-in-All): A term coined to depict the suffusion and inseparability of the individual into his/her community and environment.

BEC: Bio-eco-communalism just like one-in-all, refers to the inseparability of the individual within his/her community and environment.

Ecosystem: A biological system composed of a community of organisms and the nonliving environment with which it interacts [same for Environment and Ecology].

GMM: Genetically modified mosquitoes, also called genetically engineered mosquitoes, transgenic mosquitoes, or living modified mosquitoes – mosquitoes that have heritable traits derived through use of recombinant DNA technology, which alter the strain, line, or colony in a manner usually intended to result in reduction of the transmission of mosquito-borne human diseases.

Global North: Also known as the industrialized world, Western, or Euro-American – refers to the 57 countries with high human development that have a Human Development Index above .8. Most, but not all, of these countries are in the Northern Hemisphere.

Global South: The industrializing world or The Global South refers to the countries of the rest of the world, most of which are in the Southern Hemisphere. Most of the Global South is in South and Central America, Africa, and Asia.

Holism: The interconnectivity and interdependence of all things.

One Health: One Health is the collaborative effort of multiple disciplines—working locally, nationally, and globally—to attain optimal health for people, animals and the environment.

ENDNOTES

1 Holism, communalism, bio-eco-communalism (BEC), interconnectedness and interdependence are all used interchangeably.

2 Sponsored by the World Health Organization, the *2014 WHO Guidance Framework for Testing of Genetically Modified Mosquitoes* compendium is the product of the meeting of the minds of some of the best experts in the field. However, not all aspects of this dense report will pertain to this chapter, hence the chapter will be referencing only the relevant parts. Special tribute is here paid to Paul B. Thompson, a member of the think tank which formulated the report, and who made the report available to the author early as it was still receiving reviews and comments prior to its publication.

3 The four principles of bioethics (a.k.a., principlism) for mainstream practice are: respect for autonomy (i.e., what is best for the individual or a norm of respecting the decision-making capacities of autonomous person); non-maleficence (avoid harm towards the person or a norm of avoiding the causation of individual harm); beneficence (that we do good rather than bad or a group of norms for providing benefits and balancing benefits against individual risks and costs); and, justice/fairness (equal access under the law to information and treatment or a group of norms for distributing individual benefits, risks, and costs fairly).

4 Credit to Tangwa's (2004) ingeniousness in smithing the original term 'eco-biocommunalism.' There, he fuses eco-ethics, environmental ethics, developmental ethics, medical ethics, and bioethics under one label. Though related, but the BEC nomenclature here is however different.

5 The WHO think tank drew people with expertise in molecular biology, medical entomology, ecology, law, ethics, sociology, culture, epidemiology, biostatistics, economics, biology, chemistry, agriculture, toxicology, and psychology.

6 It is here suggested that considerations for ethics and engagement activities should commence at the planning stage (long before Phase 1). The advantage of this early application is to test the waters, meet with third party (outside) groups and individuals, and gauge the strategies in order to tweak any areas that might need improvements. It is at this stage that the GMM acknowledgment makes complete sense: "Engagement and involvement with the communities hosting the GMM trials must be guided by detailed knowledge of the local community, its institutions and common practices. Finding out what kinds of concerns the community might have, any past engagements around science that went badly, or determining what the community wants/expects in terms of engagement or consent [and assent] will be important," p. 70.

7 This chapter is authored from within the domain of bioethics. It is a branch of philosophy which itself is an intellectual and cultural phenomenon that rose from the ashes of medical scandals in the U.S. and elsewhere that seemed to culminate in the late 1960s and the 1970s, leading to the emergence of bioethics as a discipline.

8 Potter, Van. 1971. *Bioethics: Bridge to the Future*. Englewood Cliffs, New Jersey: Prentice-Hall, Inc. There is little wonder why he dedicated this work to the memory of Aldo Leopold who he says anticipated the extension of ethics to bioethics. More of the author's exegesis on this subject matter are available in the following publications: *Global Bioethics: Building on the Leopold Legacy*. East Lansing Michigan: Michigan State University Press, 1988; "Getting to the Year 3000: Can global bioethics overcome evolution's fatal flaw?" *Perspectives in Biology and Medicine*, 34, 1:89-98, 1990; Potter, Van and Potter, Lisa. 1995. "Forum: Global Bioethics: Converting Sustainable Development to Global Survival." *Medicine and Global Survival*, 2, 3:185-91; Porter, Van and Whitehouse, Peter. 1998. "Deep and Global Bioethics for a Livable world." *The Scientist*, 12: 9; and, "Fragmented Ethics and 'Bridges Bioethics.'" *Hastings Center Report* 29, 1:38-40, 1999.

9 In Verheren's words, the *Nun* is sometimes called water, but this translation makes the principle too much like Thales's principle of water. The difference is that for the Kemetians (old name for Egyptians), the Nun is neither physical nor spiritual, but includes both. From this original principle of Nun flows the universe, the gods, humans, heavens, and the earth. Some analogues for this holism are Heraclitus's fire, the Hindu's Brahman, Spinoza's God or Nature, Hegel's Spirit, and contemporary cosmology's hydrogen atoms, quarks, or strings.

10 All African communities, with a varying wealth of symbolism, have akin interpretations. The author could have used any ethnic group anywhere on the African continent to make this point, but Kelbessa's research of the world view of the Oromo ethnic group, the largest in Ethiopia, is representative of a typical perspective that can easily be replicated across Africa. Kelbessa used a combination of desk research, descriptive methods, and field investigation to analyze primary and secondary data.

Chapter 3
One Health Study Design

Punit Jhandai
Lala Lajpat Rai University of Veterinary and Animal Sciences, India

ABSTRACT

One health is an integrated approach that considers human, animal, and environmental health components that can improve prediction. One health implies that data on man and animal health and environmental indicators are studied and interpreted together. This chapter focuses on population-based quantitative and qualitative one health study designs with an emphasis on field surveys to understand disease dynamics and how to control measures being tested. The aim is not on early diagnoses of emerging diseases but instead of that on endemic zoonosis. It first describes examples on joint monitoring and surveillance to control diseases and then practical information on planning of a field study design, and concludes on the advantages of one health study designs. Also discussed are possible constraints for their implementation. For the examples, single sector approach could not explain the main epidemiological considerations.

DOI: 10.4018/978-1-5225-6304-4.ch003

WHAT IS A ONE HEALTH STUDY?

Human and animal health epidemiological studies done by field surveys or secondary data analyses. During different periods data is collected within human and animal health sector and interpreted and also when an identical health topic is approached, which leads to unwanted duplication of field studies. Studies on zoonoses and foodborne pathogens are mainly led by public health veterinarian. Risk assessment along the production and marketing chain of food borne pathogen in livestock sector approach allows the identification of the point of greatest leverage of control measures. Human health hazards are identified and impacts on human health are interpolated from numbers. New integrated disease surveillance systems are under evaluation (Wendt *et al.*, 2014). From separated studies it is difficult to draw coherent conclusions on linkages between human and animal health. Knowing the main source of human infection is important to achieve the greatest leverage in reduction of human infections. A One Health study implies that data on human and animal health, possibly also on ecological indicators, are analysed in an integrated way and are interpreted together. Sometimes these data are from different studies or data sources, but they should be comparable in terms of location, time, level of aggregation, details and quality, and a multidisciplinary team should publish their results together. A One Health study should lead to insights that would not be visible without intersectoral collaboration such as impacts of multi-host infections on humans, animal and ecosystem health and economics (Zinsstag *et al.*). Rabinowitz *et al.* (2013) have defined a One Health approach similarly: 'Integrated approaches that consider human, animal, and environmental health components that can improve prediction and control of certain diseases'. This is not only true for infectious diseases, but also for non-communicable diseases and health system strengthening. The aim is not necessarily improved human health or averted human burden of disease. Messenger *et al.* (2014) showed that an increasing number of reports indicate that humans are transmitting pathogens to animals. Recent examples include methicillin-resistant *Staphylococcus aureus*, influenza A virus, *Cryptosporidium parvum* and *Ascaris lumbricoides*.

A One Health study would show bi- and multidirectional relations between human and animal health and their health in relation to the health of their ecosystem (Zinsstag, 2012). Thus the aim is ideally improved human, animal and ecosystem health. The most difficult step of a One Health study remains the initiation of a process that leads to change and health improvement. To successfully control neglected zoonoses we must extend our vison outside the health sectors; for example policies may need to be focussed into poverty reduction strategies and continuous training to build health service skills and competences. Networking and regional approaches have been successfully used for zoonoses control (Parkes *et al.*, 2012). Avian influenza led to the establishment of highly recognized networks for exchange of information and lessons such as from the Asian Partnership for Emerging Infectious Diseases Research and the Mekong Basin Disease Surveillance (Grace *et al.*, 2011). For most zoonoses, one country alone can hardly implement successful control measures without the neighbouring countries doing likewise. Disease-control programmes designed in developed countries for industry-wide application cannot be transferred without appropriate adaptation to other settings (Randolph *et al.*, 2007). Many factors critical to successful disease control cannot be assessed quantitatively. The way forward is to enhance interdisciplinary cooperation between the social and health-related sciences (Whittaker). Note that the literature is richer on studies describing broader socio-cultural considerations for emerging zoonoses. These are, for example, human encroachment into forests with potential exposure to new pathogens, global travel and eating of bush meat. While One Health recognizes the importance of understanding the social and cultural factors in disease transmission dynamics and the planning of control interventions, anthropological studies on zoonoses are sparse and limited (Bardosh and Thys, 2012). Socio-cultural One Health surveys and the role of social sciences are described elsewhere in this book (Whittaker). In this chapter we focus on population based quantitative One Health study designs with emphasis on planning of field surveys. Such studies are central to the understanding of disease dynamics and for evaluating evidence based testing of control measures. In addition, data for cost–benefit and cost-effectiveness calculations (Zinsstag *et al.*, 2007) are hardly available at central level alone and good quality field data is needed. Therefore, laboratory- based studies used to improve and create new vaccines against zoonoses and comparative pathology. We do not focus on early detection of emerging diseases but rather on endemic zoonoses. The incidences of the latter are believed to be much higher, however are under-reported due to low capacity to recognize and diagnose the causative agents of zoonoses. Health of ecosystems is difficult to define. They are inherently dynamic and changing (Cumming and Cumming,). The simultaneous assessment of human and animal health is beneficial in understanding of the context and associated different disciplines. A key discipline in One Health field studies is epidemiology, thus the study of health and disease in populations.

Epidemiology derives from Greek and literally means 'the study of what is upon the people'; 'demos' meaning 'people, district' (Omran, 1971). This may suggest that epidemiology applies only to human populations. Most veterinary epidemiologists believe, however, that it is pointless to use different terms such as epizootiology, epizootic, or enzootic when referring to a disease in an animal population. The words 'epidemiology', 'epidemic' and 'endemic' should be used to describe disease occurrence in all host species. Epidemiology has also been applied to studies of plant populations (Bartlett and Judge, 1997; Nutter, 1999). Common in epidemiology is that a health-related question leads to a hypothesis and defines an objective, which leads to the appropriate study design to use. We first provide examples on joint surveys and surveillance, then on practical information on planning of a field study design and conclude on the advantages of One Health study designs. We also mention possible constraints for their implementation given that there are only a few One Health studies to date. For the examples, the main epidemiological considerations and the results that could not be achieved with single sector approaches are highlighted.

One Health Surveys and Surveillance

Joint human and animal health surveys are either done during the same period or in the same geographical area and at different levels of aggregation. Levels of aggregation are vary from individual, for example an owner– pet relation, household and village levels, and also communities and their animals, districts, provinces or countries.

Simultaneous Human and Animal Health Assessment

A simultaneous assessment of livestock milk and human sera vitamin levels, combined with a 24 h nutrition recall study, showed that milk was the most important source of vitamin A for the person involved in herding of animal, but 17% of tested women were severely retinol-deficient. Therefore the consumption of more vegetables and fruits needs to be promoted (Zinsstag *et al.*, 2002). The latter survey could show the linkages between livestock and human nutrition, but was only done in one specific community. A mixed team composed of medical and veterinary staff assessed during repeated cross-sectional surveys health and health-related issues of mobile pastoralists and their livestock using standardized clinical examination forms and questionnaires. The main diseases and conditions found among mobile pastoralists did not differ substantially from morbidity typical for the diseases such as respiratory diseases, malaria and diarrhoea. Despite frequent diarrhoea and fevers, respiratory infections including lower tract infections in children and tuberculosis in adults, and malaria, had more impact on individual and community health than food-poisoning and zoonotic diseases such as brucellosis. Therefore, a programme on control of zoonoses should not ignore other prevailing health problems of the communities. This simultaneous health assessment also showed that there was no fully immunized pastoralist child in the study population. In contrast, livestock had been vaccinated by veterinarians visiting the pastoralist camps during compulsory vaccination campaigns (Schelling *et al.*, 2005). Based on this finding and in agreement with the communities and the Chadian national and local authorities, joint human and animal vaccination services were conducted and evaluated (Schelling *et al.*, 2007;). Health impact assessments of industrial development projects (Winkler *et al.*, 2012) could be extended to simultaneously assess livestock health, if veterinarians were associated. Projects such as construction of dams and mining can adversely affect the health of the livestock kept by the surveyed households and have implications on their livelihoods and income. Hence health impact assessment could be extended to One Health Impact Assessment (OHIA).

Field Surveys on Zoonoses

Simultaneous assessment of zoonotic incidences and prevalence in animals and people at the same levels and same quality, for example regarding selection, helps to establish epidemiologic links. In Chad, human Q-fever seropositivity was associated with keeping of camels but not of cattle (Schelling *et al.*, 2003); in Kyrgyzstan and Egypt human brucellosis sero-prevalences were most closely related to keeping of sheep (El Sherbini *et al.*, 2007; Bonfoh *et al.*, 2012) and thus small ruminants cannot be excluded in a control programme. In Togo, human seropositivity was astonishingly low (below 1%), although cattle seropositivity was high (9% in village and 7% in transhumant cattle) (Dean *et al.*, 2013). The isolated *Brucella abortus* strains from cattle harboured a large deletion in a gene (*bruAb2_0168*) encoding for a putative autotransporter. This gene is of particular interest because it is used as a target for PCR in the identification of the species *B. abortus* and it encodes for a putative autotransporter, which might be involved in virulence and/or host predilection (Dean *et al.*, 2014). Further laboratory-based virulence studies will likely better explain the observations from the field (Zinsstag *et al.*). In Ethiopia, *Mycobacterium bovis* in human TB infection is very low (4 *M. bovis* isolates compared to 1000 *M. tuberculosis* isolates from clinical suspects of pulmonary and extra-pulmonary TB) (Firdessa *et al.*, 2013). Interestingly, *M. tuberculosis* was isolated from cattle and one camel (Gumi *et al.*, 2012). The latter study was a combined field, slaughterhouse and hospital study with data collection during the same period (Tschopp). In 2006, the Health for Animals and Livelihood Improvement (HALI) project was initiated to test the feasibility of a One Health approach to find creative solutions to health problems in communities living in the water-limited Ruaha ecosystem of Tanzania. Simultaneous investigations of medical, ecological, socio-economic and policy issues driving the ecosystem were implemented. Based on input from local stakeholders, waterborne diarrhoeal diseases and cattle diseases were also assessed to identify geographic areas with varying water availability, where risk of transmission may be highest (Mazet *et al.*, 2009). The researchers could show with the example of bovine tuberculosis that there was livestock–wildlife pathogen transmission in the Ruaha ecosystem (Clifford *et al.*, 2013).

Food- and Water-Borne Zoonoses

Control of foodborne and waterborne infections requires input from public health, environmental health and veterinary public health practitioners as well as regulatory authorities responsible for safe food and water. They also require a deep understanding of how social, economic, environmental and cultural factors interact with dynamics of disease transmission and the acceptability of control measures (VWB/VSF Canada, 2010). The Caribbean Eco-Health Program (CEHP) has supported interdisciplinary training, particularly of human and environmental health agents and assisted to identify regional knowledge gaps in environmental health threats such as pesticide residues, which were important to users and policy makers. The Atlantis Mobile Laboratory could move throughout the Caribbean and be able to respond to calls for specific research concerns and capacity-building opportunities (Forde *et al.*, 2011). Total bacteria, *Streptococcus/Enterococcus*, yeast and mould, Enterobacteriaceae and *Staphylococcus* counts all increased along the chain from milk at milking to marketed milk in Kenya, indicating a human health hazard according to Kenyan quality standards. To test this, an unmatched nested case-control study – constructed from a cross-sectional survey – confirmed that gastrointestinal illness was significantly associated with consumption of certain vegetables and camel milk (Kaindi *et al.*, 2012). This study led to revitalizing the past efforts of seeing that milk collectors use containers that can be easily washed with water and soap (Bonfoh *et al.*, 2003). High levels of pathogens and other hazards in milk and milk products are reported from both the formal and informal dairy sectors. The role of food safety in dairy policy potentially constrains the shift of policy to more pro-poor policies because informal markets are prior excluded.

Survey and Surveillance of Antimicrobial Resistance

Pets are often companions used for psychological support in the therapy of nursing home residents but have also been described as reservoirs for antibiotic-resistant bacteria. To investigate the role of healthy pets as reservoirs of multidrug-resistant staphylococci or Extended Spectrum Beta-Lactamase (ESBL) producing Enterobacteriaceae, several studies have assessed these with the same approach in both people and pets in nursing homes and the general population (reviewed in Messenger *et al.*, 2014). Although identical genomic patterns from people and from animals have been found, the direction of transmission often remains unclear. The same issues arose for example in tuberculosis. Cattle were infected with *M. tuberculosis* and could have acquired infection from people or from other cattle (Gumi *et al.*, 2012). Likely the question on 'who infects whom' is not necessarily the primary question since people and animals share the same ecosystem and evolve together, but rather which control measure has highest leverage in both people and animals (Tschopp). The Canadian Integrated Program for Antimicrobial Resistance Surveillance (CIPARS) unifies surveillance components, which can be linked to examine the relationship between antimicrobials used in food-animals and humans and the associated health impacts. Analysis of CIPARS data identified a link between ceftiofur (an antimicrobial of high importance to human medicine) usage in poultry and ceftiofur resistant *Salmonella,* Heidelberg isolates obtained from people and chicken meat in Quebec. Communication of this information led to a voluntary ban on the use of ceftiofur in 2005 (CIPARS, 2007). It would be interesting to have more information on costs of running this nationwide programme, which, in turn, can inform other countries on investing in a shared intersectoral system for evidence based guidance to physicians and veterinarians in their selection of appropriate antimicrobials.

Joint Disease Surveillance Systems and Use of Routine Data

In the Q-fever outbreak in the Netherlands (2007–2010), there were 4000 confirmed human Q-fever cases with 11 deaths and huge economic losses among dairy goat herds given the 40,000 slaughtered pregnant goats (Enserink, 2010). Could the outbreak have been controlled earlier if the health and veterinary sectors had exchanged data and communicated at an earlier stage? Most abnormal disease events are seen rather late in the human health and veterinary sectors, despite the fact that early detection is a core objective of surveillance systems. The cohort study set up in the Netherlands between 2007 and 2011 (van Loenhout *et al.*, 2012) included only people. A parallel cohort in goats may have led to additional links seen between events in people and goats. Surveillance and monitoring efforts are major components and central to disease prevention and control programmes. Joint human and animal surveillance networks could be more effective in terms of earlier detection or lower fixed costs than active surveys. Currently such surveillance systems are being tested. Since they have been set up more recently, the results on possible added value are not yet available. Wendt *et al.* (2014) have reviewed these recent systems and found that the majority of the 27 identified human and animal surveillance systems world-wide were established for the purpose of early detection and tend to focus predominantly on emerging pandemic threats. Most systems use different data sources, and secondary data, methods and frameworks on the integration of disparate and secondary data are of great interest. Information integration is possible to achieve despite the fact that data have been collected in different surroundings and often for different purposes and thus differ in content, quality and terminology and are stored in different locations or formats. However, transforming and cleaning procedures have to be applied and this requires time and effort as long as the different data sources have not been standardized or prepared for an easy linkage. Above all, cross-sectoral structures, trust and good communication networks are required (Wendt *et al.*, 2014). Regional and national intersectoral data exchange cannot be expected to work if there are no collaborations at all levels of data reporting, at least to briefly cross-check reports. There is a need for consistent, reliable data at a national level – over a longer term – but also – in the shorter term – the need for reliable data to demonstrate the neglected status of the diseases. The lack of diagnostic facilities and regional reference laboratories for diagnosis of zoonoses in many parts of the world is a constraint to this, since most current joint surveillance systems rely on routine data from diagnostic laboratories (WHO *et al.*, 2009; Wendt *et al.*, 2014). In future more alternative surveillance systems will be evaluated – such as syndromic surveillance, participatory

epidemiology and risk-based joint surveillance systems. However, these systems still need to show that they can be effective in detection of abnormal events and are not too costly to be maintained. Also, to achieve added value of integrated surveillance systems requires shared objectives and strategies for institutional integration at the appropriate level (Mariner *et al.*, 2011). Use of modern mobile technology for near real-time reporting will be used more frequently in future, for One Health and other surveillance systems (Karimuribo *et al.*, 2012; Jean-Richard and Crump). But no near real-time reporting system should be established without giving possibilities of reacting to reported events. The lack of response capacity has stopped several surveillance systems in the past, because reporting ceased when the communities did not see any result to their reporting efforts (Karimuribo *et al.*, 2012). Also, monitoring can include other parameters than diseases or antimicrobial resistances. Stakeholders in zoonoses control and response capacity of the health and veterinary sectors can and should be monitored. For Rift Valley fever (RVF) in Kenya, a stakeholder analysis showed that the 28 relevant agencies in prevention/control of RVF go beyond the line of the livestock and public health sectors. A survey just after the RVF outbreak in 2006/2007 showed that the veterinary sector is understaffed to respond adequately to such an epidemic. The public health sector could deploy five times more staff than the veterinary sector, although the latter had more tasks during the outbreak situation (Schelling and Kimani, 2007). Routine data is often compared with Survey data to estimate under-reporting. For example, Cleaveland *et al.* (2002) found that active detection of human rabies deaths is difficult due to low incidence and the need to set up specific detection studies such as collection of verbal autopsy data from household surveys. Passive surveillance may be insufficient, leading to vast under-reporting of human rabies cases. However, animal bites can be surveyed given their rather high incidence and the likelihood of victims to seek professional care. Cleaveland *et al.* (2002) used a probability decision tree to estimate human mortality from information provided by animal bite victims. After validation with field studies, the authors estimated that in rural Tanzania the true incidence of human rabies was 10–100 times higher than the officially reported human rabies incidence. Good routine data can be used for mathematical models (Zinsstag *et al.*,) – for example avian influenza. A mathematical model of avian influenza transmission between wild birds and domestic poultry was used to provide proof of concept for a proposed integrated intervention involving human, animal and environmental health to interrupt such transmission (Guan *et al.*, 2007). However, modelling of prediction is only possible where suitable primary (fieldbased) data are available. No model can improve data of doubtful quality.

PRACTICAL CONSIDERATIONS FOR ONE HEALTH STUDIES STUDY TYPES IN PUBLIC HEALTH AND VETERINARY EPIDEMIOLOGY

Epidemiological research can be broadly classified into field-based and hospital-based studies. In veterinary epidemiology, studies at veterinary clinics are less common than in public health at health centres, and the main categories are field-based and abattoir/ slaughterhouse-based studies. Obviously, field-based studies represent the general population much better than studies conducted in slaughterhouses, since the age distribution of the animals is different. Reviews found significantly higher prevalence's in slaughterhouses compared to field-based surveys (Agrawal, 2012). In some settings, animal producers preferentially send their old, unproductive or infertile cattle for slaughter, which increases the chance of detecting more chronic infections than in the population. Conversely, farmers may prefer home slaughter if they fear condemnation of carcasses at abattoirs. Another constraint is the limited amount of additional information on the animals. Since intermediary traders are common in many parts of the world, information about origin, herd size or farming system is missing. On the other hand, field-based studies are much more resource intensive in terms of costs, time and administration. Besides more time and needed transportation, they also require higher logistical skills such as storage of samples until processing in laboratories. Besides the study population, the study design is strongly linked to the associated level of evidence. For example, cross-sectional studies have a high risk of bias, which raises questions about the validity of the findings. One considers a systematic review of high quality studies as having a high level of evidence. In 1972, Archie Cochrane highlighted the lack of reliable reviews of available evidence and established the concept of evidence-based medicine. It was soon recognized that there was a need to develop also systematic approaches to assess the study quality in other health sectors. Consequently, evidence-based veterinary medicine and evidence-based public health evolved. Unfortunately, until today no attempt has been made to adapt the evidence base concept into the

One Health context. However, numerous tools and checklists for assessing study quality are available and the main aspects apply also to One Health studies. The main constraints that prevent a causal interpretation are bias, confounding and chance. One of the seminal papers on this subject was by Sir Austin Bradford Hill (Hill, 1965). The highest level of evidence is provided by experiments, i.e. cluster randomized controlled clinical trials. However, such trials are often not feasible for ethical, operational or financial reasons. Properly designed large cohort studies are usually graded as high quality. It is noteworthy that not only the level of evidence defines the most suitable study design, but also disease and exposure characteristics. For example, cohort studies are inappropriate if the outcome of interest is rare.

Sampling and Sampling Frame

In particular, young researchers commonly underestimate the complexity of planning and conducting sampling in resource-limited settings. However, an improperly drawn and not representative sample might introduce serious bias, which can easily double or halve the observed effective size. Unfortunately, only if controversial publications are published, will the importance of proper sampling attract more attention (for example, Burnham *et al.*, 2006, which led to numerous discussions on 'main street bias' and showed the difficulties associated with proper sampling in urban settings). Next to a careful sampling, a detailed description of the sampling approach used is mandatory. There are too many publications with an incomplete description of the sampling procedure. Likewise, research on sampling approaches and theory has been neglected by the scientific communities in both human health and veterinary epidemiology. There are only a few studies investigating appropriateness or bias associated with common but non-random sampling techniques such as 'spin the bottle' (i.e. spinning a bottle on the ground to select a direction). The potential of as unbiased as possible sampling using modern techniques using GIS and satellite images also remains underexploited. Most statistical techniques require the theoretical assumption of a simple random sample, i.e. each individual from the population has the same probability to be selected and enrolled in the study. The sampling frame is a list of all members – or as complete as possible – from the population. Individuals are randomly drawn from the sampling frame and all individuals have the same chance to be enrolled in the study. Where no complete registries of humans or animals exist, as is the case in most studies a multi-stage cluster sampling is commonly used. In a first stage, clusters, i.e. administrative units such as villages or neighbourhoods, are randomly selected. If a nationwide study is done, selection may start at a higher level, such as provinces. Afterwards households or animal-keeping households are randomly selected within each cluster. In a final step, either all animals or a random subset of animals is selected. Cluster sampling is the natural sampling design in veterinary epidemiology, since livestock populations are typically clustered into herds or flocks. Surprisingly, cluster sampling is often confused with stratified sampling. Cluster sampling requires a higher sample size, which is not the case for stratified sampling compared to simple random sampling. The differences are explained in Figure 1.

Random Selection of Clusters

In contrast to lists with individuals, a sampling frame at cluster level, like a list of all villages in a certain district, is usually available or can be established. There are two main approaches to select the clusters, either by simple random sampling, or, if the number of individuals within each cluster is known, sampling with probability proportional to size (PPS). For the former approach, the probability of individuals to be selected is higher in smaller clusters. Almost all statistical software packages are able to perform a weighted sampling. If there is no software available, the method can also be applied without computer assistance. The main advantage of sampling proportional to size is that each individual in the population has the same probability of being selected. Since the risk of infectious diseases is usually density dependent, this approach provides an unbiased prevalence estimate. A challenge in a One Health study is that humans and animals are investigated simultaneously. One needs to consider that selection probabilities can only be assigned to one population, thus either to the number of humans of interest or animals at the same time. One could argue to select the main presumptive reservoir host as sampling frame. During data analysis, sampling weights can be used to produce representative estimates. If a list of villages or neighbourhoods cannot be established – for example slums are challenging in this context because they are very dynamic – alternative approaches have to be applied. But the approach needs to be selected carefully, given that virtually all are subject to selection bias. One methodology that is assumed to be tolerably unbiased is the random generation of geo-coordinates within the study area using GIS or alternative software and selection of the community closest to the generated point. However, bias may be introduced because villages in sparsely populated areas have a higher probability to be selected compared to villages from densely populated areas. As for humans and animals, inclusion and exclusion criteria must be clearly stated in the study protocol, e.g. villages must be accessible by car during the rainy season or must have at least one cattle-keeping household. Likewise, the study area must be clearly defined. This is not the case with statements like 'villages within X hours driving time'. Sampling procedures like 'villages were selected on the basis of proximity to' is clearly a purposive selection approach and, therefore, unsuitable for quantitative data collection.

Sampling of Humans Within Villages or Communities

The by far most common approach in selection of people in a rural community is via random selection of eligible households, but this approach requires a list of all households as the sampling frame. Such a list can usually be compiled together with the village head, who needs to be informed about the research activities anyway. To draw a map or to use a satellite image might be worth considering in longitudinal studies. Which households are eligible, e.g. only animal-keeping households or all households, depends on the disease, the cultural setting and the research question. When the priority is to cover as many villages as possible, e.g. for estimation of vaccination coverage, alternative procedures such as segmentation techniques and random transects (spin the bottle) are commonly applied, but especially the latter approach is more prone to bias.

After random selection of households, the next step is to sample persons living within the households. For certain research questions only people with intense animal contacts may be of interest, but for a detailed understanding of the epidemiology and transmission pathways all family members are often considered eligible (whereby for ethical and practical reasons sometimes children or young children are excluded). In the ideal case, all family members are enrolled. But if the diagnostic procedures are time consuming or costly, it may be better to sample only some household members to ensure that the number of households will not be compromised. If only a single or few household members are selected, it is important to be aware of the 'household

Figure 1. Stratified random sampling versus cluster sampling

In a *stratified random sampling*, the individuals of the target population are first divided into subgroups called strata. Each individual belongs to one stratum. Then a random sample is drawn from each stratum, e.g. 10% of the population. This approach is advantageous if subpopulations vary greatly and the estimates in each subgroup or the differences between subgroups are of particular interest. *Cluster sampling* is an approach in which clusters of individuals rather than individuals are randomly selected. Like stratified random sampling, the population is divided into separate groups such that each individual belongs to exactly one cluster. Clusters are usually defined by geographic boundaries or administrative units (in contrast, strata can be defined as age groups, sex, etc., Fig .1). Natural clusters are herds and households or villages. Depending on the research question, the cluster can be selected via simple random sampling or with a probability proportional to their size. Cluster sampling requires rather sophisticated analytical methods and a larger sample size.

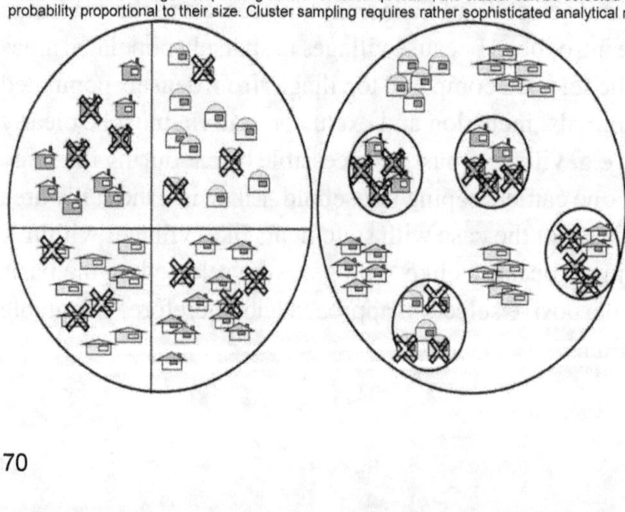

size bias'. Since all households have the same probability to be selected and a single person per household is randomly chosen, individuals in small households have obviously a higher selection probability compared to households with many family members. Since household size is associated with the age structure – and many diseases have age-dependent distribution – the bias might be substantial.

Random Selection of Animals

Informed consent is sought before the sampling from all animal owners (see ethical considerations below). The investigator must be in charge of the random selection of animals. Animal owners have the tendency to catch less healthy animals hoping that the present veterinarian would provide a treatment and thus one should make sure that owners influence the selection as little as possible. If the owner has a complete list of all eligible animals, a simple random selection can be drawn. However, the most common sampling method is that livestock owners are asked to drive the animals into an enclosure or pen. The total number of the herd (e.g. 100 sheep) is divided by the sample size (e.g. 10), which gives the sampling interval (in our case 10). Every tenth sheep coming out of the pen is then sampled, whereby the first sheep is selected with a random number from 1 to the sampling interval, for example by drawing a number from a bag or a dice if the sampling interval is smaller or equal to 6.

Herd-Level Prevalence

For many diseases, not only the animal-level prevalence, but also the herd-prevalence is of interest. When all animals of the herd are sampled and a perfect diagnostic test is applied, no bias derives from the calculation of the herd-level prevalence. It becomes more complicated if the estimate needs to be corrected for imperfect test sensitivity and specificity and when only a small fraction of all animals is sampled. If animals were randomly chosen from each herd, the animal-level prevalence estimate will be unbiased, but this is not true for the herd-level prevalence. Formulae are available to calculate the corresponding herd-level prevalence's (Faes *et al.*, 2011).

Statistical Analysis

Since cluster sampling is a study design feature and the outcome of interest is likely to be correlated within clusters, the data analysis has to take this into account. A comprehensive introduction goes beyond the scope of this chapter. We present some key aspects, which should be considered in the analysis. Theoretically, modern statistical software is in most cases able to handle several levels of clustering, i.e.

animals within herds, herds within villages, villages within administrative units. However, in practice, only one level of clustering is considered in the analysis. The main question in this context is: which is the ecological unit? If all animals within a certain village are free roaming and mixing at water points and during grazing, all animals from this village should be considered as one herd. If animals are held in fenced and dispersed pastures, the ecological unit is more likely the individual herd. An increasingly popular statistical method that accounts for the cluster level sampling is the generalized linear mixed model (GLMM). This method also handles multi-stage cluster sampling. The disadvantage of this method is that it relies on strong assumptions, which are difficult to assess and rarely checked in practice. In particular, if there are many clusters with zero prevalence, the assumptions likely to be violated. Alternatively, generalized estimating equation models (GEE) can be used. They are relatively easy to apply, but result in too narrow confidence intervals if the number of clusters is small (e.g. less than 30). In addition it is not possible to estimate the intra- cluster correlation coefficient (see below) and the interpretation is slightly different. The combined analysis of human and animal data is challenging, since a certain person can only be linked to a certain animal under certain conditions. A joint analysis usually requires some level of aggregation or abstraction. However, for many research questions like evaluating the impact of an intervention simultaneously on humans and animals, the joint statistical analysis is less important than the joint presentation and interpretation of the results.

Sample Size Considerations

The sample size determination in cluster sampling is more sophisticated, since individuals within the same cluster may be correlated. This seems obvious for infectious diseases, but can also be due to the fact that individuals within one cluster are more similar with respect to environmental exposure, nutrition, cultural behavior or genetic factors. This similarity is expressed by the intra-cluster correlation coefficient rho (r). Rho is calculated from the within-cluster variance and the between-cluster variance. Rho and the average cluster size (*b*) can be used to calculate the design effect, which can be interpreted as a correction factor. The sample size calculated for simple random sampling has to be multiplied by the design effect (DE) to get the final sample size (Bennett *et al.*, 1991).

$$DE = 1 + (b - 1) \times r$$

Rho is most often unknown at the planning stage and difficult to predict. If no information from previous comparable studies in similar settings is available, rho is usually set to 0.2. This value is chosen because it has been shown that rho seldom exceeds 0.3 and is often below 0.2. Unless the number of individuals sampled is low, increasing the number of clusters will usually have a stronger effect on the sample size than increasing the number of individuals per cluster. With the exception of very rare outcomes, it rarely makes sense to sample more than 30 to 50 individuals per cluster. Still, practical considerations should be taken into account. Where the distance between clusters is high, the number of individuals per cluster should be chosen so that the data collection can be completed in 1 or 2 full days. Finally, non-consent and, in longitudinal studies, loss to follow-up should be considered when determining the final sample size.

Ethical Considerations in One Health Studies

The common goal of veterinarians and physicians is to promote the health and well-being of their patients and to provide treatment where possible. There is overlap between the two sectors regarding individual versus community ethics such as cost containment, best use of resources (priority to most cost-beneficial and cost-effective approaches), herd immunity, sanitation and high risk groups. Public health ethics has a broad scope that includes ethical and social issues arising in health promotion and disease prevention, epidemiologic research and public health practice (Coughlin, 2006). Ethical concerns in public health often relate to the dual obligations of public health professionals to acquire and apply scientific knowledge aimed at restoring and protecting the public's health while respecting individual autonomy. In veterinary medicine, the client (normally the owner of the animal) making the choice for treatment is not the patient. Nevertheless, there is a duty to communicate and disclose risks as in human medicine (Johnston, 2013). Epidemics affect not only farmers, but also the entire agricultural sector and even the national economy. Van Vlissingen (2001) published a list summarizing factors that play a role in the ethical evaluation of policies and actions on suspected cases of animal diseases. The list includes aspects of animals' interests, owners' interests, veterinarians' interests, interests of an animal population, public health interests and economic interests (Zinsstag *et al* Wettlaufer *et al.*). Any survey raises ethical considerations, which is also true for surveys on zoonoses without sampling or testing of people. Informed consent is needed from all interviewees. Participants have the right to know the results of the testing of their animals since a positive result can present a health risk for themselves, their families and the consumers of their livestock products. A study on zoonoses requires close collaboration with governmental bodies. It cannot be, for example, that the government would slaughter animals (without compensation) that have tested positive for brucellosis in the framework of a survey. Collaboration with authorities can also better ensure that the results are used to identify interventions that are fully carried by the communities. Appropriate protective measures must be promoted and their application facilitated by the project

ADVANTAGES OF AND POSSIBLE BARRIERS TO ONE HEALTH STUDIES

Rabinowitz *et al.* (2013) concluded that all studies qualifying as 'proof of concept' of One Health did not use the term 'One Health' in their publications. Others, in turn, may refer to One Health, but do not necessarily comply with our criteria above. The pressure to publish in high impact journals – and the highest impact journals are disciplinary – forces researchers to split their findings and publish them according to the disciplinary strengths. Interdisciplinary/intersectoral efforts can get lost in this publication context. It is currently easier than in the past to publish interdisciplinary findings. But in one interdisciplinary manuscript, the disciplinary rigour of respective disciplines can only be sketchily presented, which, in turn, often does not satisfy reviewers of a given disciplinary background. Also, interdisciplinary journals may not reach the primary target audience. For example, a veterinarian more likely consults veterinary journals and not, for example, an ecohealth journal, despite the fact that these may have articles relevant to his/her work. Most One Health studies are driven by veterinarians. Historically, the veterinary medical profession has held a focus on protecting and improving animal and human health. Unlike their contemporary human medicine counterparts, veterinarians must have multiple species knowledge (Kahn *et al.*, 2007). Doctors are rather strictly trained to do clinical work, and less to consider interactions with the closer and broader environment. Above we have presented only a few examples of projects considering ecosystem factors, although there should be a greater incorporation of environmental and ecosystem factors into disease assessments and interventions (Rabinowitz *et al.*, 2013). An evaluation of the social-ecological systemic impacts of agricultural developments on human, animal and ecosystem health and well-being may lead to more balanced assessments of the value of changes in one sector, and possible unintended consequences that need to be guarded against (Zinsstag *et al.*, 2011). Joint surveillance systems should ensure that the data between the sectors are harmonized from local to national levels. Surveillance systems should also be in a position to react to reported abnormal disease events. Existing systems are currently under evaluation and new approaches such as syndromic surveillance and risk-based surveillance or use of alternative sources of information are being evaluated, but likewise need to show that they can generate useful information – and that they can use synergies between sectors and thus save costs. Using existing data, which have been previously collected for another purpose, makes data integration more time consuming. Too often, people are still sentinels for zoonotic disease outbreaks, despite the fact that zoonoses could be picked up earlier in animals. To note, surveillance and monitoring is not carried out on diseases alone. There is and should also be monitoring of stakeholders, demographic health indicators and response capacity. Since One Health studies most often feature concurrent sampling of humans and animals, proper planning and implementation needs more attention, and may require more funding. Data acquired from different sources are associated with more causes of variation and possibly bias and confounding. Data quality is always paramount and a particular challenge in a One Health study because every chain is only as strong as its weakest link and there are more links. Potential sources of errors range from selection bias to misclassification due to poor diagnostic test performance, all compromising the validity of the findings.

We see the following advantages of a One Health study design.

1. Simultaneous studies of human and animal health can better assess epidemiological linkages of zoonoses, including foodborne pathogens and antibiotic resistances that would otherwise not be seen.
2. Joint field research by mixed teams can serve as a nucleus for intersectoral collaboration and enhanced sharing of information in a country and a region.
3. A One Health perspective enhances intersectoral surveillance and communication, for example for rabies, and zoonotic disease outbreaks can be detected earlier if animals are used as sentinels.
4. Joint monitoring of an intervention, for example on brucellosis, can indicate if corrective actions are needed in the implementation of the livestock intervention and a decrease of human brucellosis incidence over time may be the most sensitive outcome of successful livestock vaccination.
5. Assessment of response and service provision capacity can lead to revived discussions on human and financial needs of sectors to manage zoonotic outbreaks.

REFERENCES

Agrawal, M. (2012). *Schistosomes and Schistosomiasis in South Asia.* New Delhi: Springer. doi:10.1007/978-81-322-0539-5

Bardosh, K., & Thys, S. (2012). *Socio-cultural research on neglected zoonoses in Africa: a literature review analysis.* Poster presented at the Ecohealth conference, Kunming, India.

Bartlett, P. C., & Judge, L. J. (1997). The role of epidemiology in public health. *Revue Scientifique et Technique OIE*, *16*(2), 331–336. doi:10.20506/rst.16.2.1020 PMID:9501345

Bennett, S., Woods, T., Liyanage, W. M., & Smith, D. L. (1991). A simplified general method for cluster-sample surveys of health in developing countries. *World Health Statistics Quarterly*, *44*, 98–106. PMID:1949887

Bonfoh, B., Kasymbekov, J., Durr, S., Toktobaev, N., Doherr, M. G., Schueth, T., ... Schelling, E. (2012). Representative seroprevalences of brucellosis in humans and livestock in Kyrgyzstan. *EcoHealth*, *9*(2), 132–138. doi:10.100710393-011-0722-x PMID:22143553

Bonfoh, B., Wasem, A., Traoré, A. N., Fané, A., Spillmann, H., Simbé, C. F., ... Zinsstag, J. (2003). Microbiological quality of cows' milk taken at different intervals from the udder to the selling point in Bamako (Mali). *Food Control*, *14*(7), 495–500. doi:10.1016/S0956-7135(02)00109-3

Burnham, G., Lafta, R., Doocy, S., & Roberts, L. (2006). Mortality after the 2003 invasion of Iraq: A cross-sectional cluster sample survey. *Lancet*, *368*(9545), 1421–1428. doi:10.1016/S0140-6736(06)69491-9 PMID:17055943

Canadian Integrated Program for Antimicrobial Resistance Surveillance (CIPARS). (2007) *Salmonella Heidelberg ceftiofur-related resistance in human and retail chicken isolates*. Available at: http://www.phac-aspc. gc.ca/cipars-picra/heidelberg/heidelberg-eng.php

Cleaveland, S., Fevre, E. M., Kaare, M., & Coleman, P. G. (2002). Estimating human rabies mortality in the United Republic of Tanzania from dog bite injuries. *Bulletin of the World Health Organization*, *80*, 304–310. PMID:12075367

Clifford, D. L., Kazwala, R. R., Sadiki, H., Roug, A., Muse, E. A., Coppolillo, P. C., & Mazet, J. A. (2013). Tuberculosis infection in wildlife from the Ruaha ecosystem Tanzania: Implications for wildlife, domestic animals, and human health. *Epidemiology and Infection*, *141*(07), 1371–1381. doi:10.1017/S0950268813000836 PMID:23601163

Coughlin, S. S. (2006). Ethical issues in epidemiologic research and public health practice. *Emerging Themes in Epidemiology*, *3*(1), 16. doi:10.1186/1742-7622-3-16 PMID:17018147

Dean, A. S., Bonfoh, B., Kulo, A. E., Boukaya, G. A., Amidou, M., Hattendorf, J., ... Schelling, E. (2013). Epidemiology of brucellosis and Q Fever in linked human and animal populations in northern Togo. *PLoS One*, 8.

Dean, A. S., Schelling, E., Bonfoh, B., Kulo, A. E., Boukaya, G. A., & Pilo, P. (2014). Deletion in the gene Bru-Ab2_0168 of Brucella abortus strains: Diagnostic challenges. *Clinical Microbiology and Infection*, *20*, 550–553.

El Sherbini, A., Kabbash, I., Schelling, E., El Shennawy, S., Shalapy, N., Elnaby, G. H., ... Eisa, A. (2007). Seroprevalences and local variation of human and livestock brucellosis in two villages in Gharbia Governorate, Egypt. *Transactions of the Royal Society of Tropical Medicine and Hygiene*, *101*(9), 923–928. doi:10.1016/j.trstmh.2007.04.020 PMID:17604066

Enserink, M. (2010). Infectious diseases. Questions abound in Q-fever explosion in the Netherlands. *Science*, *327*, 266–267. PMID:20075230

Faes, C., Aerts, M., Litiere, S., Meroc, E., Van der Stede, Y., & Mintiens, K. (2011). Estimating herd prevalence on the basis of aggregate testing of animals. *Journal of the Royal Statistical Society. Series A, (Statistics in Society)*, *174*(1), 155–174. doi:10.1111/j.1467-985X.2010.00652.x

Firdessa, R., Berg, S., Hailu, E., Schelling, E., Gumi, B., Erenso, G., ... Aseffa, A. (2013). Mycobacterial lineages causing pulmonary and extrapulmonary tuberculosis, Ethiopia. *Emerging Infectious Diseases*, *19*(3), 460–463. doi:10.3201/eid1903.120256 PMID:23622814

Forde, M., Morrison, K., Dewailly, E., Badrie, N., & Robertson, L. (2011). Strengthening integrated research and capacity development within the Caribbean region. *BMC International Health and Human Rights*, *11*(Suppl. 2), S7. doi:10.1186/1472-698X-11-S2-S7 PMID:22166013

Grace, D., Gilbert, J., Lapar, M. L., Unger, F., Fevre, S., Nguyen-Viet, H., & Schelling, E. (2011). Zoonotic emerging infectious disease in selected countries in southeast Asia: Insights from ecohealth. *EcoHealth*, *8*(1), 55–62. doi:10.100710393-010-0357-3 PMID:21174223

Guan, Y., Chen, H., Li, K., Riley, S., Leung, G., Webster, R., ... Yuen, K. (2007). A model to control the epidemic of H5N1 influenza at the source. *BMC Infectious Diseases*, *7*(1), 132. doi:10.1186/1471-2334-7-132 PMID:17999754

Gumi, B., Schelling, E., Berg, S., Firdessa, R., Erenso, G., Mekonnen, W., ... Zinsstag, J. (2012). Zoonotic transmission of tuberculosis between pastoralists and their livestock in South-East Ethiopia. *EcoHealth*, *9*(2), 139–149. doi:10.100710393-012-0754-x PMID:22526748

Hill, A. B. (1965). The environment and disease: Association or causation? *Proceedings of the Royal Society of Medicine*, *58*, 295–300. PMID:14283879

Johnston, C. (2013). Lessons from medical ethics. In C. M. Wathes, S. A. Corr, S. A. May, S. P. McCulloch, & M. C. Whiting (Eds.), *Veterinary & Animal Ethics*. Oxford, UK: Blackwell Publishing Ltd.

Kahn, L. H., Kaplan, B., & Steele, J. H. (2007). Confronting zoonoses through closer collaboration between medicine and veterinary medicine (as 'one medicine'). *Veterinaria Italiana*, *43*, 5–19. PMID:20411497

Kaindi, D. W., Schelling, E., Wangoh, J. M., Imungi, J. K., Farah, Z., & Meile, L. (2012). Towards one health disease surveillance: The Southern African Centre for Infectious Disease Surveillance approach. *The Onderstepoort Journal of Veterinary Research*, *79*, 454. PMID:23327374

Mariner, J. C., Pfeiffer, D. U., Costard, S., Knopf, L., Zingeser, J., Chibeu, D., & Mehta, P. (2011). *Surveillance for the Present and the Future. Challenges of Animal Health Information Systems and Surveillance for Animal Diseases and Zoonoses*. FAO.

Mazet, J. A., Clifford, D. L., Coppolillo, P. B., Deolalikar, A. B., Erickson, J. D., & Kazwala, R. R. (2009). A 'one health' approach to address emerging zoonoses: The HALI project in Tanzania. *PLoS Medicine*, 6.

Messenger, A. M., Barnes, A. N., & Gray, G. C. (2014). Reverse zoonotic disease transmission (zooanthroponosis): A systematic review of seldom-documented human biological threats to animals. *PLoS One*, *9*(2), e89055. doi:10.1371/journal.pone.0089055 PMID:24586500

Nutter, F. W. (1999). Understanding the interrelationships between botanical, human, and veterinary epidemiology: The Ys and Rs of it all. *Ecosystem Health*, *5*(3), 131–140. doi:10.1046/j.1526-0992.1999.09922.x

Omran, A. R. (1971). The epidemiologic transition. A theory of the epidemiology of population change. *The Milbank Quarterly*, *49*(4), 509–538. doi:10.2307/3349375 PMID:5155251

Parkes, M. W., Charron, D. F., & Sanchez, A. (2012). Better together: field-building networks at the frontiers of ecohealth research. In D. F. Charron (Ed.), *Ecohealth Research in Practice: Innovative Applications of an Ecosystem Approach to Health*. Ottawa: Springer and International Development Research Centre. doi:10.1007/978-1-4614-0517-7_21

Rabinowitz, P. M., Kock, R., Kachani, M., Kunkel, R., Thomas, J., Gilbert, J., ... Rubin, C. (2013). Toward proof of concept of a one health approach to disease prediction and control. *Emerging Infectious Diseases*, *19*(12). doi:10.3201/eid1912.130265 PMID:24295136

Randolph, T. F., Schelling, E., Grace, D., Nicholson, C. F., Leroy, J. L., Cole, D. C., ... Ruel, M. (2007). Invited review: Role of livestock in human nutrition and health for poverty reduction in developing countries. *Journal of Animal Science*, *85*(11), 2788–2800. doi:10.2527/jas.2007-0467 PMID:17911229

Schelling, E., Bechir, M., Ahmed, M. A., Wyss, K., Randolph, T. F., & Zinsstag, J. (2007). Human and animal vaccination delivery to remote nomadic families, Chad. *Emerging Infectious Diseases*, *13*(3), 373–379. doi:10.3201/eid1303.060391 PMID:17552089

Schelling, E., Daoud, S., Daugla, D. M., Diallo, P., Tanner, M., & Zinsstag, J. (2005). Morbidity and nutrition patterns of three nomadic pastoralist communities of Chad. *Acta Tropica*, *95*(1), 16–25. doi:10.1016/j.actatropica.2005.03.006 PMID:15866506

Schelling, E., Diguimbaye, C., Daoud, S., Nicolet, J., Boerlin, P., Tanner, M., & Zinsstag, J. (2003). Brucellosis and Q-fever seroprevalences of nomadic pastoralists and their livestock in Chad. *Preventive Veterinary Medicine*, *61*(4), 279–293. doi:10.1016/j.prevetmed.2003.08.004 PMID:14623412

Schelling, E., & Kimani, T. (2007). *Human and animal health response capacity and costs: a rapid appraisal of the 2007 Rift Valley fever outbreak in Kenya*. International Livestock Research Institute.

van Loenhout, J. A., Paget, W. J., Vercoulen, J. H., Wijkmans, C. J., Hautvast, J. L. A., & van der Velden, K. (2012). Assessing the long-term health impact of Q-fever in the Netherlands: A prospective cohort study started in 2007 on the largest documented Q-fever outbreak to date. *BMC Infectious Diseases*, *12*(1), 280. doi:10.1186/1471-2334-12-280 PMID:23110336

van Vlissingen, M. (2001). Professional ethics in veterinary science – considering the consequences as a tool for problem solving. *Veterinary Sciences for Tomorrow*, *1*, 1–8.

VWB/VSF Canada. (2010). *One Health for One World: A Compendium of Case Studies*. Available at: https:// www.vetswithoutborders.ca/images/pdfs/OHOW%20 Compendium%20Case%20Studies.pdf

Wendt, A., Kreienbrock, L., & Campe, A. (2014). Zoonotic Disease Surveillance – Inventory of Systems Integrating Human and Animal Disease Information. *Zoonoses and Public Health*, n/a. doi:10.1111/zph.12120 PMID:24712724

WHO, EU, ILRI, DBL, FAO, OIE, & AU. (2009). *Integrated Control of Neglected Zoonotic Diseases in Africa / Applying the 'One Health' Concept*. Available at: http://whqlibdoc. who.int/hq/2008/WHO_HTM_NTD_NZD_2008.1_eng.pdf

Winkler, M. S., Krieger, G. R., Divall, M. J., Singer, B. H., & Utzinger, J. (2012). Health impact assessment of industrial development projects: A spatio-temporal visualization. *Geospatial Health*, *6*(2), 299–301. doi:10.4081/gh.2012.148 PMID:22639132

Zinsstag, J. (2012). Convergence of EcoHealth and One Health. *EcoHealth*, *9*(4), 371–373. doi:10.100710393-013-0812-z PMID:23392841

Zinsstag, J., Schelling, E., Daoud, S., Schierle, J., Hofmann, P., Diguimbaye, C., ... Tanner, M. (2002). Serum retinol of Chadian nomadic pastoralist women in relation to their livestocks' milk retinol and beta-carotene content. *International Journal for Vitamin and Nutrition Research*, *72*(4), 221–228. doi:10.1024/0300-9831.72.4.221 PMID:12214559

Zinsstag, J., Schelling, E., Roth, F., Bonfoh, B., de Savigny, D., & Tanner, M. (2007). Human benefits of animal interventions for zoonosis control. *Emerging Infectious Diseases*, *13*(4), 527–531. doi:10.3201/eid1304.060381 PMID:17553265

Zinsstag, J., Schelling, E., Waltner-Toews, D., & Tanner, M. (2011). From 'one medicine' to 'one health' and systemic approaches to health and well-being. *Preventive Veterinary Medicine*, *101*(3-4), 148–156. doi:10.1016/j.prevetmed.2010.07.003 PMID:20832879

Section 2

Chapter 4
One Health and Parasites

Said Sajjad Ali Shah
Veterinary Research Institute, Pakistan

Adnan Khan
Wildlife Department, Khyber Pakhtunkhwa, Pakistan

ABSTRACT

One health is a collective term used to address human and animal health issues under one platform. More than half of the diseases of humans are directly or indirectly related to animal health and spread from animals to humans or vice versa. Etiological agents of zoonotic diseases may be bacterial, viral, or parasitic in origin. Among them, parasitic agents are very important because they are either directly involved as etiological agents or as vectors of other pathogenic organisms. Parasitic zoonoses are transmitted to humans through vectors, food, or drinking water, and thus categorized as vector borne, food borne, and water borne parasitic zoonoses. Food borne and water borne parasitic zoonoses include all those parasitic diseases which are transmitted to humans by consuming contaminated food and water. An extensive alliance is necessary amongst physicians, veterinarians, and public health workers for timely response and approach to guarantee the prevention and management of infections.

DOI: 10.4018/978-1-5225-6304-4.ch004

INTRODUCTION

One health is a collective term used to address human and animal health issues under one platform. One of the key goals of one health is to link physicians and veterinarians all over the world and work synergistically for resolving the health problems of man and animals. More than half of the diseases of humans are directly or indirectly related to animal health and spread from animals to humans or vice versa. i.e. zoonotic disease. Zoonotic diseases can be classified on the basis of environment and ecosystem in which disease circulate. Zoonotic disease might be synanthropic, where infection spread from livestock to humans or it might be exoanthropic where wild and feral animals are source of infection for humans. Initially, zooanthroponoses and anthropozoonoses were the terms used for disease transmission from humans to animals and animals to humans, respectively. But later on both of these terms were abandoned by an expert committee and the term zoonosis was recommended for diseases transmitted from animals to humans (WHO). Apart from zoonosis, two other terms are also used for transmission of diseases i.e. anthropnoses and sapronoses. Anthropnoses is the term used when source of infection is humans while in sapronoses source of infection are abiotic agents i.e. soil, water, decaying plants, corpse etc (Pavlovsk, 1966; Miller et al, 2009).

Number of zoonotic infections increased worldwide in the near past and certain factors are responsible for the emergence of infections. These factors include increase in population, military operations, mass migration of people to natural or man-made disasters, increase in urbanization and inadequate food and water supplies. Similarly, global warming, deforestation, displacement of wildlife results in overflow of infections into domestic animals and humans.

THE LINK IN HUMAN AND ANIMAL HEALTH

There are 1,415 infectious agents and 868 (61%) could be transmitted between animals and humans (Taylor et al, 2001). It has also been found that zoonotic diseases were twice as likely to be associated with emerging or newly discovered infections than nonzoonotic pathogens and that viruses and protozoa (parasites) were the zoonotic pathogens most likely to emerge (Cleaveland et al, 2001). As an academic discipline, comparative medicine or one-health is not a new concept; the first chair in it was established in 1862 in France. The field has an illustrious history. In 1893, Theobald Smith, a physician, and F.L. Kilbourne, a veterinarian, published a paper establishing that an infectious agent, *Babesia bigemina*, the cause of cattle fever, was transmitted by an arthropod vector. Their seminal work helped set the stage for Walter Reed's discovery of yellow fever transmission (Wilkinson, 1992).

Another physician-veterinarian team, Drs. Rolf Zinkernagel and Peter C. Doherty, won the 1996 Nobel Prize in physiology or medicine for their discovery of how the immune system distinguishes normal cells from virus-infected cells (Zinkerngel et al, 1974). This illustrate that medicine and veterinary medicine are complementary; they are synergistic in generating new scientific insights across species. In essence, the 2 disciplines epitomize the philosophy of one health.

The combined efforts of several fields are required to devise innovative disease control and prevention strategies as most of the diseases occur inter-species. Much understanding and closer working relationship is required between veterinarians, physicians, and public health professionals for improvements in individual health, population health, and comparative medicine research. The collaborative research between physicians and veterinarians, under the umbrella of one health concept, would improve our understanding of zoonotic agent-host interactions.

There are several reports in the recent past that certain individuals were infected with diseases of animal's origin however, the physicians involved overlooked the role of animals in the transmission of Zoonoses. Nonetheless, most patients do not view veterinarians as a source of information for human health. It has been found that only 21% of HIV patients asked their veterinarians about the health risks of pet ownership (Grant et al, 1995). Another individual who was already suffering from rheumatoid arthritis became infected with *Cryptococcus neoformans* after cleaning a cockatiel's cage a week before hospitalization (Shrestha et al, 2004). Human lymphocytic choriomeningitis virus (LCMV) infection is associated with pet rodents and also causes serious infections in immunocompromised persons (Wilson, 2004). These risks extend beyond the pet owners and can involve the recipients of the animal owners' donated organs. For example, LCMV has been responsible for the deaths of 3 organ transplant recipients who received their organs from donors who had owned infected pet rodents (Kahn, 2006).

Salmonellosis was reported to have developed in 4 children, 1 mother, and an 80-year-old woman after exposure to small pet turtles ("CDC", 2004). A research organisation in US has found 28 matching human-case isolates of *Salmonella enterica* serovar Typhimurium while comparing the data from December 2003 to October 2004. Of the 22 patients who were interviewed, 13 (59%) had been exposed to rodents during the 8 days before onset of illness ("DCD, 2003-2004).

Exotic animals can accidently introduce newer pathogen in an area. For example, the 2003 monkeypox outbreak in the Midwestern United States originated after imported African rodents infected prairie dogs in pet distribution facilities. Laboratory-confirmed monkeypox developed in 35 persons ("CDC", 2003). Similarly, farmers, butchers and other occupational personnel are at the risk of zoonotic infections e.g. *Streptococcus suis* can cause meningitis in pig farmers (Bartelink et al, 1995). *Campylobacter* and *Streptobacillus moniliformis* infection are occupational risks for packers in poultry factories and for pet shop employees (Wilson, 2004; "CDC", 2003). It has been illustrated that animals can significantly affect human health and vice versa.

There are certain avenues that can be jointly explored and practiced under the concept of one health for the benefit of mankind and its animals. Like, veterinarians could provide an overview of an animal's health status to a physician whose patient is immunocompromised and still wants to work in an animal facility or keep his companion animal. Such collaborative approach between the 2 professions would be invaluable to patients. Joint medical and veterinary medical workshops on zoonotic risks to human and animal health could help forge ties and facilitate opportunities to establish these types of collaborative efforts.

Apart from individual health, population health is also a function of one health concept. The identification of the pathogens involved and devising control strategies depends on establishing the fact that whether human and animal outbreaks were simultaneous. For example, physicians treating the initial West Nile virus (WNV) patients in New York City in 1999 might have benefited if they knew that for the previous month and concurrently, veterinarians in the surrounding area had been seeing dozens of dying crows with neurologic symptoms similar to those of the affected humans ("US General Accounting Office", 2000). There are several other reports where population health has been compromised due to lack of cooperation between agencies and organizations. E.g. In US, no local or state agency assumed full responsibility for the large wildlife die-off investigation in 1999 since which agency was responsible was not initially clear ("US General Accounting Office", 2000). This situation hindered communications between the veterinarians, public health officials, and physicians who were involved in the outbreak response at the local level (Kahn, 2006).

During the 1999 WNV outbreak, the presumptive diagnoses for the initial human cases was St. Louis encephalitis (SLE) until a veterinary pathologist at the Bronx Zoo linked the animal and human outbreaks ("US General Accounting Office", 2000). She realized that crows and other birds ordinarily resistant to SLE were dying, so the agent was not likely SLE. Her work helped set the stage for the discovery of WNV in the Western Hemisphere ("US General Accounting Office", 2000; Asnis et al, 1999). The magnitude of the problem illustrates why the efforts of medicine, veterinary medicine, and public health need to overlap under the umbrella of one health concept.

Joint surveillance of animal and human zoonotic disease outbreaks is already reaping benefits worldwide. For example, recognition of the first human case of H5N1 avian influenza in Hong Kong in 1997 was facilitated by the surveillance of ducks, geese, and chickens in southern China during the preceding decades (Shortridge et al, 2003). In 1999, the US Centers for Disease Control and Prevention has established, a cooperative surveillance system that monitors the geographic spread of WNV in humans, mosquitoes, birds, and other animals in response to the outbreak of WNV disease (Marfin et al, 2000). These types of surveillance systems need to be continued and expanded to include other serious diseases of similar nature. Physician and veterinarian teams could conduct serosurveys of humans who live and work near high-risk animal populations to assess their risk of acquiring Zoonoses (Kahn, 2006).

IMPORTANCE OF PARASITE: A PUBLIC HEALTH PERSPECTIVE

Healthier animals can guarantee the nourishment of salubrious community. Etiological agents of zoonotic diseases may be bacterial, viral and parasitic in origin. Among them, parasitic agents are very important because they are either directly involved as etiological agents or as vectors of other pathogenic organisms and thus playing havoc across the globe, both in humans and livestock and causing heavy losses in the form of poor economic development and quality of life. Parasites are broadly divided into ecto and endo parasites, affecting humans and animals equivocally. Ecto-parasites i.e. ticks, flies etc may cause disease directly by bites but mostly these parasites act as vector for other pathogenic organism i.e. arboviruses, tick borne infections (TBIs). On the other hand, endo-parasites invade the internal organs of the body i.e. intestines, liver, muscles, lungs, blood and hampering normal functioning of the body, thus causing diseases of economic importance.

Parasitic zoonoses are transmitted to humans through vectors, food or drinking water and thus categorized as vector borne, food borne and water borne parasitic zoonoses. Vector borne zoonosis can be sub categorized into those in which vector is involved in transmission of parasite of zoonotic importance e.g. Chagas disease, Human African Trypanosomiasis (Sleeping sickness), Leishmaniasis, Human granulocytic anaplasmosis (HGA) etc. while other are those which are involved in the transmission of pathogenic virus, bacteria e.g. Cremian Congo Hemorrhagic Fever (CCHF), Borreliosis, Bartonellosis.

FACTORS AFFECTING INCIDENCE OF ZOONOTIC DISEASES

There is growing trend in the emergence of zoonotic infections worldwide in the near past and certain factors deemed responsible for the increase of zoonotic infections. These factors can be broadly related to infectious agent (pathogen), host (humans and animals), vectors of the diseases and climatic changes (Naicker, 2011). Human population is increasing with a tremendous pace and thus affecting every corner of the world, either directly or indirectly (Lindahl et al, 2015). Increase in population cause scarcity of food and water, increasing risk of natural disaster, displacement of population and increasing the incidence of infections. These factors along with other (global warming, deforestation, displacement of wildlife, military operations) contribute in overflow of infections into domestic animals and humans.

Climatic Change

It is considered as one of the most important determinant responsible for the recent upsurge in emergence of zoonotic diseases. Due to variations in certain climatic parameters i.e. temperature, rainfall, soil condition and harsh environment favor the growth of the vectors in one way or the other and hence contribute in the occurrence of zoonotic diseases. Most of the etiological agents i.e. bacteria, virus and protozoa of zoonotic importance require certain vectors for the transmission and spread of the disease to humans.

Temperature

Due to certain factors i.e. pollution, increase in population etc, there is gradual increase in atmospheric temperature. Intergovernmental panel on climatic change has projected an increase of 0.2°C per decade in atmospheric temperature ("IPCC", 2007). Arthropod vectors are temperature dependent and its distribution and population is affected by change in atmospheric temperature. Most of the vectors i.e. ticks, mosquitoes and sandflies are ectothermic and grow well at temperature 25-32°C. Due to increase in global temperature, densities of vectors are expected to rise which ultimately leads to increase in incidence of zoonotic diseases. At high temperature, arthropod vectors i.e. mosquitoes, ticks and sand flies grow well, are active, their frequency of blood meals and reproductive activity is also increased. Infectious agents carried by these vectors also mature faster at high temperatures and also favor the growth and development of larvae and result in increase in overall capacity of these vectors. Incidence of vector borne zoonotic disease is highest in warm months of the year.

Rainfall

Besides land temperature, rainfall is also considered as an important determinant of the climate change. Increase rainfall indirectly favors the growth of vectors by providing breeding sites for mosquitoes and also shelter to vectors in the form of dense vegetation (Githeko et al, 2000). Vector capacity and larval development is increased due to heavy rainfall and if susceptible hosts are available results in outbreak of the disease. Heavy rainfall and melting of snow glaciers due to increased atmospheric temperature also results in flooding which lead to increase water borne zoonoses.

Humidity of Soil

Soil play an important role in transmission of many parasitic zoonosis as it provide a conducive environment required for the development of parasitic ova. Humidity of soil is required not only for the viability of ova but also for the development of ova into transmissible stages (Slifoka et al, 2000; Randolph, 2008). Soil humidity may also fervor the population of many intermediate hosts e.g. Snails, which are required for the propagation and development of parasites infection e.g. Fasciolosis.

Human Factors

Alteration in human behavior due to changing demographics resulting in the emergence and spread of zoonotic diseases (Alho et al, 2018). Along with environmental factors and challenges, there are some human factors which are related to emergence of zoonotic diseases. Almost all these measures are deliberately taken by people for their economic growth and livelihood which later on become predisposing factors for the spread of infectious diseases. On one side all these are considered as economic indicators for the development of society but if not monitored properly these may become disastrous for the survival and prosperity of the community.

Globalization

It is the growing interaction of people of different nationalities through flow of ideas and culture. Globalization is considered as an important pre-requisite for the development of nation because it bring the opportunities for the cultural exchanges and transfer of scientific knowledge and skills. One can't deny the bright aspect of globalization but on the other side, it introduces the infectious agent of zoonotic importance to new area (Alho et al, 2018). Pathogens are transmitted either directly through host (humans, animals), vectors or indirectly through transport of goods.

The importance of globalization can't be denied in today's modern era and at the same time the devastating effect can't be overlooked. To minimize the damage, quarantine measures are strictly recommended so as to minimize the introduction of pathogen or infectious agent to new area.

Urbanization

Urbanization can be defined as shift of population from rural areas to urban, the increase in the number of people living in urban areas and the ways in which people adopt to this change (Jiang et al, 2008). It is one of those changes which have deep impact on human health (Patz et al, 000; Patz et al, 2005) To have better access to facilities, job and other luxuries of life, people often migrate from rural areas to cities.

According to United Nations report, almost half of the world's population is in urban areas ("United Nations Department of Economics", 2003; Satterhwaite et al, 2010) and with every passing year world's urban population is increasing and by 2050 it is estimated to be 64% and 86% in developing and developed world, respectively. Cities are congested and overcrowded which provides very conducive environment for the dissemination of disease. Mostly there is higher environmental temperature and minimal seasonal changes in urban areas which favor the growth and development of vectors and hence the transmission of vector borne diseases.

Irrigation System

Irrigation is essential for the optimum crop production but it can also favor the development of vector borne zoonotic diseases by providing the ideal habitat for the vectors (Patz et al, 2005). Mostly in developing societies, people dispose off animal wastes and carcasses in canals or open fields which may be the potential reservoir of pathogens and can be transmitted to nearby areas.

Deforestation

Deforestation is deliberately done in the developing countries of the world to fulfill the needs of growing population in the form of providing habitation, fuel wood, setting of industries and new cultivable lands. Deforestation predisposes the land to floods and washing away by rains which in turn make the environment suitable for the development of larval stages of arthropod vectors and hence vector population increases (Patz et al, 2000). Deforestation also brings wild animals, humans and domestic animals in close association and increases the risk of communicable diseases many fold. Naïve inhabitants of the deforested area are highly exposed to wildlife vectors and thus they are at great risk of acquiring the infection.

Mass Migration Due to Natural Disasters

Over a period of time, population displacements take place in certain part of the world either due to natural disasters and calamities or due to humans conflict/military operations. This mass migration results in overcrowding and poor sanitation that create very conducive and favorable environment for the spread of many infectious diseases (Keush et al, 2009). In a statement issued by UNHCR, over 68.5 million persons were displaced internally due to humans conflict in 2017 (UNHCR, 2017) and an annual average of 21.5 million people have been displaced due to natural disasters each year since 2008. Mass migration of people has significant effect not only on human health but also animal health. Migrants are at risk of contracting diseases but they may also act as vectors for introducing infectious diseases to different regions of the world. Due to overcrowding and poor status of refugees, they are highly exposed to health risks and various communicable diseases (Loutan et al, 1997; Toole et al, 1997).

Human and Animal Interface

The number of dogs and cats kept as pets has also increased, as well as the number of animals that have been imported and exported from all over the world (Abu-Madi et al, 2016). In the modern-day society, the human animal bond has become stronger with pets playing an important role as a source of companionship, entertainment and emotional support to their owners. Nevertheless, this close contact may also increase the risk of exposure to infectious diseases, as pets have been implicated in the transmission of more than 60 zoonotic agents (Machperson et al, 2005).

In the past there were only sporadic encounters between wildlife and humans but due to variety of factors there is permanent sharing of environment between wildlife and humans which has increased the frequency of parasite transmission to humans (Daszak et al, 2009; Polley, 2005).

Hunting Practices

Hunting is practiced by humans most commonly for search of food, recreational purposes or to remove predators which are dangerous for humans and animals. It may have certain impacts on the incidence of disease, as it increase the exposure of humans to wildlife animals and vectors, or it may increase or decrease the disease reservoirs, thus affecting the disease occurence (Barbour, 1998; Ostfeld, 2004).

Political Factors

Political instability, wars and insurgency may lead to destruction of health care and public health infrastructure thereby leading to increase occurrence of infectious diseases. e.g. Due to World War II, there was decreasing in the hunting of hares in the Crimea due to which there was increase in population of hares and subsequently ticks population. Later on when Russian troops entered the area, they had no immunity and thus an outbreak of Crimean haemorrhagic fever occurred resulting in the mortality of troops.

Bushmeat Consumption

Bushmeat is basically meat from non-domesticated animals hunted for food in humid tropical forests (Ostfeld, 2004). In remote areas, bushmeat is used for sustenance purposes while in cities and towns it is considered as of high value. It is considered as high source of protein for people living in remote areas but bushmeat is an important risk factor for the transmission of diseases. Many people are directly involved in handling of bushmeat as it exposes them to wildlife pathogens and may cause disease outbreaks (Karesh et al, 2005; Wilkie et al, 1999)

Etiological Agents of Zoonosis

Etiological agents of zoonotic diseases may be bacterial, viral, fungal or parasitic in origin. Important Bacterial zoonosis are Tuberculosis (*Mycobacterium bovis*), Brucellosis (Brucella species), *Escherichia coli* infection, Anthrax (*Bacillus anthracis*), Tetanus (*Clostridium tetani*), Salmonellosis (Salmonella species). Mostly bacterial diseases are transmitted either directly through contact or through infected food and water.

Viral diseases of zoonotic importance are; Rabies, Cremian Congo hemorrhagic fever (CCHF), Chickengunya, Avian Influenza, Ebola virus disease. Viral diseases are transmitted through animal bites, direct contact with infected individuals/animals and through vectors. Apart from bacterial and viral agents, some parasitic agents are also involved in the etiology of zoonotic diseases.

Parasitic agents are either directly involved as etiological agents or as vectors of other pathogenic organisms and thus causing damage all over the world in susceptible organisms and causing heavy losses in the form of poor economic growth and quality of life. Parasites are broadly divided into ecto and endo parasites, affecting humans and animals equivocally. Ecto-parasites i.e. ticks, flies and fleas damage the skin and hides directly through bites but most importantly these ectoparasites act as vectors of other pathogenic organism i.e. arboviruses, tick borne infections (TBIs). On the other hand, endo-parasites invade the internal organs of the body i.e. intestines, liver, muscles, lungs, blood and hampering normal functioning of the body either by causing physical damage or targeting the normal defense mechanism, thus causing diseases of economic importance.

Classification of Parasitic Zoonosis

On the basis of transmission of disease, parasitic zoonoses can be categorized as vector borne, food borne and water borne parasitic zoonoses. Vector borne zoonosis can be sub categorized into those in which vector (ectoparasite) is involved in transmission of parasite of zoonotic importance e.g. Chagas disease, Human African Trypanosomiasis (Sleeping sickness), Leishmaniasis, Human granulocytic anaplasmosis (HGA) etc while other are those in which vectors (ectoparasites) are involved in the transmission of pathogenic virus or bacteria e.g. Cremian Congo Hemorrhagic Fever (CCHF), Borreliosis, Bartonellosis.

IMPORTANT PARASITIC ZOONOTIC DISEASES

Trypanosomiasis

Trypanosomes are haemoprotozoan, belonging to genus Trypanosoma, family Tryanosomatidae, order Kinetoplastida and phylum Sarcomastigophora. There are number of trypanosomes specie and subspecies which infect wide variety of host, including animals and humans. Trypanosoma is derived from a Greek word *Trypano* which means borer and *Soma* mean body. On the basis of phylogenetic homology, trypanosomes are broadly divided into two clades; Salivarian trypanosomes and Stercorian trypanosomes.

In salivarian clade, the trypanosomes are transmitted to the susceptible organism through saliva of tsetse fly. Salivarian trypanosomes are further divided into subgenera; Trypanozoon, Duttonella, Pycnomonas and Nannomonas. *Trypanosoma brucei*, *Trypanosoma equiperdum* and *Trypanosoma rhodesiense* belongs to subgenera Trypanozoon, *Trypanosoma vivax* belongs to subgenera Duttonella while *Trypanosoma congolense* belongs to subgenera Nannomonas.

On the other hand, Stercorians clad of trypanosomes are transmitted to the susceptible hosts through excreta (feces) of Triatominae family of insects. There are two subgenera of Stercorians; Herpetosoma and Schizotrypanum which consists of *Trypanosoma lewisi* and *Trypanosoma cruzi*, respectively.

There is huge variation in size (8-50μm) of Trypanosome species and every species has characteristic size, shape and appearance. Most of the Salivaria group of trypanosomes are pathogenic and develop as trypomastigotes in the mammalian hosts while promastigote form in invertebrate host.

Trypanosomes cause a range of diseases in animals and humans while some species of Trypanosomes have zoonotic importance. Important diseases caused by trypanosoma are Surra (*Trypanosoma evansi*), Nagana (*Trypanosoma vivax, Trypanosoma congolense, Trypanosoma brucei*), Dourine/covering sickness in equines (*Trypanosoma equiperdum*), Chagas (*Trypanosoma cruzi*) and sleeping sickness in humans (*Trypanosoma brucei*).

Human African Trypanosomiasis (Sleeping Sickness)

It is a vector borne parasitic disease caused by *Trypanosoma brucei* and transmitted to animals and humans through bites of infected Tsetse fly. Rural populations are highly exposed to tsetse fly comparatively and therefore incidence of disease is higher in rural populations. Apart from the infected tsetse fly bite, infection can also be transmitted through needle pricks, blood transfusion, mechanical vectors and also from mother to child. There are two stages of the disease on the basis of development of clinical signs and symptoms.

Haemo-Lymphatic Stage

This is the initial stage of disease development where trypanosome harbors the subcutaneous tissue, blood and lymph results in intermittent fever, headaches and joint pain.

Neurological or Meningo Encephalic Stage

This is critical stage of the disease in which signs and symptoms are more developed and obvious. Trypanosomes cross the blood brain barrier and result in changes of behavior, confusion and lack of coordination. In this stage, normal sleep cycle of the individual is disturbed and can be fatal if not treated.

On the basis of subspecies of Trypanosoma involved, there are two main types of Sleeping sickness disease. Chronic form of the disease is most prevalent, caused by *Trypanosoma brucei gambiense*. This is an asymptomatic disease unless central nervous system is affected. The second form of disease, caused by *Trypanosoma brucei rhodesiense,* is acute and is rarely reported. In this form of the disease, central nervous system is mainly affected and results in rapid development of signs. *Trypanosoma brucei gambiense* and *Trypanosoma brucei rhodesiense* also cause mild infection in animals and can act as reservoir for the transmission of the disease.

Chagas Disease

Chagas Disease also called as American Trypanosomiasis is another trypanosome disease of zoonotic importance caused by *Trypanosoma cruzi*. Chagas disease is manifested by anemia, weakness and splenomegaly in dogs and can be fatal in dog while in cats causing convulsion and paralysis. Chagas disease is transmitted by Reduviid bugs, member of Reduviidae family. Reduviid bugs are also termed as cone-nose bug, assassin bug or kissing bugs because these bugs tends to feed on people's face during night time. There are number of local names for kissing bugs and these are known by vinchuca in Argentina, barberio in Brazil, pito in Colombia, chipo in Venezuela and chinche in Central America. Initially Chagas disease was restricted to Latin America but due to increase mobilization, this disease is also present in other parts of the world. Chagas disease is named after Brazilian physician Carlos Chagas in 1909 and is the major cause of cardiac failure in endemic regions.

There are two stages of the development of the Chagas disease i.e. initial acute stage and chronic stage. Acute stage of the disease is mostly asymptomatic or mild and nonspecific signs with high level of parasitemia. Affected individuals may have fever, headache, lymphoadenopathy, labored breathing, abdominal and muscle pain. There might be enlargement of the liver, spleen and local swelling (chagoma) may be present at the site of insect bite. Most important sign of acute stage of disease is termed as Romona's sign, in which there is unilateral swelling of the eyelids. Occasionally immunocompromised individuals develop myocarditis and meningoencephalitis which may be life threatening. Chronic stage of the disease is further divided into two forms i.e. Indeterminate chronic form and Determinate chronic form. In inderminate chronic form of the disease, symptoms are absent while in determinate chronic form of the disease, different systems of the body i.e. nervous, digestive and cardiac are affected and may be fatal in patients.

Diagnosis

Trypanosomiasis is never pathognomonic and suspicion has to be confirmed by other means i.e. laboratory methods. A variety of diagnostic tests are available and researchers are still trying to improve existing tests and to develop new ones. Current diagnostic tests vary in their sensitivity and specificity. The simplest techniques are examination of wet, thick or thin films of fresh blood; the diagnostic sensitivity of these methods is generally low but depends on the examiner's experience and the level of parasitaemia. Others include parasite concentration techniques (microhaematocrit centrifugation technique, darkground/ phase-contrast buffy coat technique, anion exchange, and in-vitro cultivation); parasite concentration techniques rely on the detection of motile, live trypanosomes but identification of trypanosome species is difficult. Tests to detect trypanosomal antigen include serological tests (indirect fluorescent antibody test, antibody-detection enzyme-linked immunosorbent assay and card agglutination test); their species specificity is generally low and they detect immune responses to current and past infections and can, therefore, only provide a presumptive diagnosis of active infection. Different molecular tests i.e. Polymerase Chain Reaction (PCR), Loop mediated isothermal amplification (LAMP) are in use nowadays for diagnosis of Trypanosomiasis. The PCR procedure is extremely sensitive as even minute quantities of parasite DNA can be amplified into a detectable quantity if the number of cycles is sufficiently high.

Leishmaniasis

Leishmaniasis, is a group of vector borne parasitic diseases caused by protozoa of the genus Leishmania. Leishmania genus belong to subgroup Salivaria of family Trypanosomatidae, order Kinetoplastida (having extranuclear DNA), class Zoomastigophora (flagellates without chloroplast), subphylum Mastigophora (having flagella), phylum Sarcomastigophora (having flagella or pseudopodia) and subkingdom protozoa. There are about 53 species in Leishmania genus, out of which 20 species have zoonotic potential. Leishmania genus is subdivided into three subgenera i.e. Leishmania, Sauroleishmania and Viannia on the basis of their location within the gut of sand fly.

Leishmaniasis is caused by number of species of leishmania worldwide and is prevalent in both humans and animals and also having zoonotic potential. In term of burden of disease, leishmania is the 3rd most important vector borne parasitic disease worldwide but it is regarded as one of the most neglected tropical disease. Due to broad and widespread prevalence of Leishmaniasis from ancient times, it is known with various names (white leprosy, black fever) in history.

Leishmania was discovered by William Leishman and Charles Donovan in 1901 as unicellular parasites present in the cells of morbid human tissues and they termed these as Leishman-Donovan bodies. Leishmania parasite requires two hosts for completion of their life cycle i.e. sand fly in which promastigote form occur and mammal host in which amastigote form is present. Promastigote form is present in gut of sand flies and is extracellular, motile due to the presence of long flagella at the anterior end of the body. Structure of promastigote is spindle shaped, elongated having nucleus in the centre and kinetoplast and basal body in front of nucleus. Size of promastigote ranges from 15-30 µm in length. Amastigote is intracellular form of leishmania parasite present in mononuclear phagocytes (monocytes) and is non-motile due to the absence of flagella. Size of amastigote ranges from 3-6 µm, having oval shape with kinetoplast and basal body at anterior end of the body.

There are numerous species of sand fly but only few are capable of transmission of leishmania parasites.

There are more than 600 species of sand fly and based on their geographical distribution they are divided into six genera i.e. Phlebotomus, Sergentomyia, Lutzomyia, Brumptomyia, Chinius and Waruleya. Phlebotomus, Chinius and Sergentomyia are present in Old world (Asia, Africa and Middle east) and Lutzomyia, Brumptomyia and Waruleya are prevalent in New World (Central America and Latin America). Human leishmaniasis is caused by species of the genera Phlebotomus and Lutzomyia in Old world and New world, respectively.

There are three forms of Leishmaniasis i.e. Visceral Leishmaniasis, Cutaneous leishmaniasis and Mucocutaneous leishmaniasis.

Visceral Leishmaniasis

Visceral leishmaniasis is known by various names i.e. *Kala-azar*, Black fever and Dumdum fever. It is one of the most severe forms of leishmaniasis and can be fatal if not treated in time. It was first diagnosed as sub type of malaria in 1824 in Jessore in Indian subcontinent and due to black discoloration of skin in different parts of the body it acquired its name *Kala azar* which means black fever in local language. Etiological agent of the disease was first isolated by William Leishman in spleen smears of soldier died of the disease in Dumdum area of India and hence also named as Dumdum fever.

Etiological agents of visceral leishmaniasis are *Leishmania infantum* (also called as *Leishmania chagasi*) in Europe and Latin America while in Indian sub continent and Africa *Leishmania donovani* are involved. Visceral leishmaniasis can be acute, sub acute and chronic with incubation period ranges from weeks to months. *Leishmania infantum* causes disease both in humans and animals (mostly dogs which act as reservoir host) and is referred as zoonotic visceral leishmaniasis. It was first recorded in Crete, Greece in 1907.

Visceral leishmaniasis is characterized by transient fever, emaciation, weight loss, hepato-splenomegaly and pancytopenia. There is overall hyperproteinemia with elevated level of globulin but lower values of albumin. Complications of visceral leishmaniasis may cause Post kala azar dermal leishmaniasis, which is characterized by hypopigmented nodules in individuals recovered from visceral leishmaniasis. This may or may not heal spontaneously but act as important reservoir of parasites and have role in transmission of leishmaniasis.

Cutaneous Leishmaniasis

Cutaneous leishmaniasis is the disfiguring and stigmatizing form of leishmaniasis caused by various species of leishmania. It is the most common form of leishmaniasis caused by *Leishmania tropica, Leishmania aethiopica, Leishmania major* in Africa and South east Asia, while in Latin and South America *Leishmania mexicana, Leishmania amazonensis* and *Leishmania braziliensis*.

Cutaneous Leishmaniasis is also known by various names as Oriental sore, Chiclero ulcer and tropical sore. Animals (most importantly dogs and rodents) may act as reservoir host for the transmission of cutaneous leishmaniasis. Chronic form of Post kala azar dermal leishmaniasis may also act as reservoir for the parasites transmission.

Skin lesions develop at bite of sand fly and may persist for months to year. Lesions develop from papules to nodules and finally ulcerative lesions may develop with central depression and raised border. Nodules are mostly painless but occasionally bacteria can invade the lesions and may be painful.

Mucocutaneous Leishmaniasis

In this form of leishmaniasis, mucous membranes of mouth, nose and throat are partially or completely affected. It results from invading of leishmania parasite form skin to mucous membranes of mouth, nose and throat. Mucocutaneous form of leishmaniasis is caused by *Leishmania braziliensis* (Subgenus Viannia).

Oral, pharyngeal or nasal symptoms (bleeding) may develop initially but later on ulcerative destruction of mucous membranes occur which may ultimately lead to perforation of nasal septum.

Poverty, environmental changes, poor nutrition, urbanization, migration of people and climatic changes are regarded as important risk factors of leishmaniasis as they contribute in increasing population of sand flies or increasing interaction of affected and healthy individuals.

Diagnosis of Leishmanis

Leishmaniasis can be diagnosed through variety of tests in combination with clinical signs and symptoms. Visceral leishmaniasis can be diagnosed through detection of leishmania parasites in bone marrow aspirates while skin lesion specimen is used for detection of cutaneous form of leishmaniasis. Serological and molecular tests can also be used for diagnosis of visceral and cutaneous leishmaniasis but serological tests can be least helpful in cutaneous form.

Human Granulocytic Anaplasmosis

It is a tick borne disease caused by *Anaplasma phagocytophilum* and transmitted to humans through bite of *Ixodes scapularis* and *Ixodes parificus* (black legged ticks). These ticks are also involved in transmission of other tick borne disease of zoonotic importance i.e. Lyme's disease and Babesiosis. Human granulocytic anaplasmosis was formerly termed as Human Granulocytic Ehrlichisosis. Human granulocytic anaplasmosis was I[st] reported in 1990 in Wisconsin, USA in a patient with severe febrile illness but its role in veterinary disease was known since 1932.

Anaplasma phagocytophilum belongs to genus anaplasma, family Ehrlichiacea, order Rickettsiales, class Alphaproteobacteria, phylum proteobacteria and domain bacteria. *Anaplasma phagocytophilum* is small gram negative obligate intracellular bacterium with size ranges from 0.2-2µm. It has the affinity to granulocytic cells mainly neutrophils where it replicates and form morula microcolony which can be visualized during microscopy in stained smears. *Anaplasma phagocytophilum* invades neutrophils and alter gene expressing thereby prolong the life span of these cells by avoiding apoptosis.

Anaplasma phagocytophilum can also cause infection in horses, ruminants, dogs and other small mammals. White footed mouse may act as reservoir host for *Anaplasma phagocytophilum.* Major clinical signs of Human granulocytic anaplasmosis include fever, headache, myalgia (muscular aches), joint pain, loss of mental status, fatigue and chills. In Human Granulocytic Anaplasmosis, mainly neutrophils are affected; results in decreased level of leukocytes and platelets. HGA may affect people irrespective of age but adults and immunocompromised individuals are at great risk. In animals most important signs and symptoms include anemia, decrease in white blood cells and lameness. Different tests like microscopy, serological test and molecular tests are used with various successes for the diagnosis of human granulocytic anaplasmosis.

Crimean Congo Hemorrhagic Fever (CCHF)

Crimean Congo hemorrhagic fever is an acute viral hemorrhagic fever caused by genus Nairovirus of the family Bunyaviridae. Bunyaviridae is one of the largest viral family containing more than 300 viruses. This family consists of five genera namely; Phlebovirus, Bunyavirus, Nairovirus, Hantavirus and Tospovirus. Size of these viruses ranges from 80-120 nm with spherical structures. Nairovirus is tick borne virus which is divided into seven sero groups, out of which CCHF sero group is most important which consists of CCHF virus and Hazara virus. Hazara virus was isolated from wild rodent ticks in Pakistan but till to no information is available about its involvement in human disease. CCHF virus like other viruses of the family Bunyaviridae, is an enveloped, single stranded negative sense RNA genome that is divided into three segments i.e. small (S), medium (M) and large (L) segment. All these segments encode for different proteins i.e. small segment encode for nucleocapsid protein (NP), medium for the envelope glycoproteins G1 and G2 and large segment for RNA dependent polymerase. Small segment consists of 1672 nucleotides, medium segment consists of over 5000 nucleotides while large segment consists of about 12000 nucleotides. All three segments are linear, single stranded and each code for 1 gene and 1 protein.

CCHF outbreak was I[st] reported in 12th century in present day Tajikistan as a severe hemorrhagic syndrome due to tick bite. First modern day outbreak of CCHF was recorded in 1944 when Soviet army were engaged in military operation for re-occupying Crimean areas from German forces. Many soldiers were hospitalized, showing signs of febrile illness, bleeding and about 20 soldiers died of the disease. Group of researchers including Mikhail Chumakov and Lev Zilber had linked the disease with tick bites. During German occupation, most of the land was uncultivated due to which Hyalomma ticks population drastically increased. Army personnel and other workers, working in field to re-cultivate the lands were exposed to large number of tick bites. At this time, they named this disease as Crimean hemorrhagic fever on the basis of their locality. Almost after a decade, in 1956 in Belgian Congo, virus was isolated from a patient showing febrile illness by Ghislaine Courtois and named the disease as Congo hemorrhagic fever. In 1969, it was reported that Crimean strain isolated by Chumakov from Moscow and Congo strain have same antigenic structure. The International committee on Taxonomy of viruses suggested the name Congo-Crimean hemorrhagic fever virus but Soviets insisted on alternate name as Crimean Congo hemorrhagic fever virus. Due to strong political pressure from Soviets and cold war, name of the virus was changed against all the norms and principles of scientific nomenclature as Crimean Congo hemorrhagic fever virus. In muslim countries, especially in Pakistan CCHF cases were reported higher in religious festival (Eid-ul-Azha) due to large number of animal movements throughout the country. Small ruminants are thought to be an important source of infection for humans with increased risk associated with their slaughter during the Eid-u-Azha festival.

Apart from tick vertebrate cycle, CCHF virus can also be transmitted from infected to healthy ticks (Hyaloma) through horizontal and vertical routes. It can affect wide range of species including wildlife species, ruminants, Ostriches (other birds are resistant) and humans. CCHF virus replicates in tissues of tick during metamorphosis form larval to adult stages. Virus is transmitted from male ticks to female during copulation and from female ticks to their eggs. This virus predominantly replicates in midgut and have highest titer in salivary gland and reproductive organs which favor the vertical transmission of virus in ticks.

CCHF is most commonly transmitted in spring and summer months of the year when ticks larvae and nymph stage required blood meals for their growth and development. After bite of infected tick, virus replicates in tissues of vertebrate host and spread in bloodstream which become source of infection for healthy ticks feeding on the vertebrate host.

CCHF virus spread to the nearby lymph nodes after entering in to the host body and then invade liver and spleen. Virus infect dendritic cells and macrophages to release certain chemokines which act as chemoattractant for new macrophages to site of infection and these naïve macrophages are also infected by CCHF virus.

Synthesis of albumin in hepatocytes is affected due to CCHF infection which results in development of edema or swelling in the body and also there is abnormal synthesis of clotting factors which is manifested by hemorrhages and bleeding.

There are four phases of development of CCHF illness i.e. incubation, pre-hemorrhagic, hemorrhagic and convalescence phase. Incubation period of the CCHF mainly depends on the route of transmission of the infectious agent. It may be fastest (1-9 days), median (5-6 days) or slower (5-13 days) in case of transmission through tick bite, blood or infected animal, respectively.

In pre-hemorrhagic phase, there is persistent high fever for 5-12 days along with dizziness, headache, body pain and vomiting. Some patients may exhibit abnormal behavior and aggression. In case of severe infection, patient from pre-hemorrhagic phase enters into the hemorrhagic phase in 3-6 days. Patients in this phase have extensive hemorrhages, petechiation, ecchymosis and bruising. There might be hemorrhages of the gastrointestinal tract manifested by black stool, hematemesis or epistaxis. Some of the patients will enter into next convalescence phase while 15-30% of the patients expire in hemorrhagic phase. This is a recovery phase and is characterized by generalized weakness, impairment in eye sight and hearing.

Only humans exhibit signs and symptoms of the diseases while animals though carrier of the CCHF, are mostly asymptomatic and thus difficult to control the spread of infection to other susceptible hosts.

Borrelliosis (Lyme Disease)

Borrelliosis or lyme disease is tick borne bacterial diseases, caused by various species of genus Borrelia. Multiple body systems get involved in lyme disease due to which broad range of symptoms developed. Similarly, Bartonellosis is another bacterial disease, either transmitted by scratches of domestic or feral cats/kittens or through bite of infected fleas.

Toxoplasmosis

Toxoplasmosis, present worldwide is a parasitic disease, is caused by *Toxoplasma gondii* which is an obligate intracellular protozoan. This is probably the most widespread protozoan infecting almost half a billion people throughout the world. *Toxoplasma gondii* belong to the subfamily Toxoplasmatinae, family Sarcocystidae, order Eucoccidiorida, class Conoidasida, phylum Apicomplexa and subkingdom Protozoa.

In 1908, Nicolle and Manceaux first identified *Toxoplasma gondii* in *Ctenodactylus gundii* (North African rodent, gundi) while at the same time Splendore described the protozoan in rabbit. In 1909, Nicolle and Manceaux named this organism as *Toxoplasma gondii* because of it curved structure (*Toxo* in Greek mean arch like or bow, and gondii because it was Ist reported in gundi ; a rodent).

Wolf, Cowen and Paige identified *Toxoplasma gondii* for the Ist time as human parasite in 1939. They successfully isolated *Toxoplasma gondii* from congenital infection of an infant girl died with encephalomyelitis. There are three major genotypes of *Toxoplasma gondii* and they differ in their pathogenicity and occurrence in people.

Type I genotype is pathogenic in both mice and humans and is mostly seen in combination with AIDS disease in people.

Type II genotype is not causing disease in mice but is mainly virulent for humans. Genotype 2 is mostly responsible for congenital toxoplasmosis in Europe and North America.

Type III genotype is mainly pathogenic for animals and is rarely seen in humans. This genotype is not pathogenic for mice.

Almost all warm-blooded animals are susceptible of acquiring Toxoplasmosis but cats (wild and domestic) are the only hosts where *Toxoplasma gondii* can develop sexual reproduction.

Cats mainly acquire the infection either by ingesting tissues from animals having cysts of *Toxoplasma gondii* which contain bradyzoites, or by ingesting tissues from acutely infected animals having tachyzoites or through ingestion of oocysts shed in feaces of other cats. *Toxoplasma gondii* develop first through asexual stages in feline intestinal epithelium or develop directly through sexual stages under certain conditions. Zygotes are developed to oocyst and enter into lumen of small intestine and then shed in faeces in unsporulated form. Time from ingestion of cysts to shedding of oocysts is about 3-10 days and shedding continues for about 7-21 days. Oocysts, once exposed to air at room temperature after shedding become sporulated and can cause infection in susceptible hosts.

Sporulated oocyst consists of two sporocysts and each sporocyst contains four sporozoites. During exposure of non-feline hosts to either sporulated oocysts or tissue containing cyst undergo a process called endodyogeny, in which tachyzoites undergo rapid and repeated multiplication until transform into bradyzoites. Bradyzoites are surrounded by cyst wall and remain infectious for long period of time. In immunocompromised hosts or when cysts are ingested by naïve hosts, bradyzoites are transformed into tachyzoites.

Feces of the cats, which are mainly deposited in gardens, field, lawns, playgrounds, are potential source of infection to humans. Oocysts of *Toxoplasma gondii* are lighter comparatively and thus can be easily dispersed through wind, water or through humans/animals.

Fasciolosis

Fasciolosis, also called as fasciolasis, distomatosis and liver rot is a parasitic disease caused by two species of fasciola i.e. *Fasciola hepatica* and *Fasciola gigantica*. This disease is water or food borne trematode zoonosis and is classified as neglected tropical disease. Cattle and sheep are susceptible to fasciolosis but humans may also acquire the infection through contaminated food or water.

Fasciola hepatica is first trematode identified and was reported for the first time in sheep. Jehan de Brie (French man) reported *Fasciola hepatica* in his publication, Le Bon Berger (The Good Shepherd) in 1379. It got its generic name Fasciola from latin word *dim of fascia* which mean band of a fillet. First human fasciolosis case was reported in 17th century and later on fasciola was isolated from gall bladder of human patient during postmortem. *Fasciola hepatica* life cycle was described later in 1883 century by Leuckart-Thomos.

Fasciola belong to subfamily fasciolinae, family fasciolidae, suborder distomata, order echinostomiformes, subclass digenea, class trematoda, sub-phylum platyhelminthes and phylum helminthes. *Fasciola hepatica* adult worm is looks like laurel leaf, having greyish brown color and range in size from 2-3cm in length and 0.8 to 1.5cm in width. Outer side of the fluke is covered by tegument which is composed of scleroprotein which protects the worm body from mechanical action of digestive system of the host. The surface of tegument is covered anteriorly with backwardly projecting spines on both dorsal and ventral sides of the body while on the posterior side tegument is smooth. The tegument plays an important role in causing fasciolosis as it suppresses the immune response of the host. Eggs of the *Fasciola hepatica* are quite large having oval shape and operculum at one pole and sometime a small stalk at the opposite pole. Eggs of *Fasciola gigantica* are comparatively larger than that of *Fasciola hepatica*. Eggs are embryonated and develop miracidium in about 2 weeks at temperature of 26-30 °C. Embryonation and development of miracidium takes about 9-12 days at optimum temperature of 26-30°C while the development is almost ceased at lower temperature. Embryonated eggs when comes in contact with water hatches and miracidium escapes through the operculum. The larvae of trematodes undergo extensive asexual multiplication parthenogenetically inside their intermediate hosts which is mollusc (snail) in case of flukes.

Miracidium of the flukes has an elongate body measuring about 150μm and is covered with cilia. Miracidium is very active, highly motile and swims in all direction to find an appropriate intermediate hosts. Miracidium penetrate the snail body within 30 min through mechanical and enzymatic means and sheds its ciliated covering and transform into sporocyst which contain germ cells to produce numerous numbers of first generation rediae. Rediae consists of mouth having tubular sac like gut and mouth is armed with sucker. Rediae are liberated from sporocyst through disintegration of the sporocyst. These liberated rediae migrate to hepatopancreas of the snail to undergo further development. Germ cells in the rediae produce another generation of daughter rediae and this process continues till it give rise to ultimate larval stage cercaria.

Cercaria consists of an oval body anteriorly while tail at the posterior side and characterizes as lophocercus type. Body of the cercaria consists of oral and ventral sucker, a pharynx, and pair of unbranched intestinal caeca while gonads are absent. The cercaria swims for short time in water and adheres to any support e.g. vegetation etc. The cercaria can infect definitive hosts through drinking of infected water or it can form cyst on vegetation, this cyst is known as metacercaria and the mammalian host can be infected while eating leaves containing metacercaria. Metacercaria may leave the cyst through mechanical action and may survive for 6 months in water. Ingested metacercaria are released from the cyst in the duodenum of the host and migrate into the peritoneal cavity and finally reach the liver. They bore through the liver capsule and in about 12 weeks enter the bile ducts where they start to lay eggs. Clinical signs and symptoms of fasciolosis is mainly divided into three phases i.e. acute, subacute and chronic phase. Acute phase of fasciolosis occurs between 14-30 days after ingestion of about 2000 metacercaria in case of *Fasciola hepatica* in sheep and 300 metacercaria for *Fasciola gigantica* while in large ruminants acute fasciolosis is caused by ingesting about 1000 metacercaria of *Fasciola gigantica.*

In this phase of fasciolosis, juvenile migrating flukes in the liver parenchyma ruptures the blood vessels and cause extensive hemorrhages. In late stage of infection, animals decline to stand or move and remain off feed. The condition may worsen more between 3-7 days and blood froth may ooze out through mouth and nostrils before death. At postmortem examination, enlarged hemorrhagic liver with migrating flukes in the necrotic tunnels may be observed. Sheep may exhibit weakness, anorexia and pain in the acute phase or may die before the onset of clinical signs.

Ingestion of relatively low doses of metacercaria for a longer period result in development of sub acute fasciolosis. Some flukes may migrate in the liver while other may reach to bile ducts and results in cholangitis. There is marked weakness, weight loss and fluid may accumulate in the abdomen and develop ascites along with submandibula and facial edema. There is marked variation in various hemato-biochemical profile i.e. anemia, eosinophilia, hypoalbuminaemia, and elevated level of alanine aminotransferase (ALT) and aspartate transaminase (AST). Sub acute fasciolosis may have fatal consequences in sheep in case of co-infection with *Clostridium novvi* in liver by developing Black disease.

Chronic fasciolisis is the most common type of infection in animals and humans caused due to the ingestion of moderate number of metacercaria. There is progressive liver cirrhosis with thickened, fibrous and calcified bile ducts. Bile ducts having flukes are distended, filled with fluke eggs and spines of fluke embedded in the epithelium result in the development of hyperplasia. Liver is pale in color and hard with irregular outlines at necropsy. There is progressive weakness, anemia, hypoalbuminaemia with submandibular edema and ascites. Fasciola eggs are demonstrated in feces or the infection may go un-noticed.

Fasciolosis in humans may be divided in to four phases i.e. incubation phase, invasive or acute phase, latent phase and chronic or obstructive phase. Damage of hepatic tissue and peritoneum occur due to the migrating juvenile flukes in acute or invasive phase. Humans may develop certain clinical symptoms i.e. fever, anemia, inappetance, urticaria, hepatomegaly, ascites, jaundice etc. In chronic or obstructive phase, there is inflammation and hyperplasia of the epithelium lining of bile ducts resulting in cholnagitis and chlocystitis. There is enlargement of gall bladder and thickening of walls in case of obstruction of biliary duct.

Fasciolosis is mainly diagnosed through detection of eggs in humans stool and animal fecal samples. More advance and sensitive techniques (copro antigen through ELISA, molecular techniques like PCR) are also in use for the detection of fasciolosis both in humans and animals.

Taeniasis/Cysticercosis

Teniasis is a parasitic disease of humans and cattle caused due to tapeworms of the genus Taenia. Taenia belong to the family Taeniiadae, order cyclophllidea, class cestodes and phylum platyhelminthes.

There are two important species of Taenia i.e. *Taenia solium* and *Taenia saginata* which causes Taeniosis in humans while cysticercosis in cattle. *Taenia saginata* infection is mostly transmitted to humans through consumption of beef infected with tapeworm's larval stage and is mostly termed as beef tapeworm while *Taenia solium* is transmitted through infected pork and is termed as pork tapeworm. Humans may acquire cysticercosis after ingestion of water/food infected with *Taenia solium* eggs.

Cysticerci of *Taenia saginata* are about 7.5 to 10 mm in width and 4 to 6 mm in length. The adult form of *Taenia saginata* have an average length of about 5 m but may reach to 25 m and consisting of 1000 proglottids. Unlike to *Taenia solium*, its scolex has no hooks but having four suckers while the scolex is slightly larger than that of *Taenia solium*. *Taenia saginata* has about 15 to 20 branches on each side.

Cysticerci of *Taenia solium* are small comparatively having 6 to 18mm width and 4 to 6 mm in length. The adult *Taenia solium* has an average length of about 3 m but may grow up to 8m in length and consists of 800 to 1000 proglottids. *Taenia solium* has about 7 to 13 branches on each side and unlike that of *Taenia saginata* scolex is equipped with double crown having 30 hooks.

Tapeworms were mentioned about 5000-1500BC in Indiana Ayurveda and in Egyptian payri (Ebers Papyrus). A book "History of Animals" written by Aristotle (384-322 BC) showed that pork with tapeworm was known to ancient Greeks at that time. Johannes Udalric Rumelr in 1555 described the Ist case of neurocysticercosis. Friedrich Kuchenmeister in 1850 fed pork contaminated with cysticerci of *Taenia solium* to prisoners awaiting execution and after their execution he had recovered the developing and adult tapeworms in their intestines. Later on in middle of the 19th century it was established that cysticercosis was caused by the ingestion of *Taenia solium* eggs. In 1869, Turnbull for the first time described the case of ocular cysticercosis.

Cysticercosis is the pathogenic form of Taeniosis and infect central nervous system causing neurocysticercosis. Normally Taeniosis is asymptomatic in humans but may develop psychological stress while neurocysticercosis form may cause neurological abnormalities such as headache, dizziness, seizures, weight loss, abdominal pain, nausea, constipation, signs of increase intracranial pressure and may be fatal. Taeniosis in animal is mostly asymptomatic but may cause economic losses to the meat industry.

The clinical signs and symptoms associated with cysticercosis depends on the organs involved and number of cysticerci present. If few cycsticerci are present in muscles or liver etc infection may be asymptomatic and go unnoticed but may cause myositis if voluntary muscles are involved. But if cysticerci are located in some sensitive organs of the body it may result in irreparable damage. It may result in blindness if cysticercus is found in the eye and paralysis if spinal cord is involved or may lead to neurocysticercosis if cysticerci is found in the brain.

Different diagnostic techniques are used for the detection of taeniosis in both humans and animals with various success. Taenia eggs and proglottids can be identified through microscopic examination but it is difficult to differentiate between species involved through microscopy. Different immunological tests may be used for the presence of cysticerci and other imaging techniques may be used for the detection of cysticerci in various tissues and organs.

Echinococcosis

Echinococcosis occurs due to infection with the larval or adult form of the tapeworm *Echinococcus granulosus (E. granulosus)* or *Echinococcus multilocularis* and occurs mostly in humans, wildlife species, and livestock. The adult form of the tapeworm is present in dogs, larval form in wild species, livestock and humans.

Echinococcosis was well known both in humans and livestock in ancient times and was recognized by Hippocrates in the 4th century AD, Arataeus in the I[st] century AD and Galen in the 2nd century AD. In 17th century Francesco Redi for the first time figured out that the cause of hydatid cysts were of animal origin. Late in 1766, a German Pierre Simon Pallas stated that these hydatid cysts were larval stages of tapeworms while in 1782 Goeze described the cysts and tapeworm heads. In 1853 Karl von Siebold demonstrated through series of experiments that cysts found in sheep may lead to adult tapeworms in dogs. In 1863, Rudolf Leuckart identified *Echinococcus multilocularis.* In the early 1900s more features of *Echinococcus granulosus* and *Echinococcus multilocularis,* their life cycle and disease pattern was described in detail.

Echinococcus belongs to the family Taeniidae, order Cyclophyllidea, class Cestode and phylum Platyhelminthes. About 10 different genotypes (G1 to G10) of *Echinococcus granulosus* have been identified using different molecular techniques. All these strains are capable of causing cystic echinococcosis (CE) in the intermediate hosts and may be referred as *Echinococuss granulosus* sensu lato (broadly speaking) while G1 to G3 strains are closely related and they are termed as *Echinococcus granulosus* sensu stricto (strictly speaking). The G1 strain of *Echinococcus granulosus* in sheep is considered as one of the most common and frequent cause of echinococcosis in humans and animals.

The life cycle of echinococcus species includes two hosts i.e. definitive hosts and intermediate hosts. Canids, felids act as definitive hosts of echinococcus while ungulates and rodents are intermediate hosts and these intermediate hosts act as prey for the definitive host. The definitive hosts shed eggs of the parasites in the feces which act as source of infection for the intermediate hosts.

The adult echinococcus is very small in size and measures about 3-6 mm in length, present in the small intestine and consists of only 3 proglottids. Eggs of echinococcus are released in feces of the definitive hosts through gravid segments. Due to resistance of eggs to environmental stress, eggs can survive for at least one year in the external environment but are very sensitive to extreme temperatures and drying however in moist and cold condition their survival time increases significantly. When the eggs are released in feces of the definitive hosts, vegetation nearby are contaminated and cause infection in the intermediate hosts when ingested. Humans acquire the infection through ingestion of contaminated food and/or water, through handling of canid hosts. Each egg consists of onchosphere which is infective stage for intermediate hosts. In the intermediate hosts, eggs hatched and release oncospheres in the small intestine. The oncospheres burrows through intestinal wall and enters into the bloodstream and eventually lodges into different organs i.e. liver, brain, lungs, kidney but most common site of infection is lungs in the cervid intermediate hosts while in humans, most common site of infection is liver.

When oncosphere or larvae is reached to their predilection site in the intermediate hosts they form hydatid cyst which is unilocular, fluid filled and lined with an inner germinal membrane that produces brood capsules. An asexual budding process is present on the inner surface of brood capsules which increases the infectivity and produces thousands of protoscolices or tapeworm's larvae. The cysts are thick walled, fluid filled and vary in size from 2-30 cm. Development of these cysts is slow and may take 1-2 years in development of protoscolices.

The definitive hosts are infected through consumption of intermediate host organs that contains hydatid cyst having protoscolices which may grow into adult tapeworm. Every cyst may contain different number of protoscolices depending on their size. After ingestion of protoscolices by canid definitive hosts, adult tapeworms are developed which results in production of eggs.

Infection of *Echinococcus granulosus* in definitive hosts is almost asymptomatic with no ill health signs but in intermediate hosts (cervid and humans), it can be fatal depending on the location and size of the cyst. In cervid intermediate hosts, most common site of infection is lungs while in humans liver is the most common site. Cyst may displace lung or liver tissue, may cause fibrosis of the surrounding area of the cyst, apply pressure on nearby organs and thus results in pathological tissue changes. In humans cyst may vary in size from 2-35 cm with numerous protoscolices and cause extensive pathological damage. Hydatid cyst is very important in humans because of the mechanical and toxic effects of the cyst. Anaphylactic shock may result when cyst burst accidentally and may be fatal.

Echinococcusis in definitive hosts can be detected through the presence of adult cestodes in the feces. ELISA can also be used for detection of the coproantigens in the feces of definitive hosts. In the intermediate hosts, echinococcusis is detected through postmortem examination and identifying the larval cyst in various organs i.e. lungs, liver or brain. ELISA can also be used for diagnosis of *Echinococcus granulosus* which uses hydatid cyst fluid as antigen for detection of antibodies.

There is also risk of infection to humans while handling animals or their fecal material but due to appropriate biosafety measures these risk can be minimized. Lab coats, gloves or mask etc should be used while handling animals or their fecal material.

CONCLUSION

The One Health concept spot human health as undividable from the health of the globe and look for attaining a decisive paradigm shift. In fact, as globalization continues apace, One Health will possibly become more and more significant. As emerging diseases and health priorities evolve into global and multi-sectoral issues, public health professionals, from interventionists to advocates to researchers, must step outside of their boxes. Since long, the notion of human and animal health interface has been accepted worldwide but both of them (human and animal medicine) were famed independently until the 20th century. Through imperative events, the concept of One Health has gained more acceptances in the health communities.

Unlike developed countries, there is huge gap and lack of cooperation in policy makers of different sectors in underdeveloped and developing countries of the world, which leads to increased frequency of parasitic zoonoses in their particular communities. There is a dire need to call attention that one health is not just a theoretical concept but an applied global stratagem to intensify interdisciplinary efforts in all facets of health biology for environment, animals and humans.

An extensive alliance is necessary amongst physicians, veterinary personnel, public health workforce and environmentalists for timely response and approach to guarantee the prevention and management of infections. Likewise, developed countries should empower in the institutionalization and escalation of surveillance systems in resource-limited countries, considering the transboundary impact of parasitic zoonoses. There need to be an emphasis to create apt knowledge and response capacity in all countries and on promoting interdisciplinary collaboration and harmonization. It is also important to work out interconnected work packages targeted at gap investigation, development of control strategies, analysis of burdens, technology transfer and report of certain parasitic zoonoses. Every one yearns to live a healthy life and this is the only way to go forward to adopt such strategies and practices to make our life free of diseases.

REFERENCES

Abu-Madi, M. A., Behnke, J. M., Boughattas, S., Al-Thani, A., Doiphode, S. H., & Deshmukh, A. (2016). Helminth infections among long-term-residents and settled immigrants in Qatar in the decade from 2005 to 2014: Temporal trends and varying prevalence among subjects from different regional origins. *Parasites & Vectors*, *9*(1), 153. doi:10.118613071-016-1433-5 PMID:26984202

Alho, A. M., Lima, C., Colella, V., Madeira de Carvalho, L., Otranto, D., & Cardoso, L. (2018). Awareness of zoonotic diseases and parasite control practices: A survey of dog and cat owners in Qatar. *Parasites & Vectors*, *11*(1), 133. doi:10.118613071-018-2720-0 PMID:29554937

Asnis, D. S., Conetta, R., Teizeira, A. A., Waldman, G., & Sampson, B. A. (2000). The West Nile outbreak of 1999 in New York: The Flushing Hospital experience. *Clinical Infectious Diseases*, *30*(3), 413–418. doi:10.1086/313737 PMID:10722421

Barbour, A.G. (1998). Fall and rise of Lyme disease and other Ixodes tick-borne infections in North America and Europe. *Br Med Bull.*, *54*, 647-58.

Bartelink, A. K., & van Kregten, E. (1995). *Streptococcus suis* as threat to pig-farmers and abattoir workers. *Lancet*, *346*(8991-8992), 1707. doi:10.1016/S0140-6736(95)92874-X PMID:8551847

(2005). Centers for Disease Control and Prevention Fatal rat-bite fever—Florida and Washington, 2003. *MMWR. Morbidity and Mortality Weekly Report*, *53*, 1198–1202. PMID:15635289

(2005). Centers for Disease Control and Prevention Outbreak of multidrug-resistant *Salmonella typhimurium* associated with rodents purchased at retail pet stores—United States, December 2003–October 2004. *MMWR. Morbidity and Mortality Weekly Report*, *54*, 429–433. PMID:15889011

(2005). Centers for Disease Control and Prevention Salmonellosis associated with pet turtles—Wisconsin and Wyoming, 2004. *MMWR. Morbidity and Mortality Weekly Report*, *54*, 223–226. PMID:15758895

Centers for Disease Control and Prevention Update. (2003). multistate outbreak of monkeypox—Illinois, Indiana, Kansas, Missouri, Ohio, and Wisconsin, 2003. *MMWR. Morbidity and Mortality Weekly Report*, *52*, 642–646. PMID:12855947

Chevalier, V., de la Rocque, S., Baldet, T., Vial, L., & Roger, F. (2004). Epidemiological processes involved in the emergence of vector-borne diseases: West Nile fever, Rift Valley fever, Japanese encephalitis and Crimean-Congo haemorrhagic fever. *Rev sci tech Off Int Epiz, 23*(2), 535-555.

Cleaveland, S., Laurenson, M. K., & Taylor, L. H. (2001). Diseases of humans and their domestic mammals: Pathogen characteristics, host range and the risk of emergence. *Philosophical Transactions of the Royal Society of London. Series B, Biological Sciences*, *356*(1411), 991–999. doi:10.1098/rstb.2001.0889 PMID:11516377

Daszak, P. (2000). Emerging infectious diseases of wildlife— Threats to biodiversity and human health. *Science*, *287*(5452), 443–449. doi:10.1126cience.287.5452.443 PMID:10642539

Githeko, A. K., Lindsay, S. W., Confalonieri, U. E., & Patz, J. A. (2000). Climate change and vector-borne diseases: A regional analysis. *Bulletin of the World Health Organization*, *78*(9), 1136–1147. PMID:11019462

Grant, S., & Olsen, C. W. (1995). Preventing zoonotic diseases in immunocompromised persons: The role of physicians and veterinarians. *Emerging Infectious Diseases*, *5*(1), 159–163. doi:10.3201/eid0501.990121 PMID:10081686

Intergovernmental Panel on Climate Change (IPCC) – Climate Change. (2007). Synthesis report - Summary for policymakers. Available: http://www.ipcc.ch/pdf/assessment-report/ar4/syr/ ar4_syr_spm.pdf

Jiang, & Young, & Hardee. (2008). Population, Urbanization, And The Environment. *World Watch*, *21*(5), 34–39.

Kahn, L. H. (2006). Confronting Zoonoses, Linking Human and Veterinary Medicine. *Emerging Infectious Diseases*, *12*(4), 556–561. doi:10.3201/eid1204.050956 PMID:16704801

Karesh, W. B., & Robert, A. (2005). Wildlife Trade and Global Disease Emergence. *Emerging Infectious Diseases*, *11*(7), 1000–1002. doi:10.3201/eid1107.050194 PMID:16022772

Keusch, G. T. (2009). Sustaining Global Surveillance and Response to Emerging Zoonotic Diseases. Academic Press.

Lindahl & Grace. (2015). Article. *Infection Ecology and Epidemiology, 5*. doi:10.3402/iee.v5.30048

Loutan, L., Bierens de Haan, D., & Subilia, L. (1997). The health of asylum seekers: From communicable disease screening to post-traumatic disorders. *Bulletin de la Société de Pathologie Exotique*, *90*(4), 233–237. PMID:9479457

Macpherson, C. N. (2005). Human behaviour and the epidemiology of parasitic zoonoses. *International Journal for Parasitology*, *35*(11-12), 1319–1331. doi:10.1016/j.ijpara.2005.06.004 PMID:16102769

Marfin, A. A., Peterson, L. R., Eidson, M., Miller, J., Hadler, J., Farello, C., & ... . (2000). Widespread West Nile virus activity, eastern United States. *Emerging Infectious Diseases*, *7*(4), 730–735. doi:10.3201/eid0704.017423 PMID:11585539

McMichael, A.J. (2002). Population, environment, disease, and survival: past patterns, uncertain futures. *Lancet, 359*, 1145-8.

Miller, L., & Hurley, K. (2009). *Infectious Disease Management in Animal Shelters*. John Wiley and Sons.

Naicker, P. R. (2011). The impact of climate change and other factors on zoonotic diseases. *Archives of Clinical Microbiology, 2*(4).

Nasi, R., Brown, D., Wilkie, D., Bennett, E., Tutin, C., Van Tol, G., & Christophersen, T. (2008). Conservation and use of wildlife-based resources: the bushmeat crisis. In CBD Technical Series no. 33. Secretariat of the Convention on Biological Diversity and Center for International Forestry Research (pp. 1–50). CIFOR.

Ostfeld, R.S., & Holt, R.D. (2004). Are predators good for your health? Evaluating evidence for top-down regulation of zoonotic disease reservoirs. *Front Ecol Environ., 2*, 13-20.

Patz, Graczyk, Geller, & Vittor. (2000). Effects of environmental change on emerging parasitic diseases. *Int J Parasitol., 30*, 1395-406.

Patz, J. A., Confalonieri, U. E. C., Amerasinghe, F. P., Chua, K. B., Daszak, P., & Hyatt, A. D. (2005). Human health: ecosystem regulation of infectious diseases. In Millennium ecosystem assessment. Condition and Trends Working Group. Ecosystems and human well-being: current state and trends. Vol. 1: Findings of the Condition and Trends Working Group. Washington, DC: Island Press.

Pavlovsky, E. N. (1966). *Natural nidality of transmissible diseases*. Urbana, IL: University of Illinois Press. doi:10.1097/00000441-196611000-00067

Polley, L. (2005). Navigating parasite webs and parasite flow: Emerging and re-emerging parasitic zoonoses of wildlife origin. *International Journal for Parasitology, 35*(11-12), 1279–1294. doi:10.1016/j.ijpara.2005.07.003 PMID:16168994

Randolph, S.E. (2008). Dynamics of tick-borne disease systems: minor role of recent climate change. *Rev sci tech Off Int Epiz, 27*(2), 367-381.

Satterthwaite, D., McGranahan, G., & Tacoli, C. (2010). Urbanization and its implications for food and farming. *Philos Trans R Soc B Biol Sci., 365*, 2809-20.

Shortridge, K. F., Peiris, J. S. M., & Guan, Y. (2003). The next influenza pandemic: Lessons from Hong Kong. *Journal of Applied Microbiology, 94*(s1), 70S–79S. doi:10.1046/j.1365-2672.94.s1.8.x PMID:12675938

Shrestha, R. K., Stoller, J. K., Honari, G., Procop, G. W., & Gordon, S. M. (2004). Pneumonia due to *Cryptococcus neoformans* in a patient receiving infliximab: Possible zoonotic transmission from a pet cockatiel. *Respiratory Care*, *49*, 606–608. PMID:15165294

Slifkoa, Huw, Smith, & Rose. (2000). Emerging parasite zoonoses associated with water and food. *International Journal for Parasitology*, 1379-1393.

Taylor, L. H., Latham, S. M., & Woolhouse, M. E. J. (2001). Risk factors for human disease emergence. *Philosophical Transactions of the Royal Society of London. Series B, Biological Sciences*, *356*(1411), 983–989. doi:10.1098/rstb.2001.0888 PMID:11516376

Toole, M. J., & Waldman, R. J. (1997). The public health aspects of complex emergencies and refugee situations. *Annual Review of Public Health*, *18*(1), 283–312. doi:10.1146/annurev.publhealth.18.1.283 PMID:9143721

UNHCR. (2017). *Global trends: Forced displacements in 2017*. UNHCR.

United Nations Department of Economics and Social Affairs. (2003). *World Population Prospects*. United Nations.

US General Accounting Office West Nile virus outbreak. (2000). *Lessons for public health preparedness*. Washington, DC: The Office. GAO/HEHS-00-180.

Wilkie, D. S., & Carpenter, J. F. (1999). Bushmeat hunting in the Congo Basin: An assessment of impacts and options for mitigation. *Biodiversity and Conservation*, *8*(7), 927–955. doi:10.1023/A:1008877309871

Wilkinson, L. (1992). *Animals and disease. An introduction to the history of comparative medicine*. Cambridge, UK: Cambridge University Press.

Wilson, I. G. (2004). Airborne *Campylobacter infection* in a poultry worker: Case report and review of the literature. *Communicable Disease and Public Health*, *7*, 349–353. PMID:15779805

Zinkernagel, R. M., & Doherty, P. C. (1974). Immunological surveillance against altered self components by sensitized T lymphocytes in lymphocytic choriomeningitis. *Nature*, 251.

Chapter 5
Veterinary Public Health:
The Planetary Path to One Health

Utpal Das
The Kolkata Municipal Corporation, India

ABSTRACT

Health and disease have always co-existed with man and animal. One medicine concept was developed in ancient times as recorded in the writings of Greek and Roman scholars. In the ecological context, animal activities tend to influence welfare of man in a number of ways and vice versa. The veterinarians are the only healthcare professionals likely to see both people and their animals and aware of the potential threat of zoonotic infections to clients. History behind conceptualization of veterinary public health to one health is discussed thoroughly, and eventually, veterinary public health is referred to as the planetary route and path to one health.

DOI: 10.4018/978-1-5225-6304-4.ch005

INTRODUCTION

The animal rearing is slowly getting transformed by the primitive system to "animal husbandry" in close human proximity and this has psychological advantages like opportunity for physical and mental occupation of millions of landless folk, marginal farmers and small holders enhancing opportunities for efficient passage of animal pathogens to human communities and vice-versa. Day by day, association of human and animal are becoming intimate, which increase exposure to risk of inter-transmissibility of diseases between man and animal (zoonoses). Veterinary and human medicine have interacted over centuries in the comparative aspects of clinical medicine, physiology, pathology and population medicine. The activities dealing with zoonoses, supply of disease-free livestock products to human community, studies pertaining to environmental health, ecology, patho-biology, toxicology and so on may be classified within the umbrella of veterinary public health activities. Zoonoses are the most significant and biologically heterogeneous group of communicable diseases that are caused by different group of pathogens. Moreover, the list of zoonotic infection is expanding with the availability of better serological techniques for identifying new pathogens of man and animal across the globe. Modern perspectives of Veterinary Public Health have evolved through the pioneering work of M. Kaplan in the WHO and J.H. Steele (regarded as Father of Veterinary Public Health) in the USA. Veterinary Public Health is a vital component of public health relates to the efforts, services and the inputs of veterinarians for finding solutions to human health problems of animal origin. The main issue of concern of veterinary public health is human health influenced by animals, whereas the central issue of veterinary medicine is only animal health and welfare. Hence, veterinary public health is a branch of public health rather than veterinary medicine. The One Health Concept is a worldwide strategy for expanding interdisciplinary collaborations and communications in all aspects of health care for humans, animals and environment. The potentiation of working together to produce an effort greater than the work of any individual discipline will advance better health care for the 21st century and beyond, by intensifying the biomedical research discoveries, aiming at the public health effectiveness, particularly extending the scientific knowledge base to meliorate the education and clinical care. When properly implemented, it will help protect and save untold millions of lives in our present and future generation.

INTEGRATIVE THINKING OF HUMAN AND ANIMAL HEALTH

In ancient times, scientific knowledge of health and disease developed due to keen observations and writings of Greek and Roman Scholars who found similarities between certain human and animal diseases. History testifies that, there existed many parallel relation between Veterinary and Human Medicine. Previously, there was no clear cut demarcation between human and animal medicines. It was customary for a person to practice both the professions. During middle ages, the service provided by Veterinary and Human doctors became somewhat distinct, although Veterinary doctors participated in medical practice especially in areas of obstetrics and orthopedics. The participation of Veterinarians in human practice was thought to be an accepted responsibility. Since the early 1930's, comparative orthopedic research has incorporated the 'One Medicine' Concept. Dr. Otto Stader, a small animal veterinarian used comparative medicine approach and developed the first form of external skeleton fixation—the Stader splint to stabilize fracture in dogs. During 2nd World War, Navy surgeons used Stader's procedure for fracture management in sailors—they used a splinting device consisting of intramedullary stainless steel pins inserted into the bone above and below a fracture and a bar joining the pins for holding the broken ends together. At the time of crisis this unique technique of sader helped the Navy surgeons alot. During 1940's and 1950's, Jacques Jenny performed first intramedullary pinning in animals and significantly advanced fracture repair in horses and humans. In 1500, Dr Jacob Nufer, a Veterinarian performed first successful caesarian operation on a woman. However, no systematic effort has been made to identify the areas of common interest between the two. Both of them developed in an isolation of each other due to negligence of functional association between animal and human physicians, also the objectives of degree of specialization in both profession are different. The evolutionary mingling of Veterinary and Human medicine is reflected through the pioneering work of Edward Jenner (1796-1798) on cow-pox vaccination against small-pox, rabies vaccination by Louis Pasteur (1885) and Robert Kochs work on tuberculosis. Studies on natural history of Anthrax, Glanders, Tuberculosis, Rabies and so on provide valuable insights into the intricacies of various types of host-parasite interactions and provide the basis of a new branch of medical science (epidemiology).

GENESIS OF CONCEPT ON VETERINARY PUBLIC HEALTH

Revival of ancient concept of 'One Medicine' began in sixteen and seventeen centuries. The famous epidemiologist, physician and Veterinarian Dr. Giovanni Maria Lancisi (1654-1720) advocated that physical environment played a great role in disease spread in human and animal. He was pioneer in control of rinderpest in cattle and malaria in human. Later on, Louis Rene Villerme and Alexandre Parent Duchatelet focused on the associative relation of both the human and animal health with environment and developed the concept of "Public Health and Hygiene". The greatest philosopher, German physician and father of cellular pathology Rudolf Virchow (1821-1902) stated 'Between animal and human medicine there is no dividing line nor should therebe'. The object is different, but the experience gained composes the basis of all medicine. This statement generated the concept of 'One Medicine'. This concept of 'One Medicine' rests on the ground that animal and human communities share identical habitat and react in nearly similar manner to various environmental and ecological forces. The term 'One Medicine' was used by veterinary epidemiologist and parasitologist Dr. Calvin W. Schwabe (1927-2006) in 1984 in his book entitled 'Veterinary Medicine and Human Health' to bring a renewed interest to synergy that can emerge when human and Veterinary doctors collaborate. The concept of 'One Medicine' has been discussed for many years, but for all practical purposes and despite discovery of numerous commonalities in physiology and patho-physiology of human and animals, this ' One Medicine' concept was lost and human and Veterinary medical disciplines developed into separate professions (Lewis, 2008). That is a vertical approach tending to consider each separately irrespective of whole context, whereas 'One Medicine' is a horizontal approach where several aspects of problems are considered (Narayan, 2011). Both may be applied in certain cases separately or may be harmonized together. The close relation between man, animal, and environment, whether biotic or abiotic is multi-dimensional having unique phenomenal association. In ecological context, animal activities tend to influence welfare of man in a number of ways and vice-versa. Hence, it is only natural that Veterinary medicine should provide expertise and contribute to protection of human health and welfare. To meet these obligations, the concept of 'Veterinary Public Health' (VPH) was evolved by Dr. James H. Stele at the Centre for Disease Control (CDC) in Atlanta, USA around 1950. This term was then adopted by World Health Organization (WHO) in 1975 as an element of public health activities devoted to application of professional skill, knowledge and resources for protecting and improving the human health. In 1999, WHO, FAO and OIE further formed a modified definition of Veterinary Public Health, as the sum of all contributions to physical, mental and social well being of humans through an understanding and application of Veterinary Science (WHO, 2002). The essence of almost all branches of Veterinary science lies in the subject of Veterinary Public Health. Veterinary Public Health is the confluence of many streams. As, a stream often changes in its directions and may sometimes bifurcate giving rise to rivulets, veterinary public health may also give birth to some new domains in its dynamic path. The domain of Veterinary Public Health mainly consists of the followings:

- Zoonosis
- Food Hygiene
- Environmental Hygiene
- Comparative Pathology
- Health Education and Extension
- Gnotobiology
- Bio-security
- Management of Public Health Emergencies
- Monitoring of wild life diseases
- Urban animal control
- Production and control of biological products and medical devices
- Biomedical research (xenotransplantation etc.)

Hence, veterinary Public Health activities are manifold and multidisciplinary in character. Briefly, they include the followings:

1. Protection of people against zoonotic diseases by diagnosis, surveillance, control, prevention and eradication
2. Safeguarding people against occupational hazards and diseases associated with live animals and their products
3. Ensuring safety to human health by keeping the environment free from pollution through wastes of animal origin, vector, water, wildlife and chemicals (antibiotic and hormonal residues, enzymes, growth promoters, etc.)
4. Identification and studies on problems of mutual veterinary and medical research interest through spontaneously occurring diseases in animals or by developing animal models
5. Conducting trials on the evaluation of new diagnostic methods, drugs, chemicals, vaccines, and other biologicals used in human and animal medicine
6. Safeguarding imports and exports of live animals and birds, animal products and byproducts from microbiological, physical and chemical contamination harmful to human health through ante-mortem and post-mortem meat and poultry inspection, laboratory investigation, legislation, quarantine and evaluation

7. Acting as liaison between veterinary and medical professions and participating in public health administration and prevention and control of food borne illness of animal origin in humans
8. Promoting human health through health educational programmes, practical demonstrations and services in rural areas, emergency situations, bio-terrorism etc
9. Participation in studies on human population problems by developing epidemiological and demographic procedures and models
10. Participation in Animal Welfare activities related to social aspects including service animals and human-animal bonding

Social, behavioral and mental aspects of human-animal relationship i.e. termed as Therapeutic Veterinary Public Health (Das, 2015a, 2015b) which is a new entity in veterinary public health. However, in a report, out of a total of 1415 pathogenic human infections, more than 61% are found to be zoonotic in nature (Clelavland et al., 2001). 868 (61%) human pathogens are yet known as zoonotic out of a total of 1415 pathogens and of them; 177 pathogens (13%) are regarded emerging or re-emerging. Origin wise distribution of zoonotic pathogens is tabulated, as follows along with emerging / reemerging pathogens:

Moreover, it is alarming that 75% of the 132 emerging human infections over the past 12 years have been caused by pathogens originating from animals and have the potential to create global problems. Estimates indicate that global population is rising at a rate of 1% per year in developed countries and 2.5% per year in the developing countries. The increase in population with consequent pressing demand for enhanced food requirement has led to a continuous search for novel sources of foods and proteins. Hence, it is of immense importance to look for alternative sources of food for catering to the demands in the years to come as there are no additional land masses to be discovered that would be available for traditional agriculture.

Table 1.

Origin Wise No. of Zoonotic Pathogens		No. of Emerging / Re-Emerging Pathogens
Viral / Prion	211	77
Bacterial	539	54
Fungal	318	22
Protozoal	58	14
Helminthic	289	10
Total	868	177

Man has exhibited his creative prowess by exploiting food animals and modifying the environment—the basis of human existinence–so as to suit his necessities. Deforestation is responsible for 10 percent of all global warming. Most trees especially those of forest absorb carbon dioxide and then release oxygen and storing the excess carbon. To compensate food requirement of ever-increasing global population, often thoughtless deforestation for agriculture purpose is inevitable resulting in many emerging zoonotic infections and diseases. (https://www.ecohealthalliance.org/2017/11/deforestation-impact-planet) Nipah Virus infection is an emerging zoonotic virus. In 1998 and 1999, about 265 people in Malaysia became ill with the signs of encephalitis. Many of them were pig farmers with sick animals and 105 of them were died. When the causal virus was isolated, scientists realized it was novel and named it Nipah after the Malaysian village where the first samples were collected. Nipah virus was found to infect cattle, cat, dog, human etc. mammals and has an extremely high fatality rate of 40 to 70 percent in man. Actually, the Nipah virus belongs to paramyxo virus group responsible for less fatal diseases in man like mumps, measles etc. In Malaysia, Singapore and Philippines, human affected from infected pigs and horses, which in term caught the infection from flying foxes (pteropid fruit bat). Fruit bats were found to be natural host of Nipah virus. Since 2000, it had also been reported almost every year in Bangladesh. There people fell sick after consuming date palm sap contaminated by the reservoir fruit bats. Nipah virus had already been reported in India twice before in 2001 and 2007 in West Bengal; recently appeared in Kerala. In infected people, Nipah virus causes a range of illness from asymptomatic subclinical infection to acute respiratory illness and fatal encephalitis. This can also be transmitted from human to human.

Overcrowding, deforestation, global warming, people migration, globalization of animal trade, animal by product, animal origin food, competition in fast food industry, changing of farming system, climate, lifestyle, food habit, global trade of wild-life, expanding international travel etc. have increased the threat of newer and emerging zoonotic infections and diseases. (Hamburg and Lederberg, 2003; Das, 2015c).

Biotechnological innovation have made a breakthrough in several areas of research and application in veterinary and human medical science, which are important in public health sustenance since they pose complex social and ethical problems. Transgenic mammals (cow, sheep or goats) are used as biofactories to produce important pharmaceuticals such as insulin, growth hormone, and tissue plasminogen activator (pharmaco-farming). A combination of genetic engineering and cloning has led to the development of animal for meat with less fat. Humanized animal cells, tissues and organs created by cross-species gene transfer are used for transplantation in human (xenotransplantation). An exciting new strategy called neo-organs is being tested for patients who need new vital structures, such as, a growth factor for wound or organ regeneration; prosthesis for bone and ligament repair; synthetic biomembranes; and dissolvable sutures. One of the most discussed and debated topics in the fields of biology and reproduction has been cloning, especially after the discovery of the somatic cell cloning techonology in sheep (Dolly) in 1997. Since then, cloning has been successfully achieved with mice, cows, horses, pigs and monkeys. There is additional evidence suggesting that even cloning of humans would be feasible.

Animal welfare activities including the lessening of burden on draught animals, betterment in animal houses, watering and veterinary assistance, advice on hygienic care in slaughterhouses, maintenance of HACCP in food plants, removal of unwanted animals, formation of rescue homes for animal and health education of people for humane treatment of animal, have become an integral component of current Veterinary Public Health activities.

Challenges of Veterinary Public Health in Developing Countries With Mitigation Strategies

In all developed western countries, veterinary public health take almost full responsibility in its domain, whereas, the significance of this subject is yet to realize and implement in most of the developing countries either in public or private level.

Following are the constraints hindering the Veterinary Public Health activities in developing countries with elucidations:-

- The developing countries have a poor public health infrastructure to face the challenges from emerging or re-emerging zoonoses and bioterrorist threats as compared to the developed countries necessitating strengthening of infrastructure
- The public health initiatives on control of zoonoses have not yielded the expected results since they have failed to focus on community participation and socio-economic benefits with little or no veterinary inputs. Success and sustainability is more likely when public health veterinarians are included as members of the health team
- Surveillance programmes on zoonoses lack coordinated national, regional or local human / animal health databases. This can be achieved by providing extensive training and inculcating commitment especially at the local level. The need for technical and financial support from international agencies is also essential. The programmes have to be prioritized on the basis of disease burden and the risk involved
- Issues of ecological, ethological, social, ethical and psychological considerations in zoonoses control and food safety programmes have not

been addressed adequately. It is necessary to organize combined animal and human health care programmes with the active involvement of communities, especially, women and youth in prevention based education, preferably through NGOs and farmers cooperatives

- There is very limited collaboration between Ministries of Health and Agriculture at all administrative levels. This, therefore, necessitates the identification and establishment of a suitable interface either within an existing Ministry or as an independent entity
- The syllabus and teaching methodologies need correction and updating. Innovative lectures using the electronic media, practical demonstrations, tutorials, and field visits should replace formal lectures. More real-life problem solving exercises for teaching are necessary
- Education on the basis of hygiene and other preventive measures are more effective if given by women to women directly since they constitute the major work force in animal husbandry operations
- Inter-university linkages and distance learning through multi-lingual CDs and Internet need to be encouraged
- There is absolutely no infrastructure for handling unforeseen emergencies following natural disasters, which need to be created

With the advent of studies on risk factors, clinical and molecular epidemiology, the holistic approach to health has changed over to focus on individualism moving away from the population perspective and bringing in a new direction to the delivery of public health care. This in turn has influenced the veterinary activities as well necessitating updating and re-orientation of the emerging and re-emerging zoonotic diseases in the continents of America, Africa and Asia, mainly caused by viruses, such as, Influenza, HIV1, Sin Nomber, Hantaan, Ebola, West Nile, Nipah, SARS-CoV, and Monkey pox have necessitated development of improved diagnostic capability and adoption of stringent public health care measures requiring a multidisciplinary approach with considerable attention to bio-security.

To be sustainable and efficient, Veterinary Public Health must be flexible and adaptable to changing trends, new challenges and the needs of human populations. This will require enhanced communication between Veterinary Public Health practitioners, national and international agencies, development partners, nongovernmental organizations and the public. Need based continuing education and training at different levels at par with international standards, career development to facilitate the recruitment of students with special attention to women and minority groups and active collaboration and support from the international and inter-country organization would be necessary for the effective implementation of Veterinary Public Health activities in the developing countries. In developing countries, however, the collaboration between medicos and veterinarians have not been realized well in public health programmes. Public health services should maintain liaison with veterinary and environment agencies (both public and private) for better veterinary public health activities. Liaison, by its very nature involves a two-way channel of communication. It facilitates cooperation, understanding and encourages creative effort. This type of liaison activity just mentioned are possible only when there is a readily identifiable public health service with well defined responsibilities in veterinary public health; but in developing countries that liaison is missing almost; hence the objectives of veterinary public health is not fulfilled in most of the instances. In developing countries, the stunted development of veterinary public health needs sufficient nourishment politically and professionally. Control of zoonoses should form a part of Primary Health Care Services. As per WHO, the most effective and economical solution has been found to be involvement of specially trained Public Health Veterinarians in health administrations at national, provincial and municipal level. It is also noted by WHO regarding deprivation of available trained Public Health Veterinarians in Health Sector (Das, 2004). The world noticed the failure of a slogan – "Health for All by 2000AD". Health for All cannot be achieved unless public health is connected with animal as well as environmental health and control of zoonoses should be a part of health care services (Das, 2006).

Genealogy of a New Conceptual Model for Veterinary and Medical Communities

Due to increasing threat and challenges of newer, emerging and re-emerging infections, a new concept of 'One World, One Health' has recently appeared. Fundamentals don't change, except the terminology. The necessity of collaborative programme of action between Veterinary medicine and human medicine has distinctly been brought out in a symposium on History of the Healing Professions (Michelle, 1993). Humans serve as a primary reservoir for only 3% of known zoonotic pathogens, though the capability to identify outbreaks of disease relies on identification of human cases. Effective surveillance of causal organisms and control of the zoonotic infections and diseases requires integration across human and animal populations. Such integration is lacking in contemporary veterinary and medical communities (Shaffer, 2008). On an average a new disease has emerged or remerged each year since the Second World War; A total of 335 pathogens emerged in between 1940 and 2004, of which about two-thirds (60.3%) of emerging infection diseases (EID) result from zoonoses; the majority of these have their origin in wild-life (71.8%) and have been increasing in recent years. It is estimated that India has lost about 14000 Sq. Km. of forests since last thirty years. Deforestation brings wild-life into direct contact with humans and domesticated animals—directly increasing the risk of zoonoses and indirectly alters weather pattern. It is found that about 54.3% of emerging infections were due to bacteria and that their database included a large number of drug resistant organisms (Jones, et. al., 2008). By 2050, it is presumed that more people will die of bacterial infections than cancer.

Growing antimicrobial resistance linked to discharge of drugs and chemicals into the environment is one of the most worrying health threat today in medical and veterinary communities (Joakim Larsson & Fick, 2009). Antimicrobial resistance occurs when a micro-organism evolves to resist effects of an antimicrobial agent. Anti microbial resistance threatens the effective prevention and treatment of infections, ultimately alarms the achievements of modern medicine. This results to global death of more than 7,00,000 people annually. (WHO, 2014).

There is clear evidence that the release of antimicrobial compounds in effluence from agricultural run-off, animal sheds, households, hospitals and pharmaceuticals into the environment combined with direct contact between natural bacterial communities and discharged resistant bacteria, is driving bacterial evolution and the emergence of more resistant strains. Once consumed, most antimicrobial agents are excreted un-metabolized along with resistant bacteria. This is a burning problem, since human antibiotic use increased 36% this century and in livestock the use of antibiotic is predicted to increase 67% by 2030. Moreover up-to 75% of antibiotics used in aquaculture may be lost into the surrounding environment. Wastewater treatment facilities (Effluent Treatment Plant) can't remove all resistant bacteria and antibiotics and may be hotspots for antimicrobial resistance. Multidrug resistance bacteria are frequently found even in marine water and sediments close to aquaculture, industrial and municipal discharges (Joakim Larsson, 2014).The use and disposal of antibiotics and antimicrobial drugs, relevant contaminants and resistant bacteria into the environment is a challenge of the joint concerns for medical, veterinary, agriculture and aquaculture communities. Also to combat pathogenic bacterial infections in man and animal with multi drug resistance issues, research on therapeutic use of bacteriophage should be focused more as possible alternative to conventional antibiotic treatment.It is also observed that there was a high corelation between origins of emerging infections and socio-economic, environmental and ecological factors – which guide to provide a mechanism in which hot-spot areas, emerging infections are most likely to originate. Moreover, country border do not exit for vector borne diseases. Microbes can travel by air across the world in time frames shorter than their incubation period. In this regard, a quotation of Lonnie King spoken in the plenary session of the World Veterinary Congress (2008) in Vancouver may be mentioned – "nowhere is remote and no one is disconnected". Global researches to combat the emergence of infections diseases are not well allotted as most of the research and surveillance activities are occurring in countries that do not fit the predicted sites from which new dieases are likely to emerge (Jones,

K.E. et. al., loc.cit).Agricultural intensification, the effects of accelerating climate change (global warming) and rapid global population explosion are impacting biodiversity and ecosystems challenging planetary boundaries for sustainability and creating new environmental health threats at the individual and community level (Horton, 2015). Changing patterns of communicable diseases throughout the world suggest the need of a new conceptual model for veterinary and medical education.

ANTECEDENT OF ONE HEALTH AND VETERINARY PUBLIC HEALTH

One Health is a new phrase; but the very concept was originated as far back as to the time of Aristotle in 500 B.C. Aristotle wrote the natural zoonotic history of animals in the "Historia Animalium." Greek physician Hippocrates (460 BC-370 BC) described the effect of environmental factors on human health in his text "On Airs, Waters and Places" and provided insight on other possible causation for human diseases.

In 2003, the term 'One Health' draw the attention across the globe since it was mentioned in Washington Post by Dr. William Karesh to describe the outbreak of Ebola haemorrhagic fever in Africa. He wrote "Human or livestock or wild life health can't be discussed in isolation anymore. There is just One Health. And the solutions require everyone working together on all the different levels" (Weiss, 2003). This was followed by a series of conferences across the globe with the theme "One World—One Health."

The principles of Veterinary Public Health is totally based on biological, physical and social sciences which are widely shared in agriculture, medicine and the environmental sciences. As it is a multidisciplinary subject, hence, besides veterinarians, other professionals from a number of disciplines are to be involved for their professional activities. As stated elsewhere Veterinary Public Health is dynamic in its scope, functions and its future perspectives are defined by the changing policy and priorities of the health and agriculture sectors. Veterinary Public Health continuously explores the horizons of public health needs for new opportunities in which One Health approaches has a comparative advantage. The One Health concept recognizes health connections between humans, animals and their shared environments (Kahn et.al., 2008). It promotes professional cooperation between physicians, veterinarians and others to address complex problems affecting multiple species and pathogens in changing environments. 'One Health' concept is defined as the collaborative efforts of multiple disciplines-working locally, nationally and globally to attain optimal health for people, animals and environment (King, 2008) in a harmonized and coordinated manner. Veterinarians in all areas of profession have opportunities and responsibilities to protect health and well being of people in which they work like food security, food safety, antibiotic sensitivity, ecosystem protection, zoonosis research, comparative medical research, pet practice and human physical / mental health. The Public Health Veterinarians are the only health care professional likely to interact both people and their animals and able to aware the potential threat of zoonotic infections to their client. Hence, Veterinarians are in a better position to discover public health threats than medical doctors. Public Health Veterinarians are also in an ideal position for establishing a disease surveillance system using pets as sentinels of disease exposure in home environment (Lewis, loc. Cit.) and in wilds (Jessup et al., 2007). Medical doctors and Veterinarians are turning to environmental health scientists to prevent and control outbreaks and other public health emergencies. 'One Health' is the perfect unifying concept to bring together human healthcare practitioners, Veterinarians and other public health professionals under one umbrella. On World Health Day, 2007, WHO Director General Dr. Margaret Chan rightly said 'when the world is collectively at risk, defense become a shared responsibility of all the nations'.The concept of One Health is the collaborative effort of multiple disciplines including physicians, veterinarians, environmental and climate scientist, together with their related disciplines and institutions—working locally, regionally, nationally and globally—to attain optimal health for people, domestic animals, wild life, plants and our environment.One Health can be thought of as having three major subcomponents: basic sciences, clinical medicine and public health. Components of public health include population health, community health, mental health, environmental / ecological health, economic health, occupational / recreational health and veterinary public health including clinical veterinary public health (Das, 2016), therapeutic veterinary public health (Das, 2015a, 2015b). Animal-human interactions can be beneficial as well as pose risks. Animal contact can pose a risk of zoonotic infections and this risk increases in infants, elderly and immune-compromised individuals. Likewise, pet allergy is an anaphylactic reaction to proteins (allergen) found in pets skin coat, saliva or urine and can result in sneezing and running nose in man. Humans develop deep bond with animals and this have enormous therapeutic value implicating human health care covering under the head 'Therapeutic Veterinary Public Health', as coined by Das(2015a). Animal act as sentinels like the "canary in the coalmine"; animals may show signs of exposure to a toxic or infectious hazard in the environment before humans, providing an early warning of environmental risk.Although a few veterinarians are directly employed in public health, but virtually all the veterinarians contribute to the overall public health effort through their work like food security, food safety, antibiotic sensitivity testing, research on zoonoses, emerging infections diseases, ecosystem protection, comparative medical research and human physical / mental health. Veterinary Public Health is multidimensional and is already connected Veterinary medicine, animal production and has potential to connect outside with global public health, wild life and environment. Veterinary Public Health is the precursor of One Health and the universal path to reach the goal of One Health. Veterinary Public Health or One Health, both has the similarities with the phrase "Unity in Diversity". Unity or oneness of the Veterinary Public Health or One Health involves multidisciplinary diversified approach—which is the uniqueness of both the subject. Hence, Veterinary Public Health is regarded as the planetary path to 'One Health'.

Transmission of diseases and infections between man and animal occurs at every moment in our day to day work around the globe. It is estimated that zoonotic infections are responsible for 2.1 billion human illness and 1.2 million global death annually (International Live Stock & Research Institute, 2012). The diseases cause in human beings range from mild and self-limiting (e.g. most cases of toxoplasmosis) to fatal (e.g. Rabies, Ebola haemorrhagic fever). Zoonotic diseases ranges from endemic zoonoses like rabies, brucellosis, anthrax, trichinellosis, cutaneous larva migrans to emerging zoonoses like avian influenza, SARS, bovine spongiform encephalopathy. Over the years, the field of veterinary public health has changed. It was reported by WHO (2002) that in many countries baseline information is often lacking on the burden of zoonoses and other animal related hazards. Moreover the public health content of veterinary curricula doesn't adequately prepare graduates having updated skills and knowledge in many aspects of veterinary public health. This problem is more acute in developing countries as discussed earlier. The objective of an enhanced veterinary public health curriculum is to provide all learning background with updated knowledge and expertise for active contribution to veterinary public health programmes. Hence, the veterinary public health professionals active in this field must have the needed clinical knowledge and skills to address the issues making use of the new insights and tools. Zoonotic infection or infestation in man and / or animal may often be clinically diagonosed observing some pathognomonic signs and symptoms by the medicos and animal health practitioners, known as Clinical Veterinary Public Health (C.V.P.H.) and may be defined as 'a branch of Veterinary Public Health that collectively deals with the study of the clinical manifestation of zoonotic infections or infestations in animal and man'. This particular branch is a balanced blend of subject of medical and veterinary profession to serve as an attractive platform of One Health. Clinical Veterinary Public Health is totally a field oriented clinical as well as an applied subject, mainly based on preventive and clinical aspect of population. Clinical Veterinary Public Health will strengthen the weak zoonotic and emerging disease surveillance system in under—developed and also in developing countries. Clinical Veterinary Public Health encourages for early detection, diagnosis and reporting of zoonotic diseases world-wide to reduce morbidity, mortality, and economic loss. Veterinary Public Health Education in this modules must be developed and continuing veterinary education in Clinical Veterinary

Public Health must be addressed at different levels of public health veterinarians and auxiliaries employed in different sectors. Public health veterinarians, because of their current knowledge and ability to link the health of the animal and human populations have become leaders in developing and implementing new methods of promoting sustainable public health which are eco-systematically grounded, culturally feasible and economically realistic. In fact the term 'herd health' is a metaphor for 'community health'. Moreover, clinical veterinary public health helps Global Early Warning System (GLEWS) for zoonotic diseases and infections. GLEWS is a joint system that builds on the added value of combining and co-ordinating alert mechanism by FAO, OIE and WHO (WHO, 2006). Tracking of zoonotic diseases will be more source-full from the veterinary public health communities with the good knowledge of Clinical Veterinary Public Health. GLEWS link with the International Food Safety Authorities Network (INFOSAN) to ensure food safety events from farm to fork continuum.

ROLE OF THERAPEUTIC VETERINARY PUBLIC HEALTH IN ONE HEALTH APPROACH

Veterinary Public Health (VPH) has the fundamental right to involve or utilize animal for the well-being of human health. Animal Assisted Therapy has the curative or therapeutic value on Public Health and is an unconventional entity in Veterinary Public Health to explore the wonders of animal human relationship for overcoming many physical, mental and social obstacle of man through cathexis.

Animal Assisted Therapy may be defined as "the therapeutic utilization of animal itself for the improvement of physical, social, emotional and cognitive function and reduce passivity of man". Depending on the utilization of animal species, Animal Assisted Therapy may be classified into Equine Therapy (Hippotherapy and Therapeutic riding), Canine Therapy, Feline Therapy, Dolphin Therapy and so on. Canine Therapy or Pet Therapy may again be subdivided into two:

1. Pet Therapy through dog ownership &
2. Pet Therapy by Therapist or Therapeutic dog.

There are many evidences that pet dogs maintain physical, mental and social health of his / her master. Das & Mukherjee (2006) considered pet dog as "Human Health Co-Therapist". Many sporadic approaches using therapeutic dogs have been documented and here some of the observations are recorded and the scope is gauzed.

Following observations of pet therapy are recorded in school children:-

- Dog is source of play and learning for child's development.
- Children who would cry before coming to school have started looking forward to school for pet visit.
- School children learn values like love, caring for others, sharing, socializing etc.
- Dog makes the child to overcome Attention Deficit Hyperactivity Disorder (ADHD).

Following observation of pet therapy is found on hospitalized patient:-

- Pet therapy ease pain of ailing patient probably by distracting or diverting the attention towards pet.

Following findings of pet therapy are observed in physically challenged children in Indian Institute of Cerebral Pulsy (I.I.C.P.), Kolkata, India as recorded by Das (2016):-

- The main problem, children with autism face is that they find it hard to relate to normal people. But with pet dog, they easily develop a bond and starts to socialize.
- Actions like gripping the dogs tail or combing the fur feeding or watering for dog help to improve motor co-ordination.
- Association or bonding with a physically challenged therapeutic dog improve the reflexes and health of spastic quadriplegic children. This is a unique observation of this study to use a physically challenged therapeutic dog as a source of inspiration for the handicapped children to rise above their disabilities and not be crippled by them.

Hence, it is opined that dog is the media "to reach, the unreachable". A symbiotic relationship is developed amongst themselves for worm emotional attachment.

Pet therapy is also found beneficial in many disorders like impairment of finger dexterity, communication disorder, learning disabilities, behavioral disorder, eating problem, speech impairment, limited voluntary movement, constraint induced movement (CIM) etc.

The response of pet therapy is amazing and the target population with special needs are inspired and awaited eagerly to come in contact with therapeutic dog for warm emotional attachment. This curative aspect of Veterinary Public Health is better to be called as "Therapeutic Veterinary Public Health". As stated by American Heart Association (2013), dog ownership may be responsible for reduction in cardiovascular disease risk (CVD) due to increased physical activity and reduced obesity (Levine et. al., 2013). The positive association with dog increases the levels of oxytocin, prolactin, dopamine, B-endorphins, B-phenyl ethylamine—which are associated with the regulation of blood-pressure, analgesia, stress, joy, pleasure and bonding behavior. Oxytocin is found to be a potentially key neuropeptide in Autism Spectrum Disorder (ASD); increased level of oxytocin, improves interaction with others, learning, trusting empathy and reduces aggression (Beetz et. al., 2012).

For successful pet therapy, intersectional approach, with One Health team consisting of public health veterinarian, psychotherapist and counselor is necessary.

It is highly cost effective and has potential to save DALY of people with special need per year at a nominal cost. One Disability Adjusted Life Years (DALY) can be thought as one lost year of healthy life. The sum of these DALYs across the population or the burden of the disease, can be thought of as a measurement of the gap between current health status and an ideal health situation where the entire population lives to an advanced age, free of disease and disability.

Though there is huge potentiality of pet therapy on human health, but all the sporadic works were without any systemic approach lacking full proof evidence of long term impact on human health. Hence, works on pet therapy is not fully gauged. An insightful analysis is necessary on meeting the growing need of Therapeutic Veterinary Public Health to evolve a guide line and a new paradigm. Therapeutic veterinary public health could be accepted world-wide, as an adjunct of treatment in many human health disorders as part of One Health Approach by the concerted effort of public health pet clinician,councilor and psychotherapist.This would light the lamp in the quality adjusted life of thousands of people with special need and leave a sustainable impact in global society exploring the wonders of "therapeutic veterinary public health" in near future.

Need to Link Human and Animal Health Care Professionals

One Health fosters mutual respect amongst medical and veterinary doctors; recognizes and acknowledges the interdependence of health in humans and animals not only in communicable infections, but also in non-communicable diseases like neoplasm, diabetes, obesity and so on. Many infections go undiagnosed, misdiagnosed or un-reported due to lack of investigating mind, careless attitude, lack of knowledge, non availability of proper diagnostic techniques, overlapping or complexity of clinical features etc. Hence, a formal link between two professionals is essential. As for example, amongst non communicable health hazards, obesity is one of the major health care problem in both human and veterinary medicine and there is an increasing prevalence of obesity in people and pets. Obesity is a complex disorder involving diet, physical activity, behavioral and socio-economic factors, environment, genetics, metabolism and microbiome. Pets and people share a number of obesity related co-morbidities. Obesity is a major risk factor for type 2 diabetes mellitus in people and in cats, but this association is not recognized in dogs (Chandler and Day, 2017). Obesity is a recognized risk factor for a number of human cancers, but few data is available describing this association with canine neoplasm. The most effective approach to addressing the problem of obesity is by taking a 'One Health prospective'. Comparative clinical research examining shared lifestyle and environmental risk factors and the reasons underlying species differences should provide new perspectives on the fundamental biology of obesity. The health programmes which are held in community levels having its objective to address the problem of obesity. The most effective approach must be taken involving both medical and veterinary doctors through One Health programmes where they present their views, opinion, nutritional requirements, BMI and above all measures to be taken to control obesity through the community participation.

In recent decades, emerging, re-emerging and resurging infectious diseases and infections, driven in large part by such environmental developments are mostly zoonotic or so called, animal origin. Zoonotic disease outbreaks and pandemics including Severe Acute Respiratory Syndrome (SARS), avian influenza, pandemic HINI influenza (2009), West Nile virus, Ebola and Middle East Respiratory Syndrome (MERS) are occurring with more severe frequently and threaten global health security and stability (Keusch et. al., 2009). Recent outbreaks of Zika, West Nile virus, MERSCoV, Ebola Haemorrhagic Fever, SARS, Monkey-Pox, KFD, Avian Influenza, Nipah Virus etc. reminds that human and animal health are intimately connected. There is increasing evidence for the changing relationship with in the environment leading to may chronic and emerging challenges e.g. malnutrition associated with food systems causing both under-nutrition and over-nutrition and diseases relating to declining quality of the air, water and soil of the environment. Antibiotic resistant bacteria are emerging in both animals and humans due to widespread and indiscreminatory use of antibiotics (Paulson & Zaoutis, 2015). An interesting and practical finding as observed by Gibbs (2014) is that some medical physicians have seen 'One Health' as a veterinary 'land-grab'. A survey amongst the physicians reveal very limited awareness regarding environmental health aspects in the patient-care setting (Hamilton et. al., 2015); in another study of Allen (2015), low levels of awareness about prevention or treatment of zoonotic diseases amongst the medical practitioners are found. Hence, to tackle emerging and re-emerging disease issue and for updating clinical veterinary public health knowledge, special training is needed for the physicians (Frankson et. al., 2016) under One Health Curriculam.

Urgency of One Health Approach in Developing Countries

It is predicted that future pathogens will emerge mostly from a wild-life source from the so called Emerging Infection Disease (EID) hot spots in tropical Africa, Latin America and Asia (Wool house, 2008). South Asia has been identified as one of the major hotspots for infectious diseases and has a wider impact for the region as a "Zoonotic hotspot" and on global health, raising questions on global preparedness, especially in the context of emerging and re-emerging diseases with epidemic potential. The lack of an existing frame-work to guide intersectoral liaison in developing and zoonotic hotspot countries has further impeded responsiveness to EID events. Hence, in developing countries, One Health must be integrated in national health policy. The introduction of a 'One Health' programme would need multi-dimensional changes in the prevailing health system.

Bangladesh has an overarching National Health Policy and a separate framework outlining the Strategic framework for One Health Approach to infectious diseases. Ministries of Health & Family Welfare, Fisheries and Livestock and Environment & Forests, Bangladesh were brought together in 2012 on a national One Health platform. This happened through two transdisciplinary workshops to develop a country-level strategy and action plan to operationalise the One Health framework in Bangladesh. The first workshop also incorporated the basics of environmental degradation and agriculture related impacts on health and environment (including food safety issues) within the framework. The framework further identified barriers to operationalisation of a One Health approach to infectious diseases while securing political support from the ministries involved in the policy framing process.

Nepal is also working towards it. India doesnot have one in place yet. India urgently needs to tweak its public health policy on eradication of endemic and emerging zoonotic diseases by replacing the pathogen centric programme with a holistic human-animal-environmental approach. In India, the emergence of the H5N1influenza during 2009and the resulting policy and public panic, led to conceptualization of multisectoral linkages with human health, animal health and wild life sectors coming together to combat the problem. The collaboration was institutionalized in the form of an Inter Ministerial Task Force and Joint Monitoring Group at the national level with co-ordination mechanisms established all the way down till the district level. Standard Operating Procedures (SOPs) in the form of avain influenza contingency plans, were developed and followed in subsequent outbreaks. The adopted protocols ensured successful stamping out of the virus from most of the locations, though some of the north eastern states of India are endemic with porous international borders playing a vital role in the continued transmission. While the preparedness and response to combat H5N1 have been success stories for India, the opportunity created for One Health Initiative strategy could not be capitalized on; it remained as an adhoc effort. The scope of these adopted nationwide system of co-ordination remain limited and have not been extended to cover zoonosis and wider sets of issues emerging at human-animal-wildlife interface. Unfortunately, India's Draft National Health Policy 2015 lacks the word One Health or zoonoses or even emerging infectious diseases.

The same situation also prevails in Africa, where some sorts of One Health Approach has been going on sporadically in West Africa and South Africa.Though all the governmental and non-governmental organizations endorsed One Health, but most of the One Health activity are limited within the seminar room. However, West African countries adopted 'One Health' approach for EID and improving health security in 2016. It is time that the political and technical leadership in the developing countries across sectors recognizes the threat from EIDs and responds suitably through One Health Approach.

Research, Education, and Clinical Aspects of One Health Concept

The One Health concept has been endorsed by a number of national and state organizations and international agencies including the American Medical Association, the Centers for Disease Control, and the World Health Organization (Kahn et. al., loc.cit). There have been calls for academic medical institutions to adopt One Health trans-disciplinary approaches to research and education (Allen Scott et. al., 2015; Shomaker et. al., 2013). Student One Health interest groups have been formed in a number of medical schools and some academic health centers have reorganized existing programs and initiated new ones around One Health Principles.

Current One Health research efforts include a global surveillance initiative to identify new pathogens with pandemic potential in wildlife animal reservoirs and the ecological factors driving zoonotic emergence (Morse et. al., 2012). Such work could enable the development of vaccines, diagnostic methods, and other measures to prevent future pandemics. While dealing with the burning problems of zoonotic disease emergence, the One Health concept not only emphasized on infectious and noninfectious organic diseases, this also highlights the benefits of the human health through human animal bond. More than 50% of US households have pets that are increasingly considered part of the family, and growing evidence suggests positive mental and physical health benefits of human-animal contact (Matchock, 2015). Active areas of research related to the human animal bond include studies of the therapeutic effect of contact with animals in the clinical setting (Das, 2015a, 2015b; Grubbs et. al., 2016), and determining the benefits and risks of companion animals in the home (Cherniack and Cherniack, 2014).One Health also considers the potential for physicians and veterinarians to learn from each other through a comparative, evolutionary approach to disease and health (Natterson et. al., 2012). For example, psychiatrists may derive insights into the causes of anxiety, eating disorders, and self-injury by learning about the spontaneous occurrence of these disorders in non-human animals. Similarly, medical oncologists may drive insights into treatments by learning about the types of cancers that occur in mammals and other species, and how veterinarians are treating these cancers in multiple species (Nass and Gorby, 2017). Moreover, biological similarities with humans make the dog an ideal model system of comparative pathology for studying new cancer treatments (Paloni and Khanna, 2008). For example, Canine transmissible venereal tumor (CTVT) is the most common cancer of dogs in many parts of the world. It is a unique, naturally transmissible, contagious tumor, where the mutated tumor cell itself is the causative agent and perpetuates as a parasitic allograft (Das and Das, 2000; Ganguly et. al., 2016). Moreover, CTVT is regarded as a model for studying the immune responses that are involved in tumor regression (Mizuno et al., 1989). Few studies have assessed the therapeutic efficacy of oncogenes against tumors in vitro; in vivo studies for oncotherapy with oncogenes against CTVT are also very limited (Bhat et. al., 2017). Hence, elaborate studies under One Health Approach is needed to find out the use of specific viral gene therapy for oncolysis of different animal and human cancers. Increasingly, clinical trials in companion animals such as dogs are becoming part of the process of developing and testing drugs that could benefit both humans as well as other species (Kaeberlein, 2016). Naturally occurring Canine Atopic Dermatitis is likely the most established animal model of human dermatology. Research collaborations between veterinarian and physician to improve the treatment for chronic itch and atopic dermatitis will result in better understanding of patho-physiology and treatment responses for humans and canine alike. This is truly the spirit of One Health. At present, One Health education efforts in medical schools are in their infancy, and lag behind many veterinary schools which have made One Health a central part of their curriculam. Recent published initiatives have included inter-professional training between human health and veterinary medical training institutions focusing on topics such as shared access to clean water (Courtenay et. al., 2015).Wider adoption of the One Health approach to clinical care will require educating and training health care providers in certain novel competencies (Table 1). These proposed competencies involve assessing and managing interactions between patients, animals, and their shared environments. Such interactions include health risks such as zoonoses, allergies, and animal injuries, but also health benefits including the human animal bond and the ability of animals to serve as sentinels for shared environmental health hazards.

Incorporating these competencies into medical and veterinary education and training will require the design and implementation of innovative curriculam in education and training (Mor et. al., 2013; Gonzalo et. al., 2014) of health institution.

Skill Sets

- Ability to elicit a history of human-animal-environment interactions
- Inter-professional communication and teamwork skills
- Ability to recognize and treat zoonotic and vector borne disease
- Ability to assess and improve patient environments

Knowledge Competencies

- Zoonotic and vector borne diseases (Clinical Veterinary Public Health)
- Animals as sentinels
- Human-animal bond and role of service animals, therapy animals, etc. (Therapeutic Veterinary Public Health)
- Prevention of animal-related injuries
- Ecosystem function and health
- Food systems, in particular animal source foods, in human health and disease
- Role of environment on human health
- Ethics and values including balance of health and environmental values and legal/ethical limits on physicians dealing with veterinary issues and veterinarians dealing with human health issues
- Comparative clinical and evolutionary medicine

Veterinary or Medical U.G. curricula must prepare students to successfully pass standardized board examinations. Since most students plan for a future career in clinical subject instead of public health; hence, it is essential to stress on the clinical subjects than on population level applications of the One Health mode. So, One Health requires to focus more on clinical aspects rather than the population or herd medicine to attract the subject to the students. An initial step is to incorporate an introduction to One Health principles in the teaching of zoonotic diseases during infectious disease coursework early in the health school. Educators can demonstrate how One Health approaches can lead to better detection and treatment of such diseases, (some of which will appear on the board examinations). Another preliminary step is to incorporate better animal contact or association histories into the teaching of clinical interviewing, including the use of standardized patients and recommended history checklists. Clinical electives for interested medical or veterinay students to explore One health approaches have been developed at zoos or health centre or infectious disease hospitals or veterinary institution or abattoir and other facilities near medical schools or veterinary institutions and show promise for reinforcing One health concepts during clinical training.

Also the existing common curriculum on Veterinary Public Health for both the medical and veterinary graduates must be modified to infuse One Health competencies for the need based benefits of the mankind. In this regard an example may be cited below:

A post-graduate Mastrer's Course in Veterinary Public Health (MVPH) has been started since 1970, in All India Institute of Hygiene and Public Health, Kolkata, India for the first time of its kind in India for both medical and veterinary graduates as per the recommendation of Calvin W. Schwabe to WHO after his visit in India. Surprisingly till date, no medical graduate continued the course and only the veterinary graduates has been accomplishing the course and trying to solve the veterinary public health hazards in their own field of work. For such, the very goal of the course will never be achieved. Now, it is the high time to modify the curriculum (as stated earlier) and change the nomenclature of the course as Masters in One Health or likewise to attract both the medical and veterinary graduates. It would product a new breed of physician-veterinarian who would be a testimony to the concept of One Health. Hence, veterinary public health and community medicine must be taught as a common subject in One Health curriculum for both medical and veterinary students together; this lay a foundation to work together avoiding ego attitudes.

TRANSLATE CONCEPT OF ONE HEALTH INTO ACTION

One Health approach is found to be productive and cost-effective. It can extend its existibility for a longer period of time and its practical approach to find problem oriented solution makes it remarkable. Its multi disciplinary approaches particularly in resource constrained countries is also gained appreciation. The One Health concept should not be restricted only to seminars or conferences, but it should spread widely all over with its headed objective and perspective to serve the society outmost. The One Health concept should not be confined within the seminar or conference. There is no other alternative to integrate One Health in National Health Policy in developing and under-developed countries. To establish and facilitate the One Health initiative in developing countries, legislation is needed primarily either under Health Ministry or as an independent entity. This would need multidimensional changes in the existing educational and health system. While there is growing recognition of One Health, it has to be translated from concept into actions through policy makers. It is the high time to recognize the threat of emerging infectious diseases in the developing and underdeveloped countries by adopting and promoting One Health Approach urgently by the national level policy makers to resist from the devastating pandemics as well as to "mark the beginning of the end of the Pandemic Era".

REFERENCES

Allen, H. A. (2015). Characterizing zoonotic disease detection in the United States: Who detects zoonotic disease outbreaks & how fast are they detected? *Journal of Infection and Public Health, 8*(2), 194–201. doi:10.1016/j.jiph.2014.09.009 PMID:25488822

Allen-Scott, L. K., Buntain, B., Hatfield, J. M., Meisser, A., & Thomas, C. J. (2015). Academic institutions and one health: Building capacity for transdisciplinary research approaches to address complex health issues at the animal-human-ecosystem interface. *Acod Med., 90*(7), 866–871. doi:10.1097/ACM.0000000000000639 PMID:25650827

Beetz, A., Uvnas-Moberg, K., Henri, J., & Kotrschal, K. (2012). Psychological and psycho-physiological effects of human-animal interactions: The possible role of oxytocin. *Frontiers in Psychology, 3*. doi:10.3389/fpsyg.2012.00234

Bhat, A. H., Ganguly, B., Tiwari, A. K., & Das, A. K. (2017). *Canine Pravovirus ns1 gene and hicken Anemia vp3 gene induce partial oncolysis of Canine Transmissible Venereal Tumor*. Scientific Reports 7. Retrieved from https://www.nature.com/articles/s41598-017-15734-6

Courtenay, M., Sweeney, J., Zielinska, P., Brown, B. S., & La Ragione, R. (2015). One Health: An opportunity For an inter-professional approach to health care. *Journal of Interprofessional Care, 29*(6), 641–642. doi:10.3109/13561820.2015.1041584 PMID:26652637

Chandler, M., & Day, M. (2017). Obesity and associated co-morbidities in people and companion animals: A One Health Prespective. *Journal of Comparative Pathology, 156*(4), 296–309. doi:10.1016/j.jcpa.2017.03.006 PMID:28460795

Cherniack, E. P., & Chernuack, A. R. (2014). The benefits of pets and animal assisted therapy to the health of older individuals. *Current Gerontology and Geriatrics Research, 2014*, 623203. doi:10.1155/2014/623203 PMID:25477957

Clelavland, S., Laurenson, M. K., & Taylor, L. H. (2001). Diseases of human and their domestic mammals: Pathogen characteristic, host range and the risk of emergence. *Philosophical Transactions of the Royal Society of London. Series B, Biological Sciences, 356*(1411), 991–999. doi:10.1098/rstb.2001.0889 PMID:11516377

Das, U., & Das, A. K. (2000). Review of canine transmissible venereal sarcoma. *Veterinary Research Communications, 24*(8), 545–556. doi:10.1023/A:1006491918910 PMID:11305746

Das, U. (2004). *Health and Environment: Challenges and Strategics*. Compendium of 6th Assoc. of Public Health Veterinarians conference, Nimpith, Sunderbans, India.

Das, U. (2006). *Community participation and rural health care with reference to role of professional organizations*. Compendium of 7th Association of Public Health Veterinarians Conference, Bhubaneswar, India.

Das, U., & Mukherjee, B. (2006). Pet therapy—A new concept in human health care. *Intas Polivet, 7*, 198–199.

Das, U. (2015a). *Therapeutic Veterinary Public Health—A new concept in Human Health Care*. Brochure of 14th World Congress on Public Health, Kolkata, India. Abs. No. 797, 75.

Das, U. (2015b). *Utilization of dog in Therapeutic Veterinary Public Health—The Subject of Tomorrow*. Compendium of 12th Convention of Indian Society for Advancement of Canine Practice, Allahabad, India.

Das, U. (2015c). Genesis of 'Veterinary Public Health'and Route to 'One Health'. *Intas Polivet, 16*, 182–186.

Das, U. (2017). *Shaping Veterinary Public Health in New Dimension. In Veterinary Public Health: One Health 1st edition* (pp. 213–217). New Delhi, India: New Delhi Publishers.

Frankson, R., Hueston, W., Christian, K., Olson, D., Lee, M., Valeri, L., ... Rubin, C. (2016). One Health core competency domains. *Frontiers in Public Health, 4*, 192. doi:10.3389/fpubh.2016.00192 PMID:27679794

Ganguly, B., Das, U., & Das, A. K. (2016). Canine Transmissible Venereal Tumour:A Review. *Veterinary and Comparative Oncology, 14*(1), 1–12. doi:10.1111/vco.12060 PMID:23981098

Gibbs, E. (2014). The evolution of One Health: A decade of progress and challenges for the future. *The Veterinary Record, 174*(4), 85–91. doi:10.1136/vr.g143 PMID:24464377

Gonjalo, J. D., Wolpaw, D. R., Lehman, E., & Chuang, C. H. (2014). Palint-centered interprofessional collaborative care: Factors associated with bedside interprofessional rounds. *Journal of General Internal Medicine, 29*(7), 1040–1047. doi:10.100711606-014-2817-x PMID:24615186

Grubbs, B., Artese, A., Schmitt, K., Cormier, E., & Panton, L. (2016). A pilot study to assess the feasibility of group exercise and animal assisted therapy in older adults. *Journal of Aging and Physical Activity*, *24*(2), 322–331. doi:10.1123/japa.2015-0107 PMID:26439234

Hamburg, M. A., & Lederberg, J. C. (2003). *Microbial threats to health.* Washington, DC: National Academy Press.

Hamilton, W., Ryder, D., Cooper, H. Jr, Williams, D., & Weinberg, A. (2015). Enviornmental Health: A survey of Texas primary care physicians. *Texas Medicine*, *101*, 62–70. PMID:17094519

Horton, R., & Lo, S. (2015). Planetary health: A new science for exceptional action. *Lancet*, *386*(10007), 1921–1922. doi:10.1016/S0140-6736(15)61038-8 PMID:26188746

International Live Stock Research Institute. (2012). Mapping of poverty and likely zoonoses hot spot. Zoonoses Project 4. Report to Deptt. of International Development. Author.

Jessup, D. A., Miller, M. A., Johnson, K., Conrad, P. A., Tinkar, M. T., Estes, J., & Mazet, J. A. (2007). Seaotters in a dirty ocean. *Journal of the American Veterinary Medical Association*, *23*, 1648–1652.

Kahn, L. H., Kaplan, B., Monath, T. P., & Steele, J. H. (2008). Teaching "One Medicine One Health". *The American Journal of Medicine*, *121*, 169–170.

Joakim Larsson, D. G. (2014). Antibiotics in the environment. *Upsala Journal of Medical Sciences*, *119*(2), 108–112. doi:10.3109/03009734.2014.896438 PMID:24646081

Joakim Larsson, D. G., & Fick, J. (2009). Transparency throughout the production chain – a way to reduce pollution from the manufacturing of pharmaceuticals. *Regulatory Toxicology and Pharmacology*, *53*(3), 161–163. doi:10.1016/j.yrtph.2009.01.008 PMID:19545507

Jones, K. E., Patel, N. G., Levy, M. A., Storeygard, A., Balk, D., Gittleman, J. L., & Daszak, P. (2008). Global trends in emerging infectious diseases. *Nature*, *451*(7181), 990–993. doi:10.1038/nature06536 PMID:18288193

Kaeberlein, M. (2016). The biology of aging: Citizen scientists and their pets as a bridge between research on model organisms and human subjects. *Veterinary Pathology*, *53*(2), 291–298. doi:10.1177/0300985815591082 PMID:26077786

Keusch, G., Pappaioanou, M., Scott, K., Tsai, P., & Gonzalez, M. (2009). *Sustaining global surveillance and response to emerging zoonotic diseases*. Washington, DC: National Academy Press.

King, L. (2008). One World, One Health. *Proceedings of the 2008 World Veterinary Congress*, 10-16.

Levine, G. N., Allen, K., Braun, L. T., Christian, H. E., Friedmann, E., Taubert, K. A., ... Lange, R. A. (2013). Pet ownership and cardiovascular Risk: A scientific statement from the American Heart Association. *Circulation*, *127*(23), 2353–2363. doi:10.1161/CIR.0b013e31829201e1 PMID:23661721

Lewis, H. B. (2008). One world, one health, one medicine: From the perspective of companion animal practice. *Proceedings of the 2008 World Veterinary Congress*, 10-16.

Matchak, R. L. (2015). Pet ownership and physical health. *Current Opinion in Psychiatry*, *28*(5), 386–392. doi:10.1097/YCO.0000000000000183 PMID:26164613

Michelle, A. R. (1993). *The Advancement of Veterinary Science: Vol. 3: History of the Healing Professions: Parallels between Veterinary and Medical History*. CAB International.

Mizuno, S., Fujinaga, T., Tajima, M., Otomo, K., & Koike, T. (1989). Role of lymphocytes in dogs experimentally re-challenged with canine transmissible sarcoma. *Jpn. J.Vet. Sci.*, *51*(1), 86–95. doi:10.1292/jvms1939.51.86 PMID:2927041

Mor, S. M., Robbins, A. H., Jarvin, I., Kaufman, G. E., & Lindenmayer, J. M. (2013). Curriculum asset mapping for One Health education. *Journal of Veterinary Medical Education*, *40*(4), 363–369. doi:10.3138/jvme.0313-0525R PMID:24072190

Morse, S. S., Mazet, J. A. K., Woolhouse, M., Parrish, C. R., Carroll, D., Karesh, W. B., ... Daszak, P. (2012). Parediction and prevention of the next pandemic zoonosis. *Lancet*, *380*(9857), 1956–1965. doi:10.1016/S0140-6736(12)61684-5 PMID:23200504

Narayan, K. G. (2011). Veterinary Public Health—A route to One Health. *Proceedings of the 9th Conference of Association of Public Health Veterinarians, Challenges and strategies for Veterinary Public Health in India*, 1-6.

Nass, S. J., & Gorby, H. (2015). The role of clinical studies for pets with naturally occurring tumors in Transational Cancer Res: Workshop Summary. National Academic Press.

Natterson, H. B., & Bowlers, K. Z. (2012). *The astonishing connection between human and animal health*. New York: A.A. Knopf.

Paloni, M., & Khanna, C. (2008). Translation of new cancer treatments from pet dogs to humans. *Nature Reviews. Cancer*, *8*(2), 147–156. doi:10.1038/nrc2273 PMID:18202698

Paulson, J. A., & Zaoutis, T. E. (2015). Council on Environmental Health, Committee on Infectious Diseases. Non therapeutic use of antimicrobial agents in animal agriculture: Implications for pediatrics. *Pediatrics*, *136*, 1670–1677. doi:10.1542/peds.2015-3630

Shaffer, L. E. (2008). Role of surveillance in disease prevention and control: Cross species surveillance contribution to one medicine. *Proceedings of Annual Meeting of American Veterinary Medical Association.*

Shomaker, T. S., Green, E. M., & Yandow, S. M. (2013). Prespective: One Health: a compelling convergence. *Academic Medicine*, *90*, 866–871. PMID:23165268

Weiss, R. (2003, April 7). African's Apes are imperiled, Researchers Warn. *Washington Post.*

Woolhouse, M. E. J. (2008). Epidemiology: Emerging diseases go global. *Nature*, *451*(7181), 898–899. doi:10.1038/451898a PMID:18288175

World Health Organization. (1975). The Veterinary contributions to public health practice. Report of a joint FAO/WHO Expert Committee on Veterinary Public Health. Geneva, WHO. *Technical Report Series (World Health Organization)*, *573*, 79.

World Health Organization. (2002). *Future trends in veterinary public health*. Report of a Joint FAO, WHO & OIE Expert Committee on Veterinary Public Health, Geneva, WHO Tech Rep. Ser., 907, p-85.

World Health Organization. (2014). *Antimicrobial resistance: global report on surveillance*. WHO.

World Health Organization. (2006). *Global Early Warning and Response System for Major Animal Diseases including Zoonoses (GLEWS)*. Final version adopted by WHO, FAO & OIE tripartite. 2006:1-26.

ADDITIONAL READING

Park, K. (2011). *Park's text book of preventive and social medicine*. India: Banarsidas Bhanot.

Saunders, L. Z. (2000). Virchow's contributions to Veterinary Medicine: Celebrated then, forgotten now. *Veterinary Pathology*, *37*(3), 199–207. doi:10.1354/vp.37-3-199 PMID:10810984

Schwabe, C. W. (1984). *Veterinary Medicine and Human Health*. Baltimore, London, USA: Williams & Wilkins.

Thapliyal, D. C. (1999). *Diseases of animal, transmissible to man* (1st ed.). Lucknow, India: International Book Distributing Co.

Chapter 6
Antibiotic Resistance in the Veterinary Perspective:
A Major Challenge in Achieving One Health

Sophia Inbaraj
Indian Veterinary Research Institute, India

Prasad Thomas
Indian Veterinary Research Institute, India

Vamshi Krishna Sriram
College of Veterinary Science, India

Abhishek Verma
Indian Veterinary Research Institute, India

Pallab Chaudhuri
Indian Veterinary Research Institute, India

ABSTRACT

Antibiotic resistance is an emerging threat to achieving one health all over the globe. The phenomenon leads to the emergence of drug-resistant microbes previously susceptible to an antibiotic. Drug-resistant microbes are the major reasons for medical complications like patient mortality and treatment failure. Unregulated use of antibiotics in animal husbandry is one of the major reasons for the emergence of antibiotic resistance. The resistance enters the human population mainly through the food chain. The genetic markers associated with drug resistance spread among different bacterial species by horizontal gene transfer mechanisms. Therefore, regulation of antibiotics use in animal husbandry and proper safety measures at farm level are necessary to check drug-resistant microbes entering the food chain. This chapter discusses the antibiotics, antibiotic resistance, genetic mechanisms involved, the spread of resistance, and also the available strategies to combat antimicrobial drug resistance.

DOI: 10.4018/978-1-5225-6304-4.ch006

INTRODUCTION

Antimicrobial resistance is the worldwide topic of discussion in the recent decades similar to climatic change as it affects the human and animal well being despite the geography and the developmental status of the countries (Robinson et al., 2016). Antimicrobials can be called as 'the magic bullets' against pathogenic microbes infecting human beings and animals. Microbes use various survival strategies such as modification of the target site for action of antimicrobials, protection of the target site, production of deactivating enzymes, overexpression of efflux pumps to escape themselves from the antibiotics resulting in antimicrobial resistance (Munita & Arias, 2016). The increased and inappropriate antibiotic use has created selection pressure among the microbes resulting in emergence of multi-drug resistant (MDR) microbes. The isolation of Extended Spectrum Beta lactamases (ESBL) producing and carbapenam resistant Enterobacteriaceae, colistin resistant *E.coli* and livestock associated - Methicillin resistant *Staphylococcus aureus* (MRSA) from farm animals are few examples (Fischer et al., 2013; Liu et al., 2016 & Price et al., 2012). Infection with MDR microbes lead to complications such as treatment failure, morbidity and mortality in humans and in animals. Animal husbandry plays a little but inevitable role in transmission of drug resistance to humans. Use of antimicrobial growth promoters in farm animal production has been reported as a very crucial factor in antimicrobial resistance development. The animal-borne resistant bacteria can get transmitted to human through direct contact, consumption of animal products, food-borne infections and through environmental contamination (FAO, 2016). The drug resistance factors carried by bacteria can be transmitted both vertically and horizontally. Horizontal gene transfer involves transfer of resistance determinants through mobile genetic elements namely plasmids, transposons and phages between closely related or unrelated microbes, among pathogenic and commensal microbes. This mechanism were observed to be the reason of widespread and uncontrollable nature of drug resistance at a faster pace creating an alarming situation, worldwide (Amábile-Cuevas, 2012, Courvalin, 2008). Various epidemiological and molecular tools like Multilocus Sequence Typing (MLST) and Pulse Field Gel Electrophoresis (PFGE) and whole genome sequencing are used to track the source and spread of drug resistant microbes (Harbottle et al., 2006; Woolhouse et al., 2014). Creating awareness among various stakeholders, strengthening surveillance procedures to track the status of antimicrobial resistance, adopting policies to check antimicrobial usage and improved management practices at the farm level will help to address the AMR issue by every country (FAO, 2016).

ANTIBIOTICS AND THEIR CLASSIFICATION

Antibiotics are compounds derived from micro-organisms which can selectively inhibit or kill other microbes. Antibiotics can be classified based on their chemical nature and mode of action. Based on the mechanism of action, antibiotics can be classified as (i) inhibitors of cell wall synthesis (ii) inhibitors of protein synthesis (iii) inhibitors of DNA synthesis (iv) inhibitors of various metabolic pathways of bacteria (Levy & Marshall, 2004). The common classification of antibiotics based on chemical nature includes Beta-lactams, Macrolides, Tetracyclines, Quinolones, Aminoglycosides, Sulphonamides, Glycopeptides and Oxazolidinones (Etebu & Arikekpar, 2016).

MECHANISM OF DRUG RESISTANCE

Drug resistance is the state of irresponsiveness of bacteria to a particular antibiotic class and its derivatives. It occurs with genetic mechanisms which are inherent or acquired expressed as various biochemical pathways. The resistance mechanisms through which bacteria act to inhibit drug action are (i) antibiotic inactivation by hydrolysis, group transfer and redox mechanisms (ii) target modification (iii) efflux pumps and outer membrane permeability changes (iv) target bypass. The genetic mechanisms include (i) intrinsic resistance (ii) acquired resistance. Intrinsic resistance is the innate property of the microbes to be unresponsive to certain classes of antibiotics. The inherent resistance of anaerobes to amino glycoside antibiotics due to the lack of oxidative mechanism required for drug uptake is a typical example. Resistance is said to be acquired when a bacteria previously sensitive to a particular antibiotic becomes resistant by exhibiting the biochemical mechanisms. Organism become resistant by (i) vertical transmission of spontaneous mutation acquired by the bacteria (ii) horizontal gene transfer mechanisms. The selection pressure induced due to increased and inappropriate antibiotic usage led to acquire various resistance factors by the bacteria. Horizontal gene transfer is the process in which gene transfer takes place between bacteria without cell division. HGT involves various agents such as plasmids, phages and naked DNA uptake to aid gene transfer in processes involving conjugation, transduction and transformation, respectively (Dzidic et al., 2008). Horizontal gene transfer involving plasmids plays a major role in dissemination of AMR. Plasmids are the extrachromosomal DNA structures that can replicate on their own, can integrate with the chromosome to impart resistance characters to the organism. Plasmids are associated with fluoroquinolone, cephalosporin, carbapenam and colistin drug resistance (Veldman et al., 2011; Chen et al., 2016; Fischer et al., 2013; Liu et al., 2016).

Table 1. Classification of antibiotics and their resistance mechanisms

Mode of Action	Antibiotic Class	Antibiotics	Mechanism of Resistance
Cell wall synthesis inhibitors	Penicillins	Benzyl penicillins • Penicillin G Aminobenzyl penicillin • Ampicillin, Amoxicillin Phenoxy penicillins • Penicillin V, Propicillin Ureidopenicillins • Mezlocillin, Piperacillin Penicillanase resistant penicillins • Oxacillin, Dicloxacillin Beta-lactamase inhibitors Tazobactam, Sulbactum	Enzymatic inactivation, acquisition of alternative pathways
	Cephalosporins	I generation • Cefazolin, Cefalexin	
		II Generation • Cefuroxime, Cefaclor, Loracarbef	
		III/IV Generation • Cefotaxime, Ceftriaxone, Cefepime, Cefpodoxime	
	Monobactams	Aztreonam	
	Carbapenems	Imipenem, Meropenem, Ertapenam	Enzymatic inactivation
	Glycopeptides	Vancomycin, Teicoplanin, Telavancin	Target modification
Inhibition of protein synthesis	Tetracyclines	Tetracycline, Doxycycline, Minocycline	Active efflux, target protection
	Macrolides	Erythromycin, azithromycin, spiramycin	Target modification, active efflux, enzymatic inactivation
	Aminoglycosides	Streptomycin, gentamicin, tobramycin, amikacin	Enzymatic inactivation, target modification
	Amphenicols	Chloramphenicol, thiamphenicol, florfenicol	Enzymatic inactivation, target modification, active efflux
	Oxazolidinones	Linezolid	Target modification
	Lincosamides	Clindamycin, Telithromycin	Enzymatic inactivation, target modification, active efflux
DNA synthesis inhibitors	Quinolones	**I Generation** • Norfloxacin **II Generation** • Ciprofloxacin, ofloxacin **III Generation** • Levofloxacin **IV Generation** • Moxifloxacin	Target modification, efflux pumps, target protection, enzymatic inactivation of antibiotics
Folic acid synthesis inhibitors	Sulfonamides	Sulphadiazine, Sulfisoxazole	Acquisition of alternative folate synthesis pathways, overproduction of target enzymes
	Diaminopyrimidines	Trimethoprim, Aditoprim, Ormetoprim	
RNA synthesis inhibitors	Ansamycins	Rifampicin	Target modification

Source: (*Marshall and Levy, 2004; FAO, 2016*)

ANTIMICROBIAL USE IN ANIMALS

In animals, antibiotics are used for therapeutic purpose and also as prophylactics, metaphylactics and growth promoters. Therapeutically antibiotics are used to treat various clinical conditions affecting animals such as mastitis, metritis, uro-genital, respiratory and enteric infections of bacterial etiology and in secondary bacterial infections which occurs after viral diseases such as foot-and-mouth disease, pesti-des petits ruminants, pox infections etc in animals and poultry (Economou & Gousia, 2015).

Metaphylaxis

During outbreaks, besides the few animals which exhibit clinical symptoms, the susceptible population is also treated with high antibiotic doses to prevent the spread of infection. This is called metaphylaxis in which antibiotics are given for a short time period (Anonymous, 2011).

Prophylaxis

Prophylaxis involves administration of antibiotics in feed or water in low doses to prevent the entry of infection. It is done when the window period of disease susceptibility or the disease risk is more. In dairy cattle, prior to onset of dry period, intra-mammary infusion of antibiotics is given as prophylaxis against mastitis. In piglets, antibiotics are administered to alleviate the stress due to weaning and to prevent infections (Landers et al., 2012).

Antibiotic Growth Promoters

Antibiotics are added in ultra-low doses as growth promoters in feed either by the manufacturer or farmer. This routine use of antibiotics may promote growth by stimulation of vitamins synthesis in intestine, reduction of total bacteria in the intestinal tract and the later reduction in nutrient competition between microorganisms and host, ultimately inhibiting the harmful bacteria (Stokstad & Jukes, 1950).

EMERGENCE OF ANTIMICROBIAL DRUG RESISTANCE IN ANIMAL HUSBANDRY

The increased and indiscriminate antibiotic use is the major reason for emergence of antimicrobial resistance in human and veterinary medicine.

1. **Increased Antibiotics Use:** In animal husbandry, antibiotics are used not only to treat individual animals with bacterial infections and prevent infections in herds or flocks, but also to promote growth. In 2010, worldwide, at least 63,200 tons of antibiotics were consumed by livestock (Van Boeckel *et al.*, 2015). By 2030, this figure is projected to rise by two-thirds, to 105,600 tons, to meet the demands of a projected 8.5 billion human population (United Nations, 2015). Increasing prosperity and population growth drive an increasing demand for animal protein. To satisfy this need, many farmers are transitioning to intensive agriculture and often use antibiotics to optimize production (Van Boeckel *et al.*, 2015).
2. **Inappropriate Antibiotic Use:** Inappropriate antibiotic use can be defined as using antibiotics when it is actually not intended or incorrect class, dosing or following a poor treatment regimen. In developing countries, over the counter use of antibiotics without proper veterinary advice is still practiced. Use of antibiotics as prophylactics, metaphylactics and as growth promoters in animal husbandry also fits into this category. In addition, poor quality control measures adopted during drug manufacturing and storing processes leads to degradation of the drug molecules, ultimately leading to inadequate drug dosage. The major drawback of sub-therapeutic levels of antimicrobials is that they can't eradicate target bacteria. This antibiotic pressure will lead to survival and emergence of drug resistant microbes (FAO, 2016).

RISK FACTORS ASSOCIATED WITH ANTIMICROBIAL RESISTANCE IN ANIMAL HUSBANDRY

The emergence of antimicrobial resistance is an interaction among the animal hosts, their management, the drugs to which they are exposed and the nature of the bacteria they harbours.

1. **Animal Factors:** During intensified animal production, there were high chances of disease risks for farm animals. Therefore, antibiotics are metaphylaxis or prophylactic measures. Sub-therapeutic doses or prolonged usage of same class of antibiotics increases AMR (Levy and Marshall, 2004). Direct or indirect contact with animals or their products increase the risk of transmission of antimicrobial resistance in either ways. Rearing of household pets such as dogs and cats has become one of the hobbies of humans from days untold. Nowadays, the quality of veterinary care to pet animals' increases with immunization coverage and regular health check-ups. These monogastric animals undergo similar clinical conditions as that of humans and require the similar antibiotic

treatment regime increasing the risk of emergence of AMR (da Costa et al., 2013).

2. **Managemental Factors:** The intense animal production combined with environmental stressors such as heat, cold and lack of nutrition convey signals to hypothalmo-pituatory –adrenal system resulting in release of stress hormones such as catecholamines and glucocorticoids. It is observed that these stress hormones increase the growth and virulence potential of the microbes. Furthermore, it has been reported that there were increased chances of antibiotic resistance in farm animals exposed to environmental stressors such as heat and cold and social stressors such as weaning (Mathew et al., 2007). In addition, drug administration through feed and water also creates individual level variation in intake and also more chances of reduced drug dosage and thus, indirectly leads to emergence of resistance strains (da Costa et al., 2013).
3. **Drug Factors:** Lack of adequate facilities during drug production and storage ultimately leads to reduced antibiotic dosage which favours AMR (Osei Sekyere, 2014). The major drawback of sub-therapeutic levels of antimicrobials is that they will create selection pressure on microbes leading to survival and emergence of drug resistant microbes. Sub-therapeutic dosage also increases the expression of virulence and biofilm formation genes in resistant bacteria which favours more chances of horizontal gene transfer more chances of acquiring AMR genes (Andersson and Hughes, 2014). Out of the 27 antimicrobial classes used in veterinary medicine, only nine classes are used exclusively in animals (Pagel and Gautier, 2012). This parallel use of antibiotics increases the chances of spillover and transfer of AMR genes in either way. Use of combination of antibiotics also creates selection pressure among pathogens and commensal flora resulting in emergence of resistant ones (Martinez and Baquero, 2009). Use of biocides such as antiseptics, disinfectants and animal feed preservatives also influence the AMR emergence through cross-resistance, co-resistance and clonal drift mechanisms (Davin-Regli & Pages, 2012). The non-metabolizable nature of major part of consumed antibiotics (75-90%) is another factor which creates resistance in environmental bacteria (Chee-Sanford et al., 2001).
4. **Organism Factors:** To certain bacteria, a minimal concentration of antibiotics is required for maintaining the resistance to that drug. In the absence of such selection pressure, the organisms become susceptible. The biological cost offered by the resistant bacteria in the form of compensatory mutations determines the maintenance of the resistance mechanisms (Courvalin, 2008). Moreover, the environmental and commensal bacteria are reported to be the hub of antimicrobial resistance. These bacteria harbor the antimicrobial resistance genes in integrons, plasmids, transposons which can be transmitted either inter-species or intra-species.

TRANSMISSION OF ANTIMICROBIAL RESISTANCE FROM ANIMALS TO HUMAN

Transmission of AMR to human occurs by direct contact with farm and companion animals, indirectly through various vehicles such as food, fomites etc. Environment acts as a significant mixing vessel of AMR bacteria and their genetic elements and disseminate them through various means such as water, air, crops, vegetables etc. The sources of AMR include the resistant bacteria, AMR genes and antimicrobial residues. The resistant bacteria may be the commensal bacteria, animal pathogens or the human pathogens for which animals act as reservoirs. Figure1represents the schematic diagram of the mode of the spread of antimicrobial resistance from animal husbandry to human food chain.

Direct Transmission

Direct transmission, can otherwise be, and called as occupational zoonoses. Persons in close contact with animals such as farm and abattoir workers (Aubry-Damon et al., 2004; Marshall and Levy, 2011), butchers, pet owners and veterinarians (Leonard et al., 2012; Paul et al., 2011) are at high risk of acquiring AMR. The secretory and excretory products such as blood, urine, faeces, milk, saliva and semen (Founou et al., 2016) are the sources of resistant bacteria.

Indirect Transmission

The major route of indirect transmission of antibiotic resistance is through contact or consumption of animal products such as meat, meat products, eggs and dairy products (Price et al., 2012; Coetzee et al., 2016; Liu et al., 2016). Improper handling and cooking of animal products act as additional risk factor in acquiring resistance. Fomites such as farm equipments also act as source of spread of resistance (Aarestrup, 2006). The unmetabolized antibiotic drug residues present in edible animal tissues can create pressure on the human gut microbiota resulting in emergence of resistant microbes (Marshall & Levy, 2011).

Environmental Pathways

The non-biodegradable nature of antibiotic is the major reason for the environment mediated spread of antimicrobial resistance. Here, the environmental pathways of AMR spread are discussed in the veterinary perspective only. As discussed, 75-90%

of antibiotics administered to animals is excreted with no metabolic changes. Even after sewage treatment, the antibiotics are released with no metabolic change (Chee-Sanford et al., 2001). Neither they are readily biodegradable in soil nor in water where they are released (Lindberg et al., 2004; Lindberg et al., 2005). In addition, the resistant bacteria excreted by the animals also transfer their resistant genetic elements to environmental bacteria (Woolridge, 2012). The final fate of the animal waste is to be fertilizer for croplands or discharged into water sources such as rivers, lakes and seas. The resistance factors can contaminate the surface and ground water sources during the irrigation processes and can be transmitted to the general public. AMR can also enter the human food chain through the crops and vegetables grown in such contaminated farm lands. In addition, the common water sources such as rivers, lakes and seas can transport the resistant factors to various ecological niches along the path of its travel (da Costa et al., 2013). Presence of AMR genes in microbiota of wild animals and birds states the environmental transmission of AMR which starts from a farm, hospital or community setting (Costa et al., 2007; Pinto et al., 2010). The contaminated air currents also spread the resistant factors (Jiménez-Arribas et al., 2001). Loss of biodiversity by human intervention is one of the environmental factors which enhance the spread of AMR (da Costa et al., 2013).Climate change and global warming also indirectly contributes to antimicrobial resistance. The heat waves generated due to climate change impose stress on the farm animals. Studies revealed that animals exposed environmental stress factors harbor more number of antimicrobial resistant bacteria (Verbrugghe et al., 2012).

ANTIMICROBIAL DRUG RESISTANCE: ONE HEALTH PERSPECTIVE

The term one health refers to the collaborative effort of multiple disciplines working locally, nationally and globally to attain optimal health for people, animals and our environment. The concepts of industrialization of animal husbandry, globalization, international trade and travel of human, animals and animal products have challenged the one health concept with increased zoonotic diseases (Robinson et al., 2016). AMR is one such factor which threatens the public health by its way of entry through animal sources and environment. The recent emergence of colistin resistance in *E.coli* of humans, livestock, meat and vegetables in China (Liu et al., 2016) followed by its spread to USA is the best example (McGann et al., 2016). It also explains that the human health is attained through maintaining animal and environmental well-being. Antibiotic use in animals ultimately affects the human microbiome resulting in emergence of resistant ones. For example, use of avoparcin as feed additive during 1990s in the European Union resulted in emergence of Vancomycin Resistant Enterococci (VRE) in animals and humans which reduced after the drug ban (Marshall & Levy, 2011). In Canada, in-ova injection of ceftiofur, a third generation cephalosporin, to chicken eggs resulted in transmission of resistance through chicken meat to humans. The withdrawal of the antibiotic resulted in decrease of ESBL producing bacteria in humans (Dutil et al., 2010).

STRATEGIES TO COMBAT ANTIMICROBIAL DRUG RESISTANCE

The success of combating antimicrobial resistance in veterinary medicine lies in the method of animal rearing. The process of using antibiotics as growth promoters, metaphylactics and prophylactics should be replaced with alternatives to antibiotics. Alternatives to antibiotics include vaccines, phage therapies, immunotherapy, probiotics, prebiotics, organic acids etc. Selective breeding involving disease resistance traits should also be followed at the farm level. In addition, improved managemental practices at the farm level help to reduce stress factors and thus infection control in farm animals. Various strategies have been proposed by various organizations like WHO, FAO and OIE to curb antibiotic resistance in humans, animals and food chain. These strategies are adopted from FAO action plan 2016-2020 on antimicrobial residues and antimicrobial resistance.

Awareness Among Various Stakeholders

Creating awareness to various stakeholders range from farm workers, abattoir handlers, food processing units, veterinarians, consumers and policy makers through awareness campaigns and advertising in social media must curb the spread of antibiotic resistance from farms to forks.

To Develop Capacity for Integrated Surveillance and Monitoring of Antimicrobial Resistance and Antimicrobial Use in Food and Agriculture

The major route of transmission of antibiotic resistance from animals is through food chain. Therefore regional and national level integrated surveillance networks involving human, veterinary, environmental and food scientists are needed to check the transmission routes at various critical control points. The critical control points may vary from region and at the country levels depending upon the social standards and health status of the people. Surveillance measures will therefore provide information about the entry route of antibiotic resistance into human food chain which needs great attention. Already the surveillance measures conducted in various European countries like Denmark, Netherlands and Sweden have helped to keep the resistance spread in control. The integrated surveillance network settings are at infancy in developing countries and in low and middle income countries of the world which to be enhanced to achieve 'one health'(Founou et al., 2016).

To Strengthen Governance Related to Antimicrobial Use and Antimicrobial Resistance in Food and Agriculture

The country adoption of policies regarding antimicrobial residues / antimicrobial usage in food animals, companion animals must be framed to avoid unrestricted antibiotic usage. In addition, regulatory frameworks on antimicrobial residues/ antimicrobial use and resistance in veterinary medicine at national level in par with the international standards of Codex Alimentarius, OIE must be formulated.

To Promote Good Practices in Food and Agriculture Systems and Prudent Use of Antibiotics

Adopting essential biosecurity measures at farm level paves a major way to reduce disease risk in farm animals. Uses of vaccines at regular intervals also control the emergence and spread of disease outbreaks in animals. Use of disinfectants and antiseptics in maintenance of farm hygiene can be practiced as a routine disease prevention measure. Research and farm trials regarding alternatives such as prebiotics, probiotics, synbiotics, phages and antimicrobial peptides to replace antibiotic growth promoters should be encouraged. Use of antibiotics by farmers or livestock owners' level without proper veterinary advice or prescription should be illegal and banned by every country (Founou et al., 2016). The national action plan on antimicrobial resistance aims at increased awareness about antimicrobial resistance, strengthening of research and surveillance, infection control, introduction of new antibiotics, diagnostics, vaccines and following biosecurity measures (NAP-AMR, 2017).

CONCLUSION

Antimicrobial resistance is a global problem to be addressed at individual level, farm level, regional and national level. Increased and indiscriminate antimicrobial drug usage is the driver of AMR. Therefore, antibiotic prescription is to be avoided whenever it is not required. Antibiotic alternatives should slowly replace the antibiotic growth promoters to avoid indiscriminate drug usage in animal husbandry. After the reach of AMR bacteria/AMR genes/AMR residues in the environment, the spread will be out of human control. Therefore proper preventive measures must be adopted at the farm level. Various steps such as improved managemental practices, sanitary measures, prompt vaccination and enhanced biosecurity set-up will ensure sustainable animal production with meager antibiotic usage.

ACKNOWLEDGMENT

The authors duly acknowledge the Director, Indian Council of Agricultural Research-Indian Veterinary Research Institute, Bareilly for providing necessary facilities for research regarding antimicrobial resistance.

REFERENCES

Amábile-Cuevas, C. F. (2012). Antibiotic Resistance: From Darwin to Lederberg to Keynes. *Microbial Drug Resistance (Larchmont, N.Y.)*, *19*(2), 73–87. doi:10.1089/mdr.2012.0115 PMID:23046150

Andersson, D. I., & Hughes, D. (2014). Microbiological effects of sublethal levels of antibiotics. *Nature Reviews. Microbiology*, *12*(7), 465–478. doi:10.1038/nrmicro3270 PMID:24861036

Anonymous. (2011). *Compassion in World Farming. Antibiotics in Farm Animal Production.* Public Health and Animal Welfare. Compassion in World Farming. Retrieved from http://www.fao.org/fileadmin/user_upload/animalwelfare/antibiotics in animal farming.pdf

Aubry-Damon, H., Grenet, K., Sall-Ndiaye, P., Che, D., Cordeiro, E., Bougnoux, M. E., ... Andremont, A. (2004). Antimicrobial resistance in commensal flora of pig farmers. *Emerging Infectious Diseases*, *10*(5), 873–879. doi:10.3201/eid1005.030735 PMID:15200822

Barber, M., & Rozwadowska-Dowzenko, M. (1948). Infection by penicillin-resistant *Staphylococci*. *Lancet*, *2*(6530), 641–644. doi:10.1016/S0140-6736(48)92166-7 PMID:18890505

Chen, W., Fang, T., Zhou, X., Zhang, D., Shi, X., & Shi, C. (2016). IncHI2 plasmids Are predominant in antibiotic resistant *Salmonella* Isolates. *Frontiers in Microbiology*, *7*, 1566. doi:10.3389/fmicb.2016.01566 PMID:27746775

Coetzee, J., Corcoran, C., Prentice, E., Moodley, M., Mendelson, M., Poirel, L., ... Brink, A. J. (2016). Emergence of plasmid-mediated colistin resistance (MCR-1) among *Escherichia coli* isolated from South African patients. *South African Medical Journal, 106*(5), 449–450. doi:10.7196/SAMJ.2016.v106i5.10710 PMID:27138657

Costa, D., Poeta, P., Saenz, Y., Vinue, L., Rojo-Bezares, B., Jouini, A., ... Torres, C. (2007). Detection of *Escherichia coli* harbouring extended-spectrum β-lactamases of the CTX-M, TEM and SHV classes in faecal samples of wild animals in Portugal. *The Journal of Antimicrobial Chemotherapy, 59*, 1311–1312. PMID:17023496

Courvalin, P. (2008). Predictable and unpredictable evolution of antibiotic resistance. *Journal of Internal Medicine, 264*(1), 4–16. doi:10.1111/j.1365-2796.2008.01940.x PMID:18397243

da Costa, P. M., Loureiro, L., & Matos, A. J. F. (2013). Transfer of multi-drug resistant bacteria between intermingled ecological niches: The interface between humans, animals and the environment. *International Journal of Environmental Research and Public Health, 10*(1), 278–294. doi:10.3390/ijerph10010278 PMID:23343983

Davin-Regli, A., & Pagès, J. M. (2012). Cross-resistance between biocides and antimicrobials: An emerging question. *Revue Scientifique et Technique (International Office of Epizootics), 31*, 89–104. PMID:22849270

Dutil, L. R., Irwin, R., Finley, L. K., Ng, B., Avery, P., Boerlin, A. M., ... Pillai, D. R. (2010). Ceftiofur resistance in *Salmonella enterica* serovar Heidelberg from chicken meat and humans, Canada. *Emerging Infectious Diseases, 16*(1), 48–54. doi:10.3201/eid1601.090729 PMID:20031042

Dzidic, S., Suskovic, J., & Kos, B. (2008). Antibiotic resistance mechanisms in bacteria: Biochemical and genetic aspects. *Food Technology and Biotechnology, 46*(1), 11–21.

Economou, V., & Gousia, P. (2015). Agriculture and food animals as a source of antimicrobial-resistant bacteria. *Infection and Drug Resistance, 8*, 49–61. doi:10.2147/IDR.S55778 PMID:25878509

FAO. (2016). *Drivers, dynamics and epidemiology of antimicrobial resistance in animal production*. Rome, Italy: FAO.

Fischer, J., Rodriguez, I., Schmoger, S., Friese, A., Roesler, U., Helmuth, R., & Guerra, B. (2013). *Salmonella enterica* subsp. *enterica* producing VIM-1 carbapenemase isolated from livestock farms. *The Journal of Antimicrobial Chemotherapy, 68*(2), 478–480. doi:10.1093/jac/dks393 PMID:23034713

Founou, L. L., Founou, R. C., & Essack, S. Y. (2016). Antibiotic resistance in the food chain: A developing country-perspective. *Frontiers in Microbiology*, *7*, 1881. doi:10.3389/fmicb.2016.01881 PMID:27933044

Harbottle, H., White, D. G., McDermott, P. F., Walker, R. D., & Zhao, S. (2006). Comparison of Multilocus sequence typing, Pulse Field Electrophoresis and antimicrobial susceptibility for characterization of Salmonella enterica serovar Newport isolates. *Journal of Clinical Microbiology*, *44*(7), 2449–2457. doi:10.1128/JCM.00019-06 PMID:16825363

Jiménez-Arribas, G., Léautaud, V., & Amábile-Cuevas, C. F. (2001). Regulatory locus soxRS partially protects *Escherichia coli* against ozone. *FEMS Microbiology Letters*, *195*(2), 175–177. doi:10.1016/S0378-1097(01)00007-6 PMID:11179648

Landers, T. F., Cohen, B., Wittum, T. E., & Larson, E. L. (2012). A Review of Antibiotic Use in Food Animals: Perspective, Policy, and Potential. *Public Health Reports*, *127*(1), 4–22. doi:10.1177/003335491212700103 PMID:22298919

Leonard, E., Pearl, D., Finley, R., Janecko, N., Reid-Smith, R., Peregrine, A., & Weese, J. (2012). Comparison of antimicrobial resistance patterns of *Salmonella* spp. and *Escherichia coli* recovered from pet dogs from volunteer households in Ontario (2005–2006). *The Journal of Antimicrobial Chemotherapy*, *67*(1), 174–181. doi:10.1093/jac/dkr430 PMID:22016151

Levy, S. B., & Marshall, B. (2004). Antibacterial resistance worldwide: Causes, challenges and responses. *Nature Medicine*, *10*(12), 122–129. doi:10.1038/nm1145 PMID:15577930

Lindberg, R., Jarnheimer, P., Olsen, B., Johansson, M., & Tysklind, M. (2004). Determination of antibiotic substances in hospital sewage water using solid phase extraction and liquid chromatography/ mass spectrometry and group analogue internal standards. *Chemosphere*, *57*(10), 1479–1488. doi:10.1016/j.chemosphere.2004.09.015 PMID:15519392

Lindberg, R., Wennberg, P., Johansson, M., Tysklind, M., & Andersson, B. (2005). Screening of human antibiotic substances and determination of weekly mass flows in five sewage treatment plants in Sweden. *Environmental Science & Technology*, *39*(10), 3421–3429. doi:10.1021/es048143z PMID:15952345

Liu, Y. y., Wang, Y., Walsh, T., Yi, L., Zhang, R., Spencer, J., ... Shen, J. (2016). Emergence of plasmid-mediated colistin resistance mechanism MCR-1 in animals and human beings in China: A microbiological and molecular biological study. *The Lancet Infectious Diseases*, *16*(2), 161–168. doi:10.1016/S1473-3099(15)00424-7 PMID:26603172

Marshall, B. M., & Levy, S. B. (2011). Food animals and antimicrobials: Impacts on human health. *Clinical Microbiology Reviews*, *24*(4), 718–733. doi:10.1128/CMR.00002-11 PMID:21976606

Martinez, J. L., & Baquero, F. (2009). *Antibiotics and the Evolution of Antibiotic Resistance*. Available online at http://onlinelibrary.wiley.com/doi/10.1002/9780470015902.a0021782/full

Mathew, A. G., Cissell, R., & Liamthong, S. (2007). Antibiotic resistance in bacteria associated with food animals: A United States perspective of livestock production. *Foodborne Pathogens and Disease*, *4*(2), 115–133. doi:10.1089/fpd.2006.0066 PMID:17600481

McGann, P., Snesrud, E., Maybank, R., Corey, B., Ong, A. C., Clifford, R., ... Schaecher, K. E. (2016). *Escherichia coli* harboring *mcr-1* and *bla*CTX-M on a novel IncF plasmid: First report of mcr-1 in the USA. *Antimicrobial Agents and Chemotherapy*, *60*(7), 4420–4421. doi:10.1128/AAC.01103-16 PMID:27230792

Munita, J. M., & Arias, C. A. (2016). Mechanisms of antibiotic resistance. *Microbiology Spectrum*, *4*(2). doi:10.1128/microbiolspec.VMBF-0016-2015 PMID:27227291

National Action Plan on Antimicrobial Resistance (NAP-AMR). (2017). Government of India.

Osei Sekyere, J. (2014). Antibiotic Types and Handling Practices in Disease Management among Pig Farms in Ashanti Region, Ghana. *Journal of Veterinary Medicine*, 8. PMID:26464936

Pagel, S. W., & Gautier, P. (2012). Use of Antimicrobial Agents in Livestock. *Revue Scientifique et Technique (International Office of Epizootics)*, *31*(1), 145–188. doi:10.20506/rst.31.1.2106 PMID:22849274

Paul, N., Moodley, A., Ghibaudo, G., & Guardabassi, L. (2011). Carriage of methicillin-resistant *Staphylococcus pseudintermedius* in small animal veterinarians: Indirect evidence of zoonotic transmission. *Zoonoses and Public Health*, *58*(8), 533–539. doi:10.1111/j.1863-2378.2011.01398.x PMID:21824350

Pinto, L., Radhouani, H., Coelho, C., Martins da Costa, P., Simões, R., Brandão, R. M. L., ... Poeta, P. (2010). Genetic detection of extended-spectrum β-lactamases *Escherichia coli* in birds of prey from Serra da Estrela Natural Reserve of Portugal. *Applied and Environmental Microbiology*, *76*, 4118–4120. doi:10.1128/AEM.02761-09 PMID:20418435

Price, L. B., Stegger, M., Hasman, H., Aziz, M., Larsen, J., Andersen, P. S., … Aarestrup, F.M. (2012). *Staphylococcus aureus* CC398: host adaptation and emergence of methicillin resistance in livestock. *MBio, 3*, 305–311. doi: .00305-11 doi:10.1128/mBio

Robinson, T. P., Bu, D. P., Carrique-Mas, J., Fevre, E. M., Gilbert, M., Grace, D., ... Woolhouse, M. E. J. (2016). Antibiotic resistance is the quintessential one health issue. *Transactions of the Royal Society of Tropical Medicine and Hygiene, 110*(7), 377–380. doi:10.1093/trstmh/trw048 PMID:27475987

Stokstad, E. L. R., & Jukes, T. H. (1950). Further observations on the "animal protein factor." *Proceedings of the Society for Experimental Biology and Medicine, 73(3)*, 523–528. 10.3181/00379727-73-17731

United Nations, Department of Economic and Social Affairs, Population Division. (2015). *World Population Prospects: The 2015 Revision, Key Findings and Advance Tables*. Working Paper No. ESA/P/WP.241.

Van Boeckel, T. P., Brower, C., Gilbert, M., Grenfell, B. T., Levin, S., Robinson, T. P., ... Laxminarayan, R. (2015). Global Trends in Antimicrobial Use in Food Animals. *Proceedings of the National Academy of Sciences of the United States of America, 112*(18), 5649–5654. doi:10.1073/pnas.1503141112 PMID:25792457

Veldman, K., Cavaco, L. M., Mevius, D., Battisti, A., Franco, A., Botteldoorn, N., ... Aarestrup, S. (2011). International collaborative study on the occurrence of plasmid mediated quinolone resistance in *Salmonella enterica* and *Escherichia coli* isolated from animals, humans, food and the environment in 13 European countries. *The Journal of Antimicrobial Chemotherapy, 66*(6), 1278–1286. doi:10.1093/jac/dkr084 PMID:21393198

Verbrugghe, E., Boyen, F., Gaastra, W., Bekhuis, L., Leyman, B., Van Parys, A., ... Pasmans, F. (2012). The complex interplay between stress and bacterial infections in animals. *Veterinary Microbiology, 155*(2-4), 115–127. doi:10.1016/j.vetmic.2011.09.012 PMID:21963418

Woolhouse, M., Ward, M., van Bunnik, B., & Farrar, J. (2015). Antimicrobial resistance in humans, livestock and the wider environment. *Philosophical Transactions of the Royal Society of London. Series B, Biological Sciences, 370*(1670), 20140083. doi:10.1098/rstb.2014.0083 PMID:25918441

Woolridge, M. (2012). Evidence for the circulation of antimicrobial-resistant strains and genes in nature and especially between humans and animals. *Revue Scientifique et Technique (International Office of Epizootics), 31*, 231–247. PMID:22849279

Section 3

Chapter 7
Risk Management and Risk Communication in the Case of Vector-Borne Disease:
Case of Macedonia - Risk Management in VBDs

Sekovska Blagica
University St. Kiril and Methodius, Macedonia

Stefanovska Jovana
University St. Kiril and Methodius, Macedonia

ABSTRACT

Change in environmental and socio-economic, emerging zoonotic diseases will be an increasing challenge for public health in Europe and in Macedonia also. The risks and consequences triggered by vector-borne diseases (VBD) for public health in Macedonia are just starting to emerge in public awareness. This is clearly shown by recent events such as spread of hemorrhagic fevers in Europe. The term "public health" in the scope of this chapter suggests re-conceptualization of public health by adapting the risk governance framework developed by the International Risk Governance Council (IRGC) for this purpose. The IRGC approach is distinguished from more classical risk governance approaches, inter alia, by an explicit inclusion of a systematic concern assessment. However, unfortunately, not all countries are adapted on this innovative public health model. This chapter shows results of a risk management study based on interview in depth with the officials regard public health risk, in frame of one health concept in the Republic of Macedonia.

DOI: 10.4018/978-1-5225-6304-4.ch007

INTRODUCTION

Vector-borne diseases (VBD), account for 17% of the estimated global burden of all infectious diseases. Their burden and economic impact continue to be very high. (Report of an informal expert consultation SEARO, New Delhi, 7-8 April 2014, WHO). Environmental and socio-economic changes mean that emerging diseases, particularly vector-borne diseases, will become an increasing challenge for the risk governance of human and veterinary health in Europe and in the Macedonia. The risks and the consequences triggered by vector-borne diseases for (veterinary) Public Health in Europe are just starting to emerge in public awareness and to be treated in spirit of in health approach. In order to meet the new challenges of Public Health, a re-conceptualization of Public Health is suggested and outlined within the EDENext "White Paper: Public Health and Vector-Borne Diseases. A New Concept for Risk Governance" (2012, see also: Schmidt et al 2013). In this frame, we were researched risk management concept in Republic of Macedonia.

Communication plays a central role and interacts with all elements. Therefore, aspects of communication were integrated on all analysed levels. Considered communication aspects in this study include the analysis of the communication process at the governmental level (internal communication between different departments), at the interface between the government and stakeholders, and between the government or stakeholders and the public (top-down approaches). Perception and communication patterns of recognized top-down approaches as well as information expectations towards authorities or stakeholders on the micro-level are analysed (bottom-up approaches).

During this, study realization, 12 experts on macro and mezzo level were interviewed. Interviews in depth with experts on vector-borne disease, will inform us about actual organizational structure and strategy about risk health management, and about experience with communication in case of possible health risk connected with vector-borne diseases in Republic of Macedonia. The person (experts) who were interviewed on macro level were representatives from:

- Ministry of health of Republic of Macedonia,
- State Crisis management center,
- State Institute for public health,
- Food and veterinary agency and
- Epidemiology institute.

On mezzo level were interviewed representatives (experts) from:

- State Clinic for infectious disease and febrile conditions in frame of State Clinical center and Medical faculty,
- Representatives from regional units of State Institute for public health, such as Center for public health - Skopje and Center for public health –Prilep,
- Doctors chamber of Republic of Macedonia,
- Veterinary chamber of Republic of Macedonia,
- Macedonian farmers' federation and
- Representative from the Veterinary institute that is in the frame of Faculty for veterinary medicine in Skopje.

THEORETICAL FRAMING: IRGC RISK GOVERNANCE FRAMEWORK

The International Risk Governance Council (IRGC) is a privately funded, independent non-profit organisation that was founded in 2003 and is based in Geneva. Its mission is to support governments, industry, non-governmental organizations and other organizations in their efforts to deal with major and global risks facing society and to foster public confidence in risk governance. In 2005, the IRGC published its first White Paper on 'Risk Governance. Towards an Integrative Approach'. The IRGC framework model encompasses five elements (IRGC 2005, 2008): (1) Pre-assessment, early warning and 'framing' of the risk; (2) appraisal (combining scientific risk assessment and concern assessment); (3) characterisation and evaluation; (4) management and (5) communication of a risk. The model shall assist decision-makers in preparing decisions that are characterised by scientific uncertainty, complexity and ambiguity – also known as systemic risks (Renn et al., 2001, IRGC, 2008). The model was designed to be compatible with competing risk analysis approaches, although it puts particular emphasis on the aspect that risk assessment should not just include scientific risk assessment, but also include a systematic analysis of public concern and perceptions. Public Health is concerned with questions of prevention, rather than healing and it is concerned with health on a population-level rather than on an individual level. Moreover, it is concerned with the facilitation of health equity in the society through the mobilisation of political, social and economic resources. Hence, Public Health considers various determinants of health, such as ecological environment, political structures, socio-cultural patterns, economic living and working conditions, social and community networks or individual lifestyle factors" (Schmidt et al 2013).

MAIN ACTORS IN RISK MANAGEMENT

Republic of Macedonia has very serious and complex system for risk management in case of outbreak. In the state exists Crisis management center that is top body. In the frame of this center are existing different units for different kind of risks and crises. Health risk is only one of the risks. In the frame of unit for health risks, there is a Commission for health risks, and if it is necessary in case of outbreaks, the center organizes body for crises. In that body are participating representatives from different institutions which are relevant for concrete health risk (Ministry of health in Republic of Macedonia, Institute for public health, Food and veterinary agency and also representatives from Ministry of foreign affairs and Ministry of interior, local governmental representatives from affected areas, different public enterprises (if it necessary), and also different public institutions like Center for public health or its units and representatives from local government Counsel for public health). This commission are considering all relevant information regarding the problem day by day. They are collecting information on daily basis from their units around the country. In the case of crisis, this is on more serious and wider basis, but daily questions regarding health problems (not big outbreak) are managed in Ministry of health. In the frame of Ministry of health a Commission for communicable diseases exists which is regular body consisted of experts with advisory but not executive role in the Ministry. The Minister of health who is reacting and giving executive decisions upon their advices and suggestions forms this commission. Members of the Commission are elected for a period of four years and are prominent experts in the field of epidemiology, infectology, microbiology, pediatrics, veterinary medicine and other specialties that implies on one health approach.

It is on top (macro) level, but if we go little bit lower we will find that Institute for public health is dealing with health risks as well in the Sector for control and prevention of contagious diseases and Center for statistical analyses of data related to health, publication and education. This institute also carries out activities as national contact point in case of some international epidemics or risks of epidemics and is responsible for implementation of health measures according the International Health regulation. As part of this institute a 10 regional centers – named as Center for public health and 21 units in each municipality named as Public health units are operating. They all are covering the territory of whole country. Also the local government of one or more municipalities together are forming Counsel for public health (according the Low for public health) who are reporting firstly to the local government and latter to the Institute for public health.

State Crisis management center has 35 regional crisis's management centers for local level – 8 main and 27 smaller covering all 85 municipalities), with obligation to take care about risks and crises in every local government office. From all this centers, they are collecting information from the field and all this information related to health risks are collected in Institute for public health. From there the healthy information assessed and analyzed go to the Ministry of health and if it necessary (Law for protection of population from infectious diseases) they are sent in the Office of World Health Organization in Skopje.

On the basic level Family doctors (general practitioners) have a form called "Report for diseases or/and death from communicable (infectious) diseases and carriers of the infectious agent" in which they have the names of all diseases they are obliged to report for including CCHF. They send this report to the Centres for public health related to the location where they work in. In addition, there is a software (alert.mk) and all the family doctors are into this net. They are obliged to inform in case of some condition that might lead to epidemics. Analyses of this data are under the responsibility of Institute for public health and Centres for public health. This is a project of WHO (EWARN) (Early warning and response system for communicable diseases).

Management of insects, such as vector control and eradication is also responsibility of the State sanitary and health inspectorate, which is working within Ministry of health, and is consisted of 15 regional units. This institution is responsible for controlling implementation of the low regulations related to DDD programs (disinfection, disinsection and deterioration) in relevant institutions.

Figure 1. Structure of crises management in the health sector in Republic of Macedonia

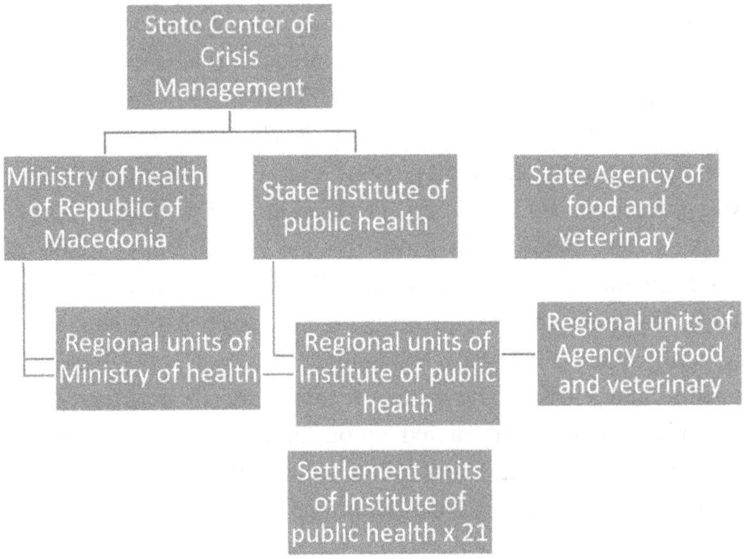

The problem is that most of the mezzo level institutions are not involved actively on this health risk management on the state level, such as Clinic for infectious diseases, Centers for public health as well as Veterinary chamber, Macedonian federation of farmers, which is the grates weaknesses of the system. Human health structures, even on the lower level are more familiar with the topic of risk management and risk communication than the veterinary structures.

RISK PERCEPTION

Experts believe that vector spread diseases will grow in future in significance due to climate changes as well as the range expansion of disease spreading i.e. the spreading of their vectors. The doctors from the primary health practice have not always suspected to some of vector born disease and not its every real appearance has been diagnostically confirmed." Very often diseases, especially some hemorrhagic fever, are confirmed later, even postmortem," says the Head of the Prilep Department for Infectious Diseases. The macro-level experts have far more knowledge that is relevant and data for these diseases to the mezzo-level experts. In addition, the mezzo-level and macro-level human doctors are far more knowledgeable about these diseases rather than the veterinarians and even more than the farmers are.

The experts reported that the public does not know sufficiently about these diseases. Even the professionals (human doctors, veterinarians, and farmers in particular) have very little or even no data regarding VBD, especially hemorrhagic fevers. Experts agree that in the Republic of Macedonia there are small or not at all chances for a VBD epidemics due to the fact they all have no knowledge of the spread of the particular vector. In addition, most of them were not aware of interhuman and nosocomial transmit ion of VBD. Representatives of the Epidemiology unit says- "there have always been sporadic cases of VBD and there always will be especially in the spring period and in the rural municipalities, but the number of infected would increase if the global warming trend persists, that is to say if the trend of increasing average yearly temperature continues in R.M.. Generally, there is a high incidents (number of cases) tendency, for diseases that are typical transmittable diseases in the humid continental climate such as the CCHF and other diseases. "Experts also concur that the danger of this disease is underestimated because as a rare disease not always the family doctor diagnose it and it appears in the form of atypical symptoms as the conventional virosis. The cases are not always confirmed by laboratory analyses and if certain tests are carried out on routinely basis the statistical number of cases may happen to increase, but that does not mean that in reality the number of cases increases in practice but just that more cases are confirmed that is to say appropriately diagnosed. There are no big differences in the experts' opinions on a mezzo-level and a macro-level regarding this particular question.

Representative of the Epidemiology Department at the Medical Faculty in Skopje stated: "General Practitioners are the first barrier that have a responsibility to care not only to cure patients. Family doctor are the pyramid's foundation therefore, they need to be more knowledgeable and pay more attention to the primary prevention as oppose to sending all cases to secondary and tertiary health care. "The general disposition of all experts on this matter is that Family doctor need constantly to upgrade their knowledge, to inform themselves due to the fact that the General Practitioner is the one whose responsibility is to register the disease or the suspicion of a disease that is subordinate to registration abiding by a decisive legal regulation of RM and to transmit the information to the Institute for Public Health. On the basis of these data gained from Family doctor the Epidemiologists follow the condition and trace the trends. The problem is with General Practitioners (family doctors) who are insufficiently aware and do not pay attention to transmittable disease. Precisely because of that, many diseases appear as conventional viroses.

REQUIREMENTS FOR PUBLIC PROTECTION

In order to protect the population from vector spread diseases especially as hemorrhagic fevers, the experts propose various methods. Still in the first place as the most significant is education of the population for ways of disease spreading and protection from vector spread diseases. Additionally the state should take care of the environment by taking care of green areas, disinfection. When vector spread and diseases appear, it is most logical to act immediately on destroying those vectors and the sources of infection. For that purpose the Insitute for public health is responsible to give professional methodological support for disinsection, disinfection and deterioration)- DDD programs to all relevant bodies in the local government especilay to their localunits such as Center for public health and their public helath units This institutions are responsible to give their professional opinion for the DDD measures that have to be undertaken in the municipality on the base of epidemiological data. All local governments (government of the municipalities) have legal responsibilities to finance and implement DDD programs. Programs for eradication of vectors include spraying with different insecticides form the ground and some times from air. This activities are controlled by the State sanitary and health inspectorate. This programs does not include treatment of animals. In case of out brake of some animal diseases Food and veterinary agency is responsible for preparing and conveying such activities. For a successful protection of the public a good communication between the Veterinary services and the Human medicine services is necessary so as, the activity is done in a timely fashion, emphasized representative of the Institute for Public Health of RM. He also adds that: "unfortunately this in-between sectors cooperation is not at the highest level, i.e. there are no established protocols and procedures. The preventive takes the most central part in the risk management as well as disinsection, disinfection and deterioration, immunization and the cooperation between the veterinary and the human medicine."

The most important measure for protection of vector spread diseases is vector eradication, stressed the representative of the Doctors chamber and she adds: "There are plans and strategies for risk management, in the Ministry of Health there are protocols and in Macedonia there is a legal responsibility to register some specific diseases. Depending on the registered number, the Ministry of Health and the Institute for Public Health of RM make analyses and reach decisions and devise plans which need to be followed by Family doctor. The Doctors chamber has a successful cooperation with the Health Insurance Fund as well as the Ministry of Health whose sectors have representatives and gathers information from all sides, but the Chamber does not get any field information."

Experts of macro-level and mezzo-level exclude the probability of an epidemic outbreak in larger proportion caused by vector spread diseases especially the hemorrhagic fevers in the Republic of Macedonia. "There is a possibility of sporadic cases in endangered rural area in the spring and summer period said the representative from Center for public health - Skopje and added: "In the Republic of Macedonia there are no special protocols for dealing with epidemics of hemorrhagic fevers, but there is an action plan for suppression of vector spread diseases, especially mosquito spread diseases. Preventive measures are necessary in terms of disinsection, education of population and bigger awareness of health workers in terms of recognition of these particular diseases and their forwarding to higher health levels as well as supply of new reagents for detection and diagnosis of as large as possible number of vector spread diseases."

If there is an epidemic outbreak and there is a crisis situation on the entire territory of RM or just in separate regions of the country then a before-hand prepared standard operative procedures shall commence in the country. For each crisis type including the health crisis there are special procedures defined. In case of a bigger risk epidemic outbreak the control of the crisis management is run by a Steering (management) committee body composed of representatives of all relevant institutions (Ministry of Interior, Ministry of Foreign Affairs, Ministry of Health, Agency for Food and Veterinary Inspection, The Institute for Public Health of RM, etc.) as well as a corresponding body from the field of Health- National committee.

Depending of the situation development a decision is reached whether to proclaim an epidemic outbreak of a certain disease on the entire territory or a portion of the territory of RM. Within the frame of the Crisis management, center 195 functions as a free of charge contact number that can be dialed by any citizen to register a crisis. The Crisis management center has its own regional centers as well as people responsible for crisis management in each municipality. In addition, the public utilities have the responsibility to have a person designated in case of a crisis. The State Crisis management center has regional centers. This area is regulated in a detailed way with the Law for Crisis Management, in which all aspects are set in a detailed manner. Since 2009 according the Law for protection of population from infectious diseases, all VBDs are reportable disease.

KEY ELEMENTS OF RISK MANAGEMENT

The main element of risk management is the fact that in the Republic of Macedonia there is a really good organization structure for the entire system for risk management. Also there is developed institutional coverage of health risk management in particular infectious diseases through the entire state system for health risks and crisis management. The Institute for public health in the RM has 10 regional and 21 local units nationwide. Whereas the State Centre for risks and crisis management has 35 regional centers in each municipality in RM. Through these centers health data, field information are collected and the same are distributed to The Institute for public health in the RM, from there they are transmitted to the Ministry of Health and when necessary (registration of infectious disease) are submitted to the offices of WHO in RM. If the situation becomes critical and a crisis situation is established on the entire territory of RM, or just in some specific areas of RM, then there is before-hand standard operational procedures execution. For each type of crisis including the health crisis there is separate defined procedures. In case of a higher risk of epidemics, the planning of the risk management is taken over by a body composed of representatives from all relevant institutions (Ministry of Interior, Ministry of Foreign Affairs, Ministry of Health, Agency for Food and Veterinary Inspection, The Institute for Public Health of RM, etc.) as well as a corresponding body from the field of Health (composed of practitioners from various clinics and other people if necessary) which on the basis of field data gives recommendations. Depending of the situations development a decision is reached whether to proclaim an epidemic outbreak of a certain disease on the entire territory, or a portion of the territory of RM. Within the frame of the Centre for Risk Management 195 functions as a free of charge contact number which can be dialed by any citizen so as to register a crisis. The State Centre for Crisis Management has its own regional centers as well as people responsible for crisis management in each municipality. Also, the public utilities have the responsibility to have a person designated in case of a crisis. The State Crisis management center has regional centers. This area is regulated in a detailed way with the Law for Crisis and Crisis Situations Management, in which all aspects are set in a detailed manner.

RISK COMMUNICATION OF EMERGING VBDs

The rules for communication in a case of risk constantly are subject to changes even legal ones. The last alteration was in the segment of communication. Namely a standard operative procedure is established in a case of establishing a crisis situation, but this is operative communication not communication with the public. Regarding the communication with the public there is a portal that transmits information to the media within the framework of the Ministry of Health, and the websites of all relevant institutions are constantly updated. Within the frame of the Centre for Risk Management 195 functions as a free of charge contact number which can be dialed by any citizen so as to register a crisis. Family doctor are under a legal obligation to register various diseases even if it is just a suspicion. Also the local units of the Institute of Public Health of RM, public utilities, as well as the municipality's offices for risk management collect and transmit data. All of these data are collected on daily basis in the Centre for Crisis Management. All diseases that could cause an epidemic outbreak are on the legal list for registration and a monthly, quarterly, and yearly report for their tracking is devised. Information between institutions is exchanged on daily basis via email and if there is a risk of a health crisis institution representatives are convened when necessary depending on the risk type that may cause a crisis. The State Centre share information with all relevant institutions and advising the public comes out of the expert meeting whose proposals and directions when needed shall be distributed to the public. There are communication systems in case of a risk that is internet based. The experiences with epidemics so far have shown how things on the field can be tracked in an easier way, thus giving opportunity for strengthening in-between institution cooperation.

„In the Institute of Public Health in the Republic of Macedonia there are procedures for various diseases and all have a place in the system. Professional manuals are distributed to 31 organization-units nationwide and a daily communication is established with them thus response information is gathered. This is vertical communication, while the horizontal communication we are located in the same facilities with the Ministry of Health and with the Offices of the WHO in RM. If some infectious disease appears and spreads there is a Crisis Headquarters for Crisis Situation Management that is a permanent body of the Centre for Crisis Management convened when necessary. According to low the hemorrhagic fevers must be registered within 24 hours, due to the fact that this disease is subordinated to mandatory registration, "notes the Head of the Sector for Infectious Diseases at the

Institute for Public Health of RM. "Communication in a case of risk is information exchange that we do horizontally and vertically on the topic that is a current risk," says the Head of the Sector for risk management at the Institute of Public Health of the Republic of Macedonia

RISK COMMUNICATION PROCESS

In the Republic of Macedonia there are crisis communication procedures. Namely, the bottom up communication flows by registering the field problem on the crisis telephone number 195. Also, in the case when the local branches of the Institute for Public Health of the RM detect a problem or crisis situation they report the same to the upper levels. All information is collected and processed in the Institute for Public Health of the RM and/or State Centre for Crisis Management and on the basis of experts' opinion measures are proposed. "The last Amendment of the Law for Crisis Management fell particularly in the communication domain. Namely, the need for establishing a standard operative procedure in a case of setting up a crisis situation in operational communication, not communication with the public has been determined, says the Head of the Sector for Analytics in the Center for Crisis Management. All the diseases that may cause epidemics are listed and on the basis of filed collected information monthly, quarterly, 6 months and yearly reports are devised for the appearance of these diseases and their easier tracking. Information exchange between relevant institutions is performed on daily basis via email and if there is danger from crisis institution representatives are called upon depending the crisis type. This is done by the Centre for Crisis Management which collects and shares information whereas the communication with the public springs out from the deductions reached from the gathering of experts in specific fields which shall be released to the public. When it comes to the Institute for Public Health of the RM there are procedures for different diseases and all have an exact place within the system. "Professional manuals are distributed to 31 organization-units nationwide and a daily communication is established with them thus response information is gathered. This is vertical communication, while the horizontal communication we are located in the same facilities with the Ministry of Health and with the Offices of the WHO in RM. If some infectious disease appears and spreads there is a Crisis Headquarters for Crisis Situation Management that is a permanent body of the Crises management center convened when necessary" says the Head of the Sector for Infectious Diseases at the Institute for Public Health of the RM. Regarding CCHF at the moment there are no rules but the hemorrhagic fevers according to the existing law must be registered within 24 hours due to the fact that this disease is subordinated to mandatory registration. All Family doctor, the local and the regional centers of the Institute for Public Health of the RM as well as the Ministry of Health are connected with the alert.mk system through which they gather and exchange information for every occurrence or suspicion of infectious disease from the positive legal list of RM. "There are plans for the health system as well as a project for early notification and prevention from infectious disease alert.mk. There are plans for development of a Health center as well as plans for preparation of each hospital in crisis situations where communication is a special segment. A soft spot is the absence of radio stations in a case of telephone failure as a backup communicational system. Due to the fact that Macedonia is a small country in case where all communicational systems fail there is a courier system, -says a member of the Committee for Infectious disease at the Ministry of Health of RM. However, according to the representative of the Institute for Epidemiology,: "In Macedonia there is a lack of awareness about the meaning of a preventive action especially among those that participate in that preventive action. At first the system is perfect, but unreliable information from Primary health care are gained, from the start bad quality information is gained, thus conclusions are reached based on unreliable health information. It is not known if what is registered is reality compatible for example, if it is written atypical pneumonia that may hide Q fever, Lyme disease or something else. It is better false alarm rather than underestimating the situation." When it comes to communicating in danger, the human medicine system is a lot more adequately prepared than the one form Veterinary medicine. Namely, in Veterinary medicine there is only one general what-to-do-plan in case of infectious diseases. It is planned to further develop the risk management and the communication in a case of risk, says the representative from Food and veterinary agency and he adds: "With the Ministry of Health there is quantitative, but not qualitative information exchange, meaning that the statistical data for specific diseases is not the only important information to us if we do not know where the disease has appeared. Regarding the communication we devise yearly reports that we publish on our website."All this information comes from the macro-level where as at the meso-level the Veterinary chamber is not part of the official body for communication in a case of risk. The representative of the Doctors chamber said: "The Ministry of Health and the Institute for Public Health of the RM are in charge for the communication with the public." All are agreeing with one segment, in-between sector cooperation is established, but the question is how and if it is implemented. There is information cascade and it always leads from top to bottom down the hierarchical scale. "Communication in a case of risk is not adequate, i.e. there are no systematic rules for communication, there needs to be information exchange between the Veterinary Service and the Human medicine services, but the problem is that the exchange is paper perfect, but it does not come to fruition in reality and appropriate implementation is amiss," believes the representative from the Veterinary Institute. He sees the fault in the bad communication in the inadequate choice of representatives in the structures, the deficient rules for information dissemination as well as the inadequate education and aptness of the people involved as well as the frequent political changes of the people who have significant role in the system.

KEY ELEMENTS OF RISK COMMUNICATION

Kay element of risk communication is shearing information with public. From the other side, shearing the information on horizontal level is seen like normal strategy of working. Experts did not consider some special characteristic in Macedonian citizen reaction on public information regarding health issues. Almost all think that Macedonian citizens did not care too much about preventive, and they are strictly following the information only if they are afraid from the situation. The expert thinks that informative cascade must be worked out with more details (who will report and inform to whom) for improvement of risk communication. Also detailed risk management and risk communication protocols about more individual diseases should be prepared . Expert from the regional unit think that: "evaluation is our biggest weakness. Communication with the public should be done by well-informed professionals. In our country very often communication is done by insufficiently informed politicians, instead of professionals. The biggest problem with Macedonian citizens is that they are very inert for accepting preventive recommendations. Professionals have not trust in the media, because very often they are building panic. However, public must be informed and we must not laying the people." Representative from the Veterinary Institute say: "There aren't any rules for communication in the Food and veterinary agency. If there are some, only macro level institutions are informed about it. There is not main pillar in the communication. It is not enough only to create ideal scheme on the paper, but you must put it in practice. The reasons are many, like inappropriate education of involved responsible, low motivation level of the people who are involved, frequent political changes of the responsible etc. Key elements of successful risk communication are human recourses and good organization. Key elements for public protection from VBD are regular research and analysis of insects, following and analyzing potential vector born disease, regular extermination of the insects, and improvement of diagnostic capacities in the country."

According to one of the experts, there are two groups of people that are hard to communicate with in case of some crisis. In the first one are the people ling in the high mountain villages and the second are gypsies that are not leaving on one location in R.M . These two groups, especially the gypsies are a risk group that can transfer the diseases on different locations and are out of control from authorities. Communication in case of a risk with these two groups need special attention.

CONCLUSION

From previous explication, we can conclude that Republic of Macedonia has very serious and complex system for risk management in case of outbreak. In order to protect the population from vector spread diseases especially as hemorrhagic fevers, the experts propose various methods. Still in the first place as the most significant is education of the population for ways of disease spreading and protection from vector spread diseases. Additionally the state should take care of the environment by taking care of green areas, disinfection. We can conclude that human, animal and environmental health is strongly connected in this risk management practice in Republic of Macedonia. From the other side, the One Health concept links human, animal and environmental health, it is "a worldwide strategy for expanding interdisciplinary collaborations and communications in all aspects of health care for humans, animals and the environment. This approach considers all global health threats to gain cross-disciplinary collaboration, especially between physicians and veterinarians. The result is a collaborative effort to enhance human and animal health between the health professions Health care authorities and systems have the responsibility to manage health system, and communication is part of the management. Therefore, the role of communication is related to the institutional setting.

In the Republic of Macedonia there are also established crisis communication procedures. Unfortunately, communication and linking between doctors and veterinarians in these state bodies is not on high level. According to one health procedures, the institutional communication in veterinary medicine gives a high contribution to public health, because of the continuous overlapping between veterinary and human medicine in public health. We can recommend straightening of this Macedonian risk communication system according to one health concept rules and requirements.

Despite the fact that health communication is a recent matter, it has a growing importance in human medicine but it is less considered in veterinary medicine. However, because of the role of veterinary medicine in public health, communication in veterinary area also has the potential to improve public health. Therefore, a One Health approach applies to communication as well, leading to the "One Communication" concept, which is the result of the synergy in communicative efforts both in human and in veterinary medicine. As One Health, One Communication is a strategy for expanding collaborations in health communication and it will enhance health care. (Cipolla et al, 2011)

REFERENCES

Cipolla, Bonizzi, & Zecconi. (2011). *From "One Health" to "One Communication": The Contribution of Communication in Veterinary Medicine to Public Health Report of an informal expert consultation.* Academic Press.

International Risk Governance Council. (2005). *White Paper on Risk Governance. Towards an Integrative Approach.* IRGC. Retrieved from http://www.irgc.org/IMG/pdf/IRGC_WP_No_1_Risk_Governance__reprinted_version_.pdf

Schmidt, K., Dressel, K. M., Niedrig, M., Mertens, M., Schüle, S. A., & Groschup, M. H. (2013). Public Health and Vector-Borne Diseases – A New Concept for Risk Governance. *Zoonoses and Public Health, 2013*(Mar), 11. doi:10.1111/zph.12045 PMID:23480672

Stefanovska, J. (2014). *Report to EDENext projet from WG16: Public Health and Vector-Borne Diseases. A New Concept for Risk Governance.* (Unpublished)

Chapter 8
A One Health Perspective on Q Fever: Part 1

Rita Cruz
Polytechnic Institute of Viseu, Portugal

Carmen Vasconcelos-Nobrega
Polytechnic Institute of Viseu, Portugal & University of Trás-os-Montes and Alto Douro, Portugal

Fernando Esteves
Polytechnic Institute of Viseu, Portugal

Catarina Coelho
Polytechnic Institute of Viseu, Portugal & University of Trás-os-Montes and Alto Douro, Portugal

Ana Sofia Ferreira
University of Oporto, Portugal

Carla Santos
Polytechnic Institute of Viseu, Portugal

Cristina Mega
Polytechnic Institute of Viseu, Portugal

Ana C. Coelho
University of Trás-os-Montes and Alto Douro, Portugal

Helena Vala
Polytechnic Institute of Viseu, Portugal & University of Trás-os-Montes and Alto Douro, Portugal

João R. Mesquita
University of Oporto, Portugal

ABSTRACT

Q fever is a worldwide zoonotic infectious disease caused by Coxiella burnetii and ruminants, namely, cattle, sheep, and goats, are known to be the main reservoir for human infection. C. burnetii infection in animals can result in epizootic abortions which are often associated with vast bacteria shedding in birth fluids and placentas. Human infections mainly occur in persons handling infected animals and their products. Here the authors describe the history, bacteriology, biosafety, and epidemiology of Q fever, now known to be a serious threat to veterinary public health.

DOI: 10.4018/978-1-5225-6304-4.ch008

Q FEVER HISTORY

Q fever was first described in 1935 by Edward Holbrook Derrick, the director of the Laboratory of Microbiology and Pathology of the Queensland Health Department, in Brisbane, Australia after the regular occurrence of sporadic cases since 1933 (Maurin & Raoult, 1999; McDade, 1990). He was assigned to investigate an outbreak of an unknown disease that occurred among the local abattoir workers, with fever as the predominant symptom (Chmielewski & Tylewska-Wierzbanowska, 2012; Derrick, 1937).

Derrick was first decided to determine the characteristics of the illness and carefully monitored the clinical features of the disease. The symptoms described included fever, lasting from seven to twenty-four days, headaches, depression, anorexia and pain in the limbs. The patient blood cultures performed, were negative and there was no detection of any antibodies for the known agents, at the time, in their sera. Because of this, it was concluded that the outbreak was the result of a new disease of unknown aetiology and called it Q fever, Q for query, English term that means doubt (McDade, 1990).

Several experiments and studies were performed, in order to determine the cause of the disease. Derrick inoculated guinea pigs with blood and urine from infected patients and observed that the animals developed fever. He also verified transmission of the disease, when the guinea pigs were inoculated with tissue suspensions prepared from infected animals. However, he failed to detect bacteria in infected tissues. As a consequence of this result, Derrick obtained the wrong conclusion that the etiologic agent of this disease was a virus (Burnet & Freeman, 1937; Chmielewski & Tylewska-Wierzbanowska, 2012).

In an attempt to clarify the aetiology of the disease, Derrick sent the livers of infected guinea pigs to Frank Macfarlane Burnet, a virologist who worked at the Walter & Eliza Hall Institute in Melbourne. After further studies, where infected tissues were inoculated in other animal species, in 1937, Burnet and his assistant Mavis Freeman were finally able to isolate organisms, from guinea pigs, of bacterial origin with similar characteristics to the members of the genus *Rickettsia* (Burnet & Freeman, 1937; Chmielewski & Tylewska-Wierzbanowska, 2012). The Q fever agent was then designated as *Rickettsia burnetii* (McDade, 1990).

In 1935, independently of Derrick's work, Gordon Davis at the Rocky Mountain Laboratory in Montana, United States of America was investigating the ecology of Rocky Mountain spotted fever, when isolated an infectious agent from *Dermacentor andersoni* ticks, collected at the Nine Mile Creek (Maurin & Raoult, 1999). He verified that guinea pigs from where ticks were feed, developed an indeterminate fever syndrome and therefore suspected that had isolated *Rickettsia rickettsi,* the etiological agent of Rocky Mountain fever. However, the following *in vivo* inoculations shown the absence of lesions usually associated with spotted fever diseases (McDade, 1990). One year later, Herald Rea Cox joined Davis to continue the studies for identify and characterize the Nine Mile agent (Maurin & Raoult, 1999). They observed properties not identified before: the agent could pass filters, it was Gram-negative, and had an extracellular and intracellular pleomorphic rickettsia-like appearance (Davis, Cox, Parker, & Dyer, 1938; McDade, 1990). The name proposed for this new etiological agent was *Rickettsia diasporica* (Cox, 1941; McDade, 1990). A major advance was obtained when Cox was succeeded in cultivated this new agent in chicken embryos (Maurin & Raoult, 1999).

Only few years late, the importance of this discovery and its pathogenicity for humans become clear. In May of 1938, Rolla Dyer, director of National Institute of Health, visited Cox at the Rocky Mountain Laboratory and about ten days later became ill. The symptoms described were retro-orbital pain, fever, chills and cold sweats. At the sixth day of symptoms, a blood sample was collected, inoculated into guinea pigs and the animals developed fever. Subsequent studies have shown that this agent was the same that had been isolated by Davis from *Dermacentor andersoni* ticks. Dyer did know the Australian reports and suggested the link between this new agent and the "Q fever" agent (McDade, 1990).

The etiological agent of Q fever disease was discovered almost simultaneously in Melbourne, Australia, by Burnet and Freeman and in Montana, United States of America, by Cox and Davis (Maurin & Raoult, 1999).

In 1948, Cornelius Philip proposed the reclassification of the etiological agent of Q fever into *Coxiella burnetii*, honoring simultaneous Burnet and Cox, to their contributions to a better understanding of the agent (McDade, 1990; Philip, 1948).

Coxiella burnetii was originally classified as rickettsia-like, in the genus *Coxiella*, family Rickettsiaceae, order Rickettsiales (Bergey, Krieg, & Holt, 1984). However, phylogenetic studies, based on 16S rRNA gene sequence and genome analysis, shown a high homology with *Legionella pneumophila* and was reclassified into a separate genus Coxiella of the gamma subdivision of Proteobacteria (Stein, Saunders, Taylor, & Raoult, 1993; Kazar, 2005).

COXIELLA BURNETTI BACTERIOLOGY

Phenotypic Features

Coxiella burnetii is a small Gram-negative, nonmotile, obligate intracellular, Gram-negative bacterium that replicates within the phagolysosome of host cells (Howe & Mallavia, 2000; Seshadri et al., 2003). It has pleomorphic coccobacilli shape (0.2–0.4 mm wide, 0.4–1.0 mm long) and produces two morphologically distinct cell types, that comprises a bi-phasic developmental cycle (Hechemy, 2012) a small cell variant (SCV) and a large cell variant (LCV), also called dormant SCV and active LCV (Howe & Mallavia, 2000). The SCV has a characteristic condensed chromatin, has a thicker peptidoglycan layer and, as the name implies, is smaller in size (Howe & Mallavia, 2000). SCV has highly resistance to environmental stress (dissecation, heat, UV radiation and osmotic pressure), allowing *C. burnetti* to survive in the extracellular environment, maintaining its infectivity: LCV is the metabolically active and replicative entity, formed after the invasion of the host by the SCV and is more sensitive to environmental stresses than the SCV. During the stationary phase of the organism's growth cycle, LCV undergoes sporogenic differentiation to produce resistant, spore-like forms, the small-cell variants (SCV) (Angelakis & Raoult, 2010). These are released when the cells lyse and can survive for long periods in the environment (Angelakis & Raoult, 2010; Hechemy, 2012; Howe & Mallavia, 2000), maintaining the developmental cycle of *C. burnetti* (Hechemy, 2012; Howe & Mallavia, 2000).

Coxiella has an extracellular matrix, similar to that of other Gram-negative bacteria (Skultety et al., 2011) and like several other Gram-negative species. *C. burnetii* can display two different lipopolysaccharide (LPS) phenotypes (Roest, Post, van Gelderen, van Zijdcrveld & Rebel, 2013), a virulent phase I and an avirulent phase II. *C. burnetii* transition from virulent-to-avirulent involves LPS truncation known as phase variation (Beare, Jeffrey, Long, Martens, & Heinzen, 2018). The virulent phase I form of *C. burnetii* has been isolated from both, lower and higher animals, and is extremely infectious, being capable to replicate in immunocompetent hosts (Roest et al., 2013). The extracellular matrix fraction of phase I cells comprises a smooth (S) lipopolysaccharide (LPS), I with an O-specific chain. Phase II is not infectious, occurs only in laboratory strains after many culture passages in either embryonated hen eggs or cell cultures and can be easily distinguished serologically from native isolates (Skultety et al., 2011). Contrasting with phase I cells, the extracellular matrix of phase II cells has an incomplete LPS II, structure that appears rough (R), and lacks the O-antigenic region (Roest et al., 2013; Skultety et al., 2011).

Both LPS phenotypes can be distinguished via phase-specific antibodies. Phase I antibodies are directed against the full-length LPS of phase I, whereas phase II antibodies are directed against common surface proteins, that although also being present on the surface of phase I *C. burnetii*, seem to be protected by the long phase I LPS (Beare et al., 2018; Roest et al., 2013).

Coxiella burnetii phase variation should not to be confused with phase variation of other Gram-negative bacteria, which is generally a reversible on-off regulatory process. This phase variation is irreversible and seems to be associated with the loss of chromosomal DNA, involving a large group of LPS biosynthetic genes, arranged in an apparent O-antigen cluster (Hoover, Culp, Vodkin, Williams, &

Thompson, 2002) and several other genes mutations as well as deletions. One of them is related to the sugars comprising the inner/outer core regions in the O-chain of galactosaminuronyl-a-glucosamide disaccharide and the repeating O-antigen subunits of LPS (Beare et al., 2018). Two unusual O-antigen sugars unique to *C. burnetii* LPS are virenose (6-deoxy-3-C-methylgulose) (vir) and dihydrohydroxystreptose (3-C-(hydroxymethyl)-L-lyxose) (strep). Genes have been identified that might be involved in the synthesis of vir and strep (Beare et al., 2018; Mori & Roest, 2018). Unlike other Gram-negative bacteria, where O-antigen generally has a defined repeat size (Aucken & Pitt, 1993), *C. burnetii* O-antigen has populations that differ in size and composition (Vadovic, Slaba, Fodorova, Skultety & Toman, 2005); consequently, its carbohydrate structure remains unresolved (Beare et al., 2018; Mori & Roest, 2018; Vadovic et al., 2005). According to Hotta and colleagues (2002), *C. burnetii* LPS has, at least, four antigenic forms, during phase variation. *C. burnetii* phase I LPS also plays a role in both host cell internalization and survival in the phagosome. Phase I *C. burnetii* bacteria are internalized and survive intracellular killing, whereas phase II bacteria are efficiently phagocytized and then killed (Raoult, Marrie, & Mege, 2005).

At this time the phylogeny of *C. burnetti* agent can be summarized as belonging to the kingdom of Bacteria, phylum of Proteobacteria, class of the Gammaproteobacteria, order of the Legionellales, family of the Coxiellaceae, with the genus *Coxiella* and the only one species (Garrity, Bell, & Lilburn, 2015; Roest et al., 2013).

C. burnetti Genome

In 2003, Seshadri and colleagues, published, for the first time, the complete genome sequence of *C. burnetti* (Seshadri et al., 2003). They analyzed the original strain isolated from ticks, by Davies and Cox, in 1938 (called Nine Mile), and revealed a circular genome of 1995 275 base pairs (Roest et al., 2013; Seshadri et al., 2003). Analysis of the *C. burnetii* genome also revealed the presence of many mobile elements, pseudogenes, and hypothetical proteins, suggesting ongoing genome reduction (Seshadri et al., 2003). During reduction, genes accumulate mutations, lose functions, and eventually disappear. It seems probable that these processes are also associated with phase variation at which time a large group of genes is lost. The genome has a G+C content of 43 mol% and 2134 coding sequences are predicted, of which 719 (33.7%) are hypothetical, with no significant similarity to other genes in the database (Seshadri et al., 2003; Angelakis & Raoult, 2010).

BIOSAFETY AND BIOSECURITY

Coxiella burnetii is listed by the United States Centers for Disease Control and Prevention (CDC), as a potential bioterrorism agent with the potential to be developed for use in biological warfare, and as a Category B pathogen, by the National Institute of Allergy and Infectious Diseases (NIAID) (Hanczaruk, Cutler, Toman, & Frangoulidis, 2012; Heppell, Egan, & Hall, 2017; Oyston & Davies, 2011). *C. burnetti* is an environmentally-persistent ubiquitous organism, considered a containment level 3 organism by the EU, that means an agent that can cause severe human disease and present a serious hazard to workers; an agent that may present a risk of spreading to the community, but there is usually effective prophylaxis or treatment available (directive 2000/54/EC of the European parliament and of the council). Jones et al. (2006), working with guinea pigs and humans, concluded that the infectious dose of *C. burnetii* is likely one rickettsia and that the probability of a single organism initiating infection is approximately 0.9. Additionally, *C. burnetii* is able to survive in the environment, even under adverse conditions (Fournier, Marrie, & Raoult, 1998; Maurin, Benoliel, Bongrand, & Raoult, 1992; Palmela, Badura, & Valadas, 2012; Reimer, 1993). To work with containment level 3 organisms, it is mandatory to work in dedicated biosafety level 3 (BSL3) laboratories and animal facilities, and with experienced and trained personnel. All the institutional and personal security measures and emergency procedures designed to prevent the loss, theft, misuse, diversion, or intentional release of pathogens and toxins must be followed (Pastorino, Lamballerie, & Charrel, 2017). Medical monitoring of personnel working with agents such as *C. burnetii* should be implemented. An efficient marker to evaluate the effectiveness of biosafety and to optimize the risk assessment in BSL3 laboratories, is the surveillance of laboratory acquired infection (LAI) (Wurtz et al., 2016). *C. burnetti* was one of the agents associated with LAI, in a 1976 study (Pike, 1976) and in another study in 2006, performed by Byers & Harding. However, current practices have minimized worker's pathogen exposition as well as the advance of safety rules and the improvements in containment equipment, engineering controls, and safety training, therefore we have been assisting to a great reduction in LAI (Kozajda, Bródka, & SzadkowskaStańczyk, 2013). Good laboratory practices, regarding biosafety and bioethics, are essential measures to avoid LAIs (Coelho & García Diez, 2015).

Isolation and Cultivation of C. burnetii

Coxiella burnetii can only be isolated using embryonated eggs, animal hosts, or mammalian cell culture (Boden, Wolf, Hermann, & Frangoulidis, 2015). The cell culture system is currently the most widely used *in vitro* system to isolate and cultivate *C. burnetii*. A number of cell lines can be used for *in vitro* cultures: Vero (African green monkey kidney epithelial) (Heinzen, Scidmore, Rockey, & Hackstadt, 1996), BHK-21 (hamster kidney fibroblast) (Miller, Wang, Mooseker, & Koleske, 2004), L-929 (murine fibroblast) (Baca & Paretsky, 1983), HEL (human embryonic lung fibroblast) (Raoult, Vestris, & Enea, 1990), HeLa (human cervical epithelial) (Berón, Gutierrez, Rabinovitch, & Colombo, 2002; Mori et al., 2013) and CHO (Chinese hamster ovary fibroblast) (Romano, Gutierrez, Beron, Rabinovitch, & Colombo, 2007) cells.

Guinea pigs were the first laboratory animals to be used in Q fever research. They develop hyperthermia of over 40°C, at five to twelve days post inoculation, and *C. burnetii* can be isolated from the spleen, indicating systemic infection (Vohl & Heinzen, 2007). There are also several mouse strains, with different susceptibilities, that can be used in these studies. In an evaluation of 47 strains of inbred laboratory mice, 33 were found to be resistant to infection with *C. burnetii*, 10 were partially susceptible and 4 were susceptible (Bewley, 2013) The A/J strain of mouse was found to have 100% of morbidity and the highest mortality (70%) but could still be protected by vaccination with formalin-inactivated *C. burnetii* whole cells (Bewley, 2013; Scott, Williams, & Stephenson, 1987). The BALB/c strain of mouse was reliably infected and displayed overt signs of illness, including ruffled fur and lethargy in all members of the group, but with no mortality (Bewley, 2013).

In natural infections, *C. burnetti* has a tropism for cells of the mononuclear phagocyte system, such as alveolar macrophages of the lung and Kupffer cells of the liver (Khavkin, & Tabibzadeh, 1988; Stein et al., 2005), with organisms also infrequently observed in pneumocytes, fibroblasts and endothelial cells (Khavkin, & Tabibzadeh, 1988). Consequently, monocyte/macrophage-like cell lines including J774A.1 (murine macrophage-like) (Brennan, Russell, Zhang, & Samuel, 2004; Howe & Mallavia, 2000), P388D1 (murine macrophage-like) (Tujulin, Lilliehöök, Macellaro, Sjöstedt, & Norlander, 1999) and THP-1 cells (human monocyte-like) (Ghigo et al., 2002) have been extensively employed to more accurately mimic the *in vivo* situation, with more recent studies focused on interactions with primary human monocytes/macrophages (Ghigo et al., 2004; Shannon & Heinzen, 2008) and dendritic cells (Shannon, Howe, & Heinzen, 2005).

Embryonated eggs were also used to grow *C. burnetii*. This technique demands time and experience. It involves the inoculation of a tissue suspension containing *C. burnetii,* into 6 to 7 day-old embryonated chicken eggs via the yolk sac, that is harvested after 10 to 15 days (OIE, 2012). On the other hand, culture results are hard to monitor and the results are comparable to cell culture isolation techniques.

A milestone in *C. burnetii* research was reached in 2009 by the development of an axenic culture system for this formerly obligate intracellular bacterium (Boden et al., 2015). This system, acidified citrate cysteine medium (ACCM), was created based on information from acid activation studies, together with analyses using transcription microarray techniques, metabolic pathway reconstruction and metabolite typing (Omsland et al., 2009). The development of this type of host cell-free medium allows the understanding of *C. burnetii* physiology and capacitates the development of advanced genetic tools for biomolecular manipulation (Sandoz, Sturdevant, Hansen, & Heinzen, 2014).

Quality Control in C. burnetii Cultivation

When working with cell cultures, one of the biggest concerns is to guarantee that there is no contamination and/or cross-contamination. A visual check, on isolate purity and contamination, is hampered by the intracellular nature of *C. burnetii*. Bacterial contamination of cell cultures is easily visible by the change in clarity of the culture medium, especially when culture medium without antibiotics is used. To control these type of contaminations, it is mandatory to implement regular checks for contaminants and monitor cultures by light microscopy at 100× magnification. To detect possible cross-contamination between cultures with different strains, there is the need to regularly identify the strains by genotyping techniques (Vincent et al., 2015).

EPIDEMIOLOGY

Hosts

Q fever is an ubiquitous zoonosis whose reservoirs include a wide variety of animal species, including arthropods, mainly ticks, wildlife, namely rodents, birds, marine mammals and wild ruminants, as well as domestic animals, like dogs and cats. However, many studies emphasize the importance of wild and domestic ruminants, being the last considered the primary animal reservoir (Fernández-Aguilar, Cabezón, Colom-Cadena, Lavín, & López-Olvera, 2016; Meredith, Cleaveland, Denwood, Brown, & Shaw, 2015; Million & Raoult, 2013; Van den Brom, van Engelen, Roest, Van der Hoek, & Vellema, 2015).

Domestic ungulates (dairy cattle dairy sheep and goats) are considered the major reservoirs of *C. burnetti* (S. Kim, E. Kim, Lafferty, & Dubovi, 2005) within these aborting domestic ruminants are the main sources of human infection (Woldehiwet, 2004; Bartelink et al., 2000) and environment contamination (Bartelink et al., 2000; Million & Raoult, 2013; Van den Brom et al., 2015; Woldehiwet, 2004).

Prevalence

Q fever has been described as a disease with worldwide distribution, except in some countries such as New Zealand (Angelakis & Raoult, 2010). However, the estimation of prevalence is depending on the methodology, body fluid or tissue used and region of the globe where the study was performed. In general, is highest in cows, followed by goats and sheep and lower in the other species indicated above. Also, it is generally higher in bulk tank milk tests (BTM). Thus, the prevalence data available in several studies are difficult to compare, being difficult to estimate accurately the real prevalence of infection (Angen et al., 2011; Astobiza et al., 2012; Guatteo, Seegers, Taurel, Joly, & Beaudeau, 2011; Kim et al., 2005; Van den Brom et al., 2012, 2015). In addition, the results of the BTM samples should be analyzed with caution and carefully correlated with other tests, namely individual tests (Astobiza et al., 2012).

Route of Transmission

Domestic ungulates (dairy cattle, sheep and goats), specially aborting domestic ruminants, shed widely highly resistant bacteria by all fluids, including feces, urine, milk, placental membranes and birth fluids, which in turn are spread by aerosols (Bartelink et al., 2000; Million & Raoult, 2013; Van den Brom et al., 2015; Woldehiwet, 2004). Once domestic ruminants undergo subclinical infection they are considered the main sources of human and environment contamination (Bartelink et al., 2000; Woldehiwet, 2004).

One Health and Occupational Hazards

Human infection has most often been attributed to contact (indirect or direct) with infected ruminants, primarily sheep, goats, and cattle, and hence, by the nature of their occupation, professions linked to animals have been identified to be at higher risk of C. burnetii infection than the non-exposed general population (Colville & Berryhill, 2007). These groups include veterinarians, veterinary technicians, livestock farmers, dairy workers, slaughterhouse workers and researchers, mainly at facilities where ruminants are housed (Colville & Berryhill, 2007). Contaminated aerosols are the main human infection source, by inhalation, affecting mainly occupational groups who deal with placental membranes or birth fluids that contain billions of agents (Colville & Berryhill, 2007; Million & Raoult, 2013; Van den Brom et al., 2015). From the occupational groups, livestock farmers are those with high seroprevalence of antibodies against *C. burnetii,* even in countries where acute Q fever are rare and without registration of outbreaks. Also people who lives close to the farms could be contaminated and are potential targets of acute outbreaks (Van den Brom et al., 2015).

Predispositions

A few reports have suggested special predisposition to the immunocompromised hosts are considered to be at risk of severe disease to the development of chronicity. Q fever is considered a rare disease in children which could be explained by the often asymptomatic or nonspecific course of infection leading to undiagnosed cases of Coxiellosis. Nonetheless, hepatitis and pneumonia have however been reported in children suffering from Q fever and can be fatal (Maltezou & Raoult, 2002; Parker, Barralet & Bell, 2006; Kuroiwa, Oyanagi, Fuse, Mori, Ueno & Tsutsumi, 2007). Furthermore, people with heart valve lesions, vascular abnormalities, liver cirrhosis, and cancer are more susceptible to developing chronic Q fever (Raoult, Brouqui, Marchou & Gastaut, 1992; Fenollar, Thuny, Xeridat, Lepidi & Raoult, 2006; Parker, Barralet & Bell, 2006).

Pathogenesis

The pathogenesis of Q fever still lacks investigation but it is known that the portal of entry is oropharynx, followed by primary multiplication in the regional lymph nodes and then bacteraemia, which lasts for 5–7 days (Woldehiwet, 2004). Once in the bloodstream, the bacteria are directed to the target organs, which are reproductive organs, including mammary glands, placenta of pregnant animals or other organs, like lung, liver, spleen, lymph nodes, intestine and bone marrow (Woldehiwet, 2004).

The virulent factors of *C. burnetii* include the LPS and plasmids, in some strains, triggering, usually, a granulomatous host response, causing variable degrees of pneumonia, granulomatous hepatitis, granulomas in bone marrow and spleen, with splenomegaly, and chronic endocarditis, affecting aortic and mitral valves, which is most commonly described in humans (Roest et al., 2013; Van den Brom et al., 2015; Woldehiwet, 2004).

This granulomatous chronic inflammatory response results from the ability of *C. burnetii* to grow and multiply within phagolysosomes, the structure of the phagocytic cells that should destroy it, and its propensity to establish persistent infection (Woldehiwet, 2004). Apparently, infected host cells are detected by the immune system and lysed by antibody dependent cellular cytotoxicity by monocytes and other effector cells, being the released organisms vulnerable to activated macrophages but its intracellular survival ability, probably due to the subversion of some macrophage functions and the impairment of T-cell responses, results in an immune deficient expression, in infections with "chronic" strains (Woldehiwet, 2004).

Relatively to the cellular response, *in vitro* studies revealed that gamma interferon (IFN-γ) limits the multiplication of *C. burnetii* and enhances its killing through apoptotic mechanisms, mediated by tumour necrosis factor (TNF-α), which induces apoptosis in infected monocytes. Also, IFN-γ mediate the killing of *C. burnetii*, through the alteration of conditions within the phagosomes and nitric oxide, up-regulated by IFN-γ and TNF-α, inhibits the multiplication of the organism *in vitro* (Roest et al., 2013; Woldehiwet, 2004).

As referred above, animals are infected from the environment and undergoes a primary infection, with discrete clinical expression. However, the organism can persist after initial acute or subclinical disease, being shed in large numbers when persistently infected female animal becomes pregnant (Woldehiwet, 2004). At pregnancy the level of antibody, probably IgG, climbs and in subsequent pregnancies the animal does not excrete again or excrete at a low titre. Whereas the *C. burnetii* may continue to be shed in the milk, particularly in dairy cattle, for long periods of time (Woldehiwet, 2004).

The bacteria have tropism and multiply in the trophoblast cells of the inter-cotyledonary allantochorion and base of the cotyledonary villi, spreading through the placenta, causing placentitis and not affecting the trophoblasts that cover the cotyledonary villi. Once these trophoblasts are involved in the exchange of gasses and nutrients, the foetal development continues until inflammation spreads and causes abortion, so aborted fetuses appear normal, occasionally autolytic, or could have only granulomatous hepatitis (Van den Brom et al., 2015; Woldehiwet, 2004).

Macroscopically, infected placenta exhibits thickening, intercotyledonary leathery and a discoloured or yellow-brownish purulent exudate of variable consistency which corresponds, microscopically, to an acute, diffuse inflammatory infiltrate in the chorion without vasculitis. The severity of inflammation varies from mild mononuclear infiltration to severe supurative exsudate or necrosis (Van den Brom et al., 2015; Woldehiwet, 2004). Intact infected chorionic epithelial cells, especially at the base of the cotyledonary villi, show cytoplasmic vacuoles, containing large numbers of basophilic granulation, highly suggestive of C. burnetii organisms (Van den Brom et al., 2015; Woldehiwet, 2004).

ACKNOWLEDGMENT

This work is financed by national funds through FCT - Fundação para a Ciência e Tecnologia, I.P., under the projects UID/Multi/04016/2016, FCOMP-01-0124-FEDER-009525, UID/AGR/04033/2013 and SBVEPS (Proc° 441.00 SERVIA); QREN/FEDER under the project Ovislab ICT-2013-05-004-5314 ID-64757; CI&DETS and CGD under projects rumDISEASE PROJ/CI&DETS/2016/0023,

SBMERGE PROJ/CI&DETS/CGD/009 and HEALTHY-ValorWhey PROJ/CI&DETS/CGD/007). This work is supported by European Investment Funds by FEDER/COMPETE/POCI– Operacional Competitiveness and Internacionalization Programme, under Project POCI-01-0145-FEDER-006958 and National Funds by FCT - Portuguese Foundation for Science and Technology, under the project UID/AGR/04033/2013. Furthermore we would like to thank to UTAD and CITAB for their support.

REFERENCES

Angelakis, E., & Raoult, D. (2010). Q fever. *Veterinary Microbiology*, *140*(3-4), 297–309. doi:10.1016/j.vetmic.2009.07.016 PMID:19875249

Angen, Ø., Ståhl, M., Agerholm, J. S., Christoffersen, A. B., & Agger, J. F. (2011). Dynamics of relationship between the presence of Coxiella burnetii DNA, antibodies, and intrinsic variables in cow milk and bulk tank milk from Danish dairy cattle. *Journal of Dairy Science*, *94*(12), 5750–5759. doi:10.3168/jds.2011-4197 PMID:22118065

Arricau Bouvery, N., & Rodolakis, A. (2005). Is Q fever an emerging or re-emerging zoonosis? *Veterinary Research*, *36*(3), 327–349. doi:10.1051/vetres:2005010 PMID:15845229

Astobiza, I., Ruiz-Fons, F., Pinero, A., Barandika, J. F., Hurtado, A., & García-Perez, A. L. (2012). Estimation of *Coxiella burnetii* prevalence in dairy cattle in intensive systems by serological and molecular analyses of bulk-tank milk samples. *Journal of Dairy Science*, *95*(4), 1632–1638. doi:10.3168/jds.2011-4721 PMID:22459811

Aucken, H. M., & Pitt, T. L. (1993). Lipopolysaccharide profile typing as a technique for comparative typing of gram-negative bacteria. *Journal of Clinical Microbiology*, *31*(5), 1286–1289. PMID:7684751

Baca, O. G., & Paretsky, D. (1983). Q fever and *Coxiella burnetii*: A model for host-parasite interactions. *Microbiological Reviews*, *47*(2), 127–149. PMID:6348504

Bartelink, A.K., Stevens, H., van Kregten, E., Meijer, J.G., Beeres, M.P., & van Deuren, M. (2000). Acute and chronic Q fever; epidemiology, symptoms, diagnosis and therapy of infection caused by Coxiella burnetii. *Ned Tijdschr Geneeskd, 144*(27), 1303-6.

Beare, P. A., Jeffrey, B. M., Long, C. M., Martens, C. M., & Heinzen, R. A. (2018). Genetic mechanisms of *Coxiella burnetii* lipopolysaccharide phase variation. *PLoS Pathogens*, *14*(3), e1006922. doi:10.1371/journal.ppat.1006922 PMID:29481553

Benson, W. W., Brock, D. W., & Mather, J. (1963). Serologic analysis of a penitentiary group using raw milk from a Q fever infected herd. *Public Health Reports*, *78*(8), 707–710. doi:10.2307/4591908 PMID:14049191

Bergey, D. H., Krieg, N. R., & Holt, J. G. (1984). *Bergey's manual of systematic bacteriology*. Baltimore, MD: Williams & Wilkins.

Berón, W., Gutierrez, M. G., Rabinovitch, M., & Colombo, M. I. (2002). *Coxiella burnetii* Localizes in a Rab7-Labeled Compartment with Autophagic Characteristics. *Infection and Immunity*, *70*(10), 5816–5821. doi:10.1128/IAI.70.10.5816-5821.2002 PMID:12228312

Berri, M., Rousset, E., Champion, J. L., Russo, P., & Rodolakis, A. (2007). Goats may experience reproductive failures and shed *Coxiella burnetii* at two successive parturitions after a Q fever infection. *Research in Veterinary Science*, *83*(1), 47–52. doi:10.1016/j.rvsc.2006.11.001 PMID:17187835

Berri, M., Souriau, A., Crosby, M., & Rodolakis, A. (2002). Shedding of *Coxiella burnetii* in ewes in two pregnancies following an episode of *Coxiella* abortion in a sheep flock. *Veterinary Microbiology*, *85*(1), 55–60. doi:10.1016/S0378-1135(01)00480-1 PMID:11792492

Bewley, K. R. (2013). Animal Models of Q Fever (*Coxiella burnetii*). *Comparative Medicine*, *63*(6), 469–476. PMID:24326221

Boden, K., Wolf, K., Hermann, B., & Frangoulidis, D. (2015). First isolation of *Coxiella burnetii* from clinical material by cell-free medium (ACCM2). *European Journal of Clinical Microbiology & Infectious Diseases*, *34*(5), 1017–1022. doi:10.100710096-015-2321-1 PMID:25876216

Brennan, R. E., Russell, K., Zhang, G., & Samuel, J. E. (2004). Both Inducible Nitric Oxide Synthase and NADPH Oxidase Contribute to the Control of Virulent Phase I *Coxiella burnetii* Infections. *Infection and Immunity*, *72*(11), 6666–6675. doi:10.1128/IAI.72.11.6666-6675.2004 PMID:15501800

Burnet, F. M., & Freeman, M. (1937). Experimental studies on the virus of Q fever. *The Medical Journal of Australia*, *2*, 299–302.

Byers, K. B., & Harding, A. L. (2006). Epidemiology of laboratory associated infections. In Biological Safety Principles and Practices (pp. 53–77). American Society of Microbiology.

Cerf, O., & Condron, R. (2006). *Coxiella burnetii* and milk pasteurization: An early application of the precautionary principle? *Epidemiology and Infection, 134*(5), 946–951. doi:10.1017/S0950268806005978 PMID:16492321

Chmielewski, T., & Tylewska-Wierzbanowska, S. (2012). Q Fever at the Turn of the Century. *Polish Journal of Microbiology, 61*(2), 81–93. PMID:23163207

Cleveland, K. O. (2017). Q Fever. *Medscape*. Retrieved December 15th, 2017 from https://emedicine.medscape.com/article/227156-overview

Coelho, A. C., & García Díez, J. (2015). Biological Risks and Laboratory-Acquired Infections: A Reality That Cannot be Ignored in Health Biotechnology. *Frontiers in Bioengineering and Biotechnology, 3*, 56. doi:10.3389/fbioe.2015.00056 PMID:25973418

Colville, J. L., & Berryhill, D. L. (2007). *Handbook of Zoonoses: Identification and Prevention.* St. Louis, MO: Mosby, Inc.

Cox, H. R. (1941). Cultivation of rickettsiae of the rocky mountain spotted fever, typhus and Q fever groups in the embryonic tissues of developing chicks. *Science, 94*(2444), 399–403. doi:10.1126cience.94.2444.399 PMID:17798222

Davies, G., Cox, H., Parker, R., & Dyer, R. (1938). A Filter-Passing Infectious Agent Isolated from Ticks. *Public Health Reports (1896-1970), 53*(52), 2259-2282. doi:10.2307/4582746

De Rooij, M. M. T., Borlée, F., Smit, L. A. M., de Bruin, A., Janse, I., Heederik, D. J. J., & Wouters, I. M. (2016). Detection of *Coxiella burnetii* in Ambient Air after a Large Q Fever Outbreak. *PLoS One, 11*(3), e0151281. doi:10.1371/journal.pone.0151281 PMID:26991094

Derrick, E. H. (1937). "Q" Fever, new fever entity: Clinical features, diagnosis and laboratory investigation. *The Medical Journal of Australia, 2*, 281–299.

Eldin, C., Mélenotte, C., Mediannikov, O., Ghigo, E., Million, M., Edouard, S., ... Raoult, D. (2017). From Q Fever to *Coxiella burnetii* Infection: A Paradigm Change. *Clinical Microbiology Reviews, 30*(1), 115–190. doi:10.1128/CMR.00045-16 PMID:27856520

Fenollar, F., Thuny, F., Xeridat, B., Lepidi, H., & Raoult, D. (2006). Endocarditis after acute Q fever in patients with previously undiagnosed valvulopathies. *Clinical Infectious Diseases, 42*(6), 818–821. doi:10.1086/500402 PMID:16477559

Fernández-Aguilar, X., Cabezón, Ó., Colom-Cadena, A., Lavín, S., & López-Olvera, J. R. (2016). Serological survey of *Coxiella burnetii* at the wildlife–livestock interface in the Eastern Pyrenees, Spain. *Acta Veterinaria Scandinavica*, *58*(1), 26. doi:10.118613028-016-0209-4 PMID:27121001

Fournier, P. E., Marrie, T. J., & Raoult, D. (1998). Diagnosis of Q Fever. *Journal of Clinical Microbiology*, *36*(7), 1823–1834. PMID:9650920

Gale, P., Kelly, L., Mearns, R., Duggan, J., & Snary, E. L. (2015). Q fever through consumption of unpasteurised milk and milk products - a risk profile and exposure assessment. *Journal of Applied Microbiology*, *118*(5), 1083–1095. doi:10.1111/jam.12778 PMID:25692216

Galiero, A., Fratini, F., Cammà, C., Di Domenico, M., Curini, V., Baronti, I., ... Cerri, D. (2016). Occurrence of *Coxiella burnetii* in goat and ewe unpasteurized cheeses: Screening and genotyping. *International Journal of Food Microbiology*, *237*, 47–54. doi:10.1016/j.ijfoodmicro.2016.08.008 PMID:27543815

Garrity, G. M., Bell, J. A., & Lilburn, T. (2015). Coxiellaceae fam. nov. In W. B. Whitman, F. Rainey, P. Kämpfer, M. Trujillo, J. Chun, P. DeVos, B. Hedlund & S. Dedysh (Eds.), Bergey's Manual of Systematics of Archaea and Bacteria. Wiley. doi:10.1002/9781118960608.fbm00223

Ghigo, E., Capo, C., Tung, C. H., Raoult, D., Gorvel, J. P., & Mege, J. L. (2002). *Coxiella burnetii* Survival in THP-1 Monocytes Involves the Impairment of Phagosome Maturation: IFN-γ Mediates its Restoration and Bacterial Killing. *Journal of Immunology (Baltimore, Md.: 1950)*, *169*(8), 4488–4495. doi:10.4049/jimmunol.169.8.4488 PMID:12370385

Ghigo, E., Honstettre, A., Capo, C., Gorvel, J. P., Raoult, D., & Mege, J. L. (2004). Link between impaired maturation of phagosomes and defective *Coxiella burnetii* killing in patients with chronic Q fever. *The Journal of Infectious Diseases*, *190*(10), 1767–7. doi:10.1086/425041 PMID:15499532

Guatteo, R., Seegers, H., Taurel, A. F., Joly, A., & Beaudeau, F. (2011). Prevalence of *Coxiella burnetii* infection in domestic ruminants: A critical review. *Veterinary Microbiology*, *149*(1-2), 1–16. doi:10.1016/j.vetmic.2010.10.007 PMID:21115308

Guidi, F., Petruzzelli, A., Ciarrocchi, F., Duranti, A., Valiani, A., Amagliani, G., & Blasi, G. (2017). Prevalence of *Coxiella burnetii* in cows' and ewes' bulk tank milk samples from selected dairy farms of Central Italy. *Italian Journal of Animal Science*, *16*(4), 673–676. doi:10.1080/1828051X.2017.1321474

Hanczaruk, M., Cutler, S. J., Toman, R., & Frangoulidis, D. (2012). Coxiella burnetii: Q Fever. In BSL3 and BSL4 Agents. In M. C. Elschner, S. J. Cutler, M. Weidmann, & P. Butaye (Eds.), Epidemiology, Microbiology and Practical Guidelines (pp. 57-69). Weinheim: Wiley-Blackwell. doi:10.1002/9783527645114.ch19

Hechemy, K. E. (2012). History and Prospects of *Coxiella burnetii* Research. In R. Toman, R. Heinzen, J. Samuel, & J. L. Mege (Eds.), *Coxiella burnetii: Recent Advances and New Perspectives in Research of the Q Fever Bacterium. Advances in Experimental Medicine and Biology* (Vol. 984). Dordrecht: Springer. doi:10.1007/978-94-007-4315-1_1

Heinzen, R. A., Scidmore, M. A., Rockey, D. D., & Hackstadt, T. (1996). Differential interaction with endocytic and exocytic pathways distinguish parasitophorous vacuoles of *Coxiella burnetii* and Chlamydia trachomatis. *Infection and Immunity, 64*(3), 796–809. PMID:8641784

Heppell, C. W., Egan, J. R., & Hall, I. (2017). A human time dose response model for Q fever. *Epidemics, 21*, 30–38. doi:10.1016/j.epidem.2017.06.001 PMID:28666604

Hoover, T. A., Culp, D. W., Vodkin, M. H., Williams, J. C., & Thompson, H. A. (2002). Chromosomal DNA Deletions Explain Phenotypic Characteristics of Two Antigenic Variants, Phase II and RSA 514 (Crazy), of the *Coxiella burnetii* Nine Mile Strain. *Infection and Immunity, 70*(12), 6726–6733. doi:10.1128/IAI.70.12.6726-2733.2002 PMID:12438347

Hotta, A., Kawamura, M., To, H., Andoh, M., Yamaguchi, T., Fukushi, H., & Hirai, K. (2002). Phase Variation Analysis of *Coxiella burnetii* during Serial Passage in Cell Culture by Use of Monoclonal Antibodies. *Infection and Immunity, 70*(8), 4747–4749. doi:10.1128/IAI.70.8.4747-4749.2002 PMID:12117996

Howe, D., & Mallavia, L. P. (2000). *Coxiella burnetii* Exhibits Morphological Change and Delays Phagolysosomal Fusion after Internalization by J774A.1 Cells. *Infection and Immunity, 68*(7), 3815–3821. doi:10.1128/IAI.68.7.3815-3821.2000 PMID:10858189

Jones, R. M., Nicas, M., Hubbard, A. E., & Reingold, A. L. (2006). The infectious dose of *Coxiella burnetii* (Q Fever). *Applied Biosafety: Journal of the American Biological Safety Association, 11*(1), 32–41. doi:10.1177/153567600601100106

Kazar, J. (2005). *Coxiella burnetii* Infection. *Annals of the New York Academy of Sciences, 1063*(1), 105–114. doi:10.1196/annals.1355.018 PMID:16481501

Khalili, M., Sakhaee, E., & Babaei, H. (2012). Frequency of anti-*Coxiella burnetii* antibodies in cattle with reproductive disorders. *Comparative Clinical Pathology*, *21*(5), 917–919. doi:10.100700580-011-1199-2

Khavkin, T., & Tabibzadeh, S. S. (1988). Histologic, immunofluorescence, and electron microscopic study of infectious process in mouse lung after intranasal challenge with *Coxiella burnetii*. *Infection and Immunity*, *56*(7), 1792–1799. PMID:3290107

Kim, S. G., Kim, E. H., Lafferty, C. J., & Dubovi, E. (2005). *Coxiella burnetii* in Bulk Tank Milk Samples, United States. *Emerging Infectious Diseases*, *11*(4), 619–621. doi:10.3201/eid1104.041036 PMID:15829205

Klemmer, J., Njeru, J., Emam, A., El-Sayed, A., Moawad, A. A., Henning, K., ... El-Diasty, M. M. (2018). Q fever in Egypt: Epidemiological survey of *Coxiella burnetii* specific antibodies in cattle, buffaloes, sheep, goats and camels. *PLoS One*, *13*(2), e0192188. doi:10.1371/journal.pone.0192188 PMID:29466380

Kozajda, A., & Bródka, K., & SzadkowskaStańczyk, I. (2013). Factors influencing biosafety level and LAI among the staff of medical laboratories. *Medycyna Pracy*, *64*(4), 473–486. PMID:24502112

Kuroiwa, Y., Oyanagi, R., Fuse, S., Mori, T., Ueno, H., & Tsutsumi, H. (2007). Persistent hepatitis and repeated wheezing in an infant. *The Pediatric Infectious Disease Journal*, *26*(8), 763–769. doi:10.1097/INF.0b013e3180f60bfe PMID:17848898

Maltezou, H. C., & Raoult, D. (2002). Q fever in children. *The Lancet Infectious Diseases*, *2*(11), 686–691. doi:10.1016/S1473-3099(02)00440-1 PMID:12409049

Mangili, P., Amagliani, G., Micci, E., Brandi, G., Foglini, M., Cinti, B., ... Schiavano, G. F. (2016). A model for *Coxiella burnetii* monitoring in a sheep dairy farm. *JSM Biotechnology & Biomedical Engineering*, *3*, 1050.

Maurin, M., Benoliel, A. M., Bongrand, P., & Raoult, D. (1992). Phagolysosomes of *Coxiella burnetii*-infected cell lines maintain an acidic pH during persistent infection. *Infection and Immunity*, *60*(12), 5013–5016. PMID:1452331

Maurin, M., & Raoult, D. (1999). Q Fever. *Clinical Microbiology Reviews*, *12*(4), 518–553. doi:10.1128/CMR.12.4.518 PMID:10515901

McDade, J. E. (1990). Historical aspects of Q fever. In T. J. Marrie (Ed.), Q Fever: The Disease (pp. 6-15). Boca Raton, FL: CRC Press.

Meredith, A. L., Cleaveland, S. C., Denwood, M. J., Brown, J. K., & Shaw, D. J. (2015). *Coxiella burnetii* (Q-Fever) Seroprevalence in Prey and Predators in the United Kingdom: Evaluation of Infection in Wild Rodents, Foxes and Domestic Cats Using a Modified ELISA. *Transboundary and Emerging Diseases, 62*(6), 639–649. doi:10.1111/tbed.12211 PMID:24479951

Miller, A. L., Wang, Y., Mooseker, M. S., & Koleske, A. J. (2004). The Abl-related gene (Arg) requires its F-actin–microtubule cross-linking activity to regulate lamellipodial dynamics during fibroblast adhesion. *The Journal of Cell Biology, 165*(3), 407–420. doi:10.1083/jcb.200308055 PMID:15138293

Million, M., & Raoult, D. (2013). 66 - Q Fever. In A. J. Magill, D. R. Hill, T. Solomon, & E. T. Ryan (Eds.), *Hunter's Tropical Medicine and Emerging Infectious Disease* (9th ed.; pp. 558–560). London: W.B. Saunders; doi:10.1016/B978-1-4160-4390-4.00066-7

Mori, M., Boarbi, M., Michel, P., Bakinahe, R., Rits, K., Wattiau, P., & Fretin, D. (2013). In Vitro and In Vivo Infectious Potential of *Coxiella burnetii*: A Study on Belgian Livestock Isolates. *PLoS One, 8*(6), e67622. doi:10.1371/journal.pone.0067622 PMID:23840751

Mori, M., & Roest, H.J. (2018). Farming, Q fever and public health: agricultural practices and beyond. *Arch Public Health., 6*, 76. doi: . doi:10.118613690-017-0248-y

Omsland, A., Cockrell, D. C., Howe, D., Fischer, E. R., Virtaneva, K., Sturdevant, D. E., & Heinzen, R. A. (2009). Host cell-free growth of the Q fever bacterium *Coxiella burnetii. Proceedings of the National Academy of Sciences of the United States of America, 106*(11), 4430–4434. doi:10.1073/pnas.0812074106 PMID:19246385

Oyston, P. C., & Davies, C. (2011). Q fever: The neglected biothreat agent. *Journal of Medical Microbiology, 60*(1), 9–21. doi:10.1099/jmm.0.024778-0 PMID:21030501

Palmela, C., Badura, R., & Valadas, E. (2012). Acute Q fever in Portugal. Epidemiological and clinical features of 32 hospitalized patients. *Germs, 2*(2), 43–59. doi:10.11599/germs.2012.1013 PMID:24432263

Parker, N. R., Barralet, J. H., & Bell, A. M. (2006). Q fever. *Lancet, 367*(9511), 679–688. doi:10.1016/S0140-6736(06)68266-4 PMID:16503466

Pastorino, B., de Lamballerie, X., & Charrel, R. (2017). Biosafety and Biosecurity in European Containment Level 3 Laboratories: Focus on French Recent Progress and Essential Requirements. *Frontiers in Public Health, 5*, 121. doi:10.3389/fpubh.2017.00121 PMID:28620600

Philip, C. (1948). Comments on the Name of the Q Fever Organism. *Public Health Reports (1896-1970), 63*(2), 58-58. doi:10.2307/4586402

Pike, R. M. (1976). Laboratory associated infections: Summary and analysis of 3921 cases. *Health Laboratory Science, 13*(2), 105–114. PMID:946794

Raoult, D., Brouqui, P., Marchou, B., & Gastaut, J. A. (1992). Acute and chronic Q fever in patients with cancer. *Clinical Infectious Diseases, 14*(1), 127–130. doi:10.1093/clinids/14.1.127 PMID:1571416

Raoult, D., Marrie, T., & Mege, J. (2005). Natural history and pathophysiology of Q fever. *The Lancet Infectious Diseases, 5*(4), 219–226. doi:10.1016/S1473-3099(05)70052-9 PMID:15792739

Raoult, D., Vestris, G., & Enea, M. (1990). Isolation of 16 strains of *Coxiella burnetii* from patients by using a sensitive centrifugation cell culture system and establishment of the strains in HEL cells. *Journal of Clinical Microbiology, 28*(11), 2482–2484. PMID:2254424

Reimer, L. G. (1993). Q fever. *Clinical Microbiology Reviews, 6*(3), 193–198. doi:10.1128/CMR.6.3.193 PMID:8358703

Rodolakis, A. (2009). Q Fever in dairy animals. *Annals of the New York Academy of Sciences, 1166*(1), 90–93. doi:10.1111/j.1749-6632.2009.04511.x PMID:19538267

Roest, H. I., Post, J., van Gelderen, B., van Zijderveld, F. G., & Rebel, J. M. (2013). Q fever in pregnant goats: Humoral and cellular immune responses. *Veterinary Research, 44*(1), 67. doi:10.1186/1297-9716-44-67 PMID:23915213

Roest, H.-J., van Gelderen, B., Dinkla, A., Frangoulidis, D., van Zijderveld, F., Rebel, J., & van Keulen, L. (2012). Q Fever in Pregnant Goats: Pathogenesis and Excretion of *Coxiella burnetii. PLoS One, 7*(11), e48949. doi:10.1371/journal.pone.0048949 PMID:23152826

Romano, P. S., Gutierrez, M. G., Beron, W., Rabinovitch, M., & Colombo, M. I. (2007). The autophagic pathway is actively modulated by phase II *Coxiella burnetii* to efficiently replicate in the host cell. *Cellular Microbiology, 9*(4), 891–909. doi:10.1111/j.1462-5822.2006.00838.x PMID:17087732

Sandoz, K. M., Sturdevant, D. E., Hansen, B., & Heinzen, R. A. (2014). Developmental transitions of *Coxiella burnetii* grown in axenic media. *Journal of Microbiological Methods, 96*, 104–110. doi:10.1016/j.mimet.2013.11.010 PMID:24286928

Scott, G. H., Williams, J. C., & Stephenson, E. H. (1987). Animal models in Q fever: Pathological responses of inbred mice to phase I *Coxiella burnetii. Microbiology, 133*(3), 691–700. doi:10.1099/00221287-133-3-691 PMID:3655728

Seshadri, R., Paulsen, I. T., Eisen, J. A., Read, T. D., Nelson, K. E., & Nelson, W. C. (2003). Complete genome sequence of the Q-fever pathogen *Coxiella burnetii. Proceedings of the National Academy of Sciences of the United States of America, 100*(9), 5455–5460. doi:10.1073/pnas.0931379100

Shannon, J. G., & Heinzen, R. A. (2008). Infection of human monocyte-derived macrophages with *Coxiella burnetii. Methods in Molecular Biology (Clifton, N.J.), 431*, 189–200. PMID:18287757

Shannon, J. G., Howe, D., & Heinzen, R. A. (2005). Virulent *Coxiella burnetii* does not activate human dendritic cells: Role of lipopolysaccharide as a shielding molecule. *Proceedings of the National Academy of Sciences of the United States of America, 102*(24), 8722–8727. doi:10.1073/pnas.0501863102 PMID:15939879

Skultety, L., Hajduch, M., Flores-Ramirez, G., Miernyk, J. A., Ciampor, F., Toman, R., & Sekeyova, Z. (2011). Proteomic comparison of virulent phase I and avirulent phase II of *Coxiella burnetii*, the causative agent of Q fever. *Journal of Proteomics, 74*(10), 1974–1984. doi:10.1016/j.jprot.2011.05.017 PMID:21616182

Stein, A., Louveau, C., Lepidi, H., Ricci, F., Baylac, P., Davoust, B., & Raoult, D. (2005). Q Fever Pneumonia: Virulence of *Coxiella burnetii* Pathovars in a Murine Model of Aerosol Infection. *Infection and Immunity, 73*(4), 2469–2477. doi:10.1128/IAI.73.4.2469-2477.2005 PMID:15784593

Stein, A., Saunders, N. A., Taylor, A. G., & Raoult, D. (1993). Phylogenic homogeneity of *Coxiella burnetii* strains as determinated by 16S ribosomal RNA sequencing. *FEMS Microbiology Letters, 113*(3), 339–344. doi:10.1111/j.1574-6968.1993.tb06537.x PMID:7505761

The Center for Food Security and Public Health (CFSPH). (2017). *Q fever*. Retrieved in April 24, 2018, from http://www.cfsph.iastate.edu/Factsheets/pdfs/q_fever.pdf

The World Organisation for Animal Health (OIE). (2012). Manual of Diagnostic Tests and Vaccines for Terrestrial Animals. *Terrestrial Manual.* Retrieved from http://www.oie.int/fileadmin/Home/eng/Health_standards/tahm/2.01.16_Q_FEVER.pdf

Tujulin, E., Lilliehöök, B., Macellaro, A., Sjöstedt, A., & Norlander, L. (1999). Early cytokine induction in mouse P388D1 macrophages infected by *Coxiella burnetii. Veterinary Immunology and Immunopathology, 68*(2-4), 159–168. doi:10.1016/S0165-2427(99)00023-9 PMID:10438316

Vadovic, P., Slaba, K., Fodorova, M., Skultety, L., & Toman, R. (2005). Structural and Functional Characterization of the Glycan Antigens Involved in Immunobiology of Q Fever. *Annals of the New York Academy of Sciences*, *1063*(1), 149–153. doi:10.1196/annals.1355.023 PMID:16481506

Van den Brom, R., van Engelen, E., Luttikholt, S., Moll, L., van Maanen, K., & Vellema, P. (2012). *Coxiella burnetii* in bulk tank milk samples from dairy goat and dairy sheep farms in The Netherlands in 2008. *The Veterinary Record*, *170*(12), 310. doi:10.1136/vr.100304 PMID:22351793

Van den Brom, R., van Engelen, E., Roest, H. I., Van der Hoek, W., & Vellema, P. (2015). *Coxiella burnetii* infections in sheep or goats: An opinionated review. *Veterinary Microbiology*, *181*(1-2), 119–129. doi:10.1016/j.vetmic.2015.07.011 PMID:26315774

Van der Hoek, W., Dijkstra, F., Schimmer, B., Schneeberger, P. M., Vellema, P., Wijkmans, C., ... van Duynhoven, Y. (2010). Q fever in the Netherlands: An update on the epidemiology and control measures. *Eurosurveillance*, *25*(12), 19520. doi:10.2807/ese.15.12.19520-en PMID:20350500

Vincent, G. A., Graves, S. R., Robsond, J. M., Nguyen, C., Hussain-Yusuf, H., Islama, A., ... Stenos, J. (2015). Isolation of *Coxiella burnetii* from serum of patients with acute Q fever. *Journal of Microbiological Methods*, *119*, 74–78. doi:10.1016/j.mimet.2015.10.008 PMID:26462766

Vohl, D. E., & Heinzen, R. A. (2007). Microreview: Lounging in a lysosome: the intracellular lifestyle of *Coxiella burnetii. Cellular Microbiology*, *9*(4), 829–840. doi:10.1111/j.1462-5822.2007.00901.x PMID:17381428

Woldehiwet, Z. (2004). Q fever (coxiellosis): Epidemiology and pathogenesis. *Research in Veterinary Science*, *77*(2), 93–100. doi:10.1016/j.rvsc.2003.09.001 PMID:15196898

Wurtz, N., Papa, A., Hukic, M., Di Caro, A., Leparc-Goffart, I., Leroy, E., ... Raoult, D. (2016). Survey of laboratory acquired infections around the world in biosafety level 3 and 4 laboratories. *European Journal of Clinical Microbiology & Infectious Diseases*, *35*(8), 1247–1258. doi:10.100710096-016-2657-1 PMID:27234593

Chapter 9
A One Health Perspective on Q Fever:
Part 2

Rita Cruz
Polytechnic Institute of Viseu, Portugal

Carmen Vasconcelos-Nobrega
Polytechnic Institute of Viseu, Portugal & University of Trás-os-Montes and Alto Douro, Portugal

Fernando Esteves
Polytechnic Institute of Viseu, Portugal

Catarina Coelho
Polytechnic Institute of Viseu, Portugal & University of Trás-os-Montes and Alto Douro, Portugal

Ana Sofia Ferreira
University of Oporto, Portugal

Carla Santos
Polytechnic Institute of Viseu, Portugal

Cristina Mega
Polytechnic Institute of Viseu, Portugal

Ana C. Coelho
University of Trás-os-Montes and Alto Douro, Portugal

Helena Vala
Polytechnic Institute of Viseu, Portugal & University of Trás-os-Montes and Alto Douro, Portugal

João R. Mesquita
University of Oporto, Portugal

ABSTRACT

Q fever, a widespread zoonotic disease caused by Coxiella burnetiid, produces a complex and polymorphic disease in humans. As a zoonotic disease, control in animals will influence the level of disease seen in humans, thus resulting in interesting one health perspectives for disease control. Here the authors describe the clinical manifestations in animals and humans, as well as the current diagnostic methods available and the strategies for disease control. A review on the published information regarding Q fever as a disease with impact for veterinary public health and public health is presented.

DOI: 10.4018/978-1-5225-6304-4.ch009

RISK FACTORS FOR COXIELLOSIS: A ONE HEALTH APPROACH

Awareness of the excretion routes of *C. burnetii* from infected domestic animals is vital to pinpoint transmission routes, and thus, prevent human infection and allow the implementation of effective and reasonable preventive measures. Transmission to humans mainly occurs through inhalation of contaminated aerosols from the environment, such as dust or tick feces (Klemmer et al., 2018), thus making Q fever, essentially, an airborne disease, although some studies refer the evidence that *C. burnetii* may be a food-borne pathogen (Benson, Brock, & Mather, 1963; Cerf & Condron, 2006; Gale, Kelly, Mearns, Duggan, & Snary, 2015) throughout experiments obtained in which contaminated milk was fed to volunteers, causing seroconversion but any clinical disease (Benson et al., 1963) or through the consumption of unpasteurized milk (Gale et al., 2015). Domestic ruminants' excretion of *C. burnetii* is considered to be the main source of environmental contamination and a key cause of human infection (Roest et al., 2012; van den Brom, van Engelen, Roest, van der Hoek, & Vellema, 2015), as referred. In the Netherlands, after one of the largest Q fever outbreaks, airborne presence of *Coxiella burnetii* showed to be associated with goat kidding season, and with spatial variation/distance/size of goat farms (de Rooij et al., 2016; van der Hoek et al., 2010).

Shedding of *C. burnetii* occurs in feces, milk, and mostly, in placental membranes and birth fluids of aborted mammal fetuses, as well as, in stillbirths and healthy infected neonates (Roest et al., 2012; van den Brom et al., 2015). Subclinically infected animals also shed the organism, but with considerably lower bacterial loads than those observed in animals that underwent abortion (Roest et al., 2012).

During abortion and parturition of infected ruminants, there is a massive excretion of bacteria from birth products. A previous study has found that around 10^9 bacteria/gram of placenta were excreted during abortions in ruminants (Khalili, Sakhaee, & Babaei, 2012), whereas birthing of healthy neonates, from infected mothers, revealed a lower quantity (Rodolakis, 2009). Infectious biological excretions are desiccated in the environment, aerosolize, thus becoming airborne and available to be inhaled, allowing for transmission and infection. Environmental surroundings, dust in windy days and fomites (inanimate objects, such as gloves, coveralls, rags, etc.), that have been exposed to contaminated materials, may also result in sources for transmission (The Center for Food Security and Public Health [CFSPH], 2017).

Although *C. burnetii* has been isolated from milk, udder tissue and corresponding lymph nodes, the transmission of Q fever to humans, via ingestion of contaminated unpasteurized dairy products, still remains controversial (Eldin et al, 2017; Galiero et al., 2016). Nonetheless, shedding of *C. burnetii* in milk should be considered an important vehicle of infection for farmers, veterinarians and for dairy workers in general. Shedding in milk seems to vary in quantity and duration between animal species (Guidi et al., 2017; Mangili et al., 2016).

When comparing two excretion routes (via vaginal mucus and milk), domestic ruminants (cattle, goats and sheep) exhibit different patterns. Milk shedding seems to be more regular in cattle and goats. Ewes shed more quantity in vaginal mucus and in a more prolonged manner than goats. Both, sheep and goats, can shed *C. burnetii* in subsequent pregnancies (Arricau-Bouvery & Rodolakis, 2005; Berri, Souriau, Crosby, & Rodolakis, 2002; Berri, Rousset, Champion, Russo, & Rodolakis, 2007).

Rare modes of transmission include tick bites, ingestion of unpasteurized milk or dairy products. Human-to-human transmission is also plausible through exposure to infected human placentas, blood transfusions and sexual contact (CFSPH, 2017; Cleveland, 2017).

In addition to being sources for disease transmission to humans, *C. burnetii* infection in animals can decrease livestock productivity and indirectly affect human health trough socioeconomic losses (Vanderburg et al., 2014).

Geographical Distribution and Seasonal Variation

Infection by *C. burnetii* has been reported almost worldwide, with New Zealand remaining an exception (Angelakis & Raoult, 2010). As Q fever is not considered a nationally notifiable diseases in most countries in the world, its epidemiology may only be extrapolated from reports of epidemics, serological surveys in humans or animals, or from data obtained from public health or rickettsial reference laboratories. While the number of Coxiellosis cases reported in humans vary greatly between regions, this may not accurately reflect the true incidence of the disease, especially since the clinical manifestations of the disease may be absent in Humans. According to data retrieved from European studies, acute Q fever cases are more frequently reported in spring and early summer (Tissot Dupont et al., 1992). The maximum incidence of Q fever during spring has been suggested to be a consequence of the "outdoors" lambing season, which can in turn be responsible to the heavy shedding of *C. burnetii* to the environment. Interestingly, the lambing season in October is not related to a higher incidence.

CLINICAL MANIFESTATION IN ANIMALS

Clinical Findings

Coxiella burnetii is capable of infecting several animal species, such as ruminants, companion animals, birds and reptiles, as well as, humans, thus being considered a widespread zoonosis (Cleveland, 2017; Roest et al., 2012; van den Brom et al., 2015). Q fever is reputed to be non-pathogenic for domestic livestock (Blood & Radostitis, 1989) and the truth is that there is very little information about the clinical signs of Q fever in domestic animals. Despite the earlier reports of respiratory disease due to *C. burnetii* in sheep, goats and cattle, anorexia was the only consistent clinical finding (Blood & Radostitis, 1989; Woldehiwet, 2004). However, it is currently recognized that *C. burnetii* causing placentitis and abortion in dairy goats and sheep. Recent studies performed in dairy cattle, reveal the possibility of a relationship between *C. burnetii* infection and an increased number of endometritis, subfertility, and retained foetal membranes (de Biase et al., 2018).

Most *C. burnetii* infections in mammals result in asymptomatic seroconversions, but when infection is clinically expressed, it displays a variety of clinical forms depending on the infected species, virulence of the strain and inoculation route. In guinea pigs and mice, pneumonia and hepatitis can be observed, as well as, occurrence of splenomegaly. In contrast, reproductive expression constitutes the highest concern in livestock, although rare cases of pneumonia can ensue after infection. Clinically infected humans may exhibit atypical pneumonia, hepatitis, flu-like symptoms, or even life-threatening endocarditis, in the presence of persistent infection (Arricau-Bouvery, & Rodolakis, 2005; Cleveland, 2017; Marrie, Stein, Janigan, & Raoult, 1996; Roest et al., 2012; Russell-Lodrigue et al. 2009; Russell-Lodrigue, Zhang, McMurray, & Samuel, 2006; van den Brom et al., 2015).

Ruminants, particularly goats and sheep, constitute the most relevant zoonotic sources since they are the main animal reservoirs of *C. burnetii*, as referred previously The most frequent clinical signs in these species are abortion, premature delivery, stillbirth, and weak offspring (de Biase et al., 2018). Abortions occur without previous warning signals and mainly during the late to end stages of pregnancy (Arricau-Bouvery, & Rodolakis, 2005; Berri et al., 2001; Berri et al., 2002; Hatchette, Campbell, Hudson, Raoult, & Marrie, 2003; Rousset et al., 2009). In dairy goat herds where Q fever abortions occurred, metritis can be present as well as neonate lambs can be equally affected, showing general weakness with low body weight and high mortality in the neonatal phase. Those that appear to be healthy may later exhibit respiratory and digestive tract disorders displaying very low viability

(Arricau-Bouvery, & Rodolakis, 2005; Roest, Post, van Gelderen, van Zijderveld, & Rebel, 2013; Wouda, & Dercksen, 2007). In dairy cattle, endemic infection is considered to reduce fertility (de Biase et al. 2018; Lang, 1990) and may predispose to sub-clinical mastitis, resulting in reduction of milk production and final break down of the quarter (Klemmer et al., 2018).

Although aborted fetuses appear grossly normal, infected placentas display unspecific alterations of intercotyledonary placentitis, showing opacity and thickening due to exudative inflammation, necrosis and intercotyledonary fibrosis, with the cotyledons exhibiting areas of grey discoloration, as mentioned previously (McGavin, & Zachary, 2007). Owing to the unspecific nature of lesions, establishing *C. burnetii* as the causal agent requires mandatory confirmation by alternative laboratory methods (Agerholm, 2013).

It is still unclear if infection always leads to abortion in ruminants. Some studies refer that in cattle and in other species, it seems that *C. burnetii* is an infrequent cause of abortion, while high abortion rates are found in goats (Agerholm, 2013; Muskens, Wouda, von Bannisseht-Wijsmuller, & van Maanen, 2012). The cause of these differences in pregnancy outcomes after infection is unknown because extensive assessments, of the effects of *C. burnetii* in each species reproductive profile, is lacking. However, there are biological indications of species differences in relation to the impact on reproduction. Recent molecular studies have already shown the existence of different strains of *C. burnetii*, these strains may be associated with different ruminant hosts despite the occurrence of cross infection (Agerholm, 2013).

Q Fever in Humans: Pathogenesis of Q Fever and Immune Response

In humans Q fever is a complex and polymorphic disease that can manifest itself in the acute form with self-limiting, mild to moderate course and therefore a benign prognosis, as well as in the persistent or chronic form of the disease (Fournier, Marrie, & Raoult, 1998).

The acute form normally appears after a period of incubation that varies between 2 and 6 weeks and may be asymptomatic or cause a "simple" flu-like illness (Bartelink et al., 2000; Kovácová, & Kazár, 2002) or could be more severe and cause a pneumonia or hepatitis (Kovácová, & Kazár, 2002). The chronic form may be mainly responsible for endocarditis, but also hepatitis and chronic fatigue syndrome (Bartelink et al., 2000; Kazar, 2005; Kovácová, & Kazár, 2002). In some cases, *C. burnetti* can be responsible for isolated cases and in outbreaks, associated with a severe or with a potentially fatal course, with important implications in public health (Santos et al., 2007b; Siciliano et al. 2008).

The primary route of infection for humans is airborne, via inhalation of aerosolized particles from animal birthing products, urine and faeces, or possibly via ingestion of raw milk (Angelakis, & Raoult, 2010; Maurin, & Raoult, 1999). After aerosol transmission, *C. burnetii* targets alveolar macrophages and other mononuclear phagocytes (Baca, Klassen, & Aragon, 1993; Ghigo, Colombo, & Heinzen, 2012). *C. burnetii* passively enters macrophages cells by actin-dependent phagocytosis (van Schaik, Chen, Mertens, Weber, & Samuel, 2013).

As an obligate intracellular pathogen, *C. burnetii* presents some challenging features to immunologists. The organism takes up residence in a lysosome-like compartment in a phagocyte (Shannon, & Heinzen, 2009). The survival of *C. burnetii* in human macrophages is based on the control of phagocytosis and the prevention of ultimate phagosome lysosome fusion (Ghigo et al., 2004). The bacteria are retained in this phagosomal compartment and the moderately acidic pH (<5) of this compartment is actually needed for its metabolism and subsequent replication (Hackstadt, & Williams, 1981; Shannon, & Heinzen, 2009).

Specific immunoglobulins are secreted following infection. IgG is mainly directed against phase II antigen, whereas IgM is directed against both phase I and II cells (Maurin, & Raoult, 1999). Once established, chronic Q fever presents defective cell-mediated immunity, highlighting the major role of cell-mediated immunity in the protection against *C. burnetii* (Koster, Williams, & Goodwin, 1985).

Diagnostic Methods

Coxiella burnetii can be detected in numerous ways, depending on the type of sample and the purpose of the analysis. The organism, or its nucleic acids, may be researched in vaginal discharge, placentas, other tissues, birth fluids, aborted foetuses, milk, colostrum, blood, urine and feces (Centers for Disease Control and Prevention [CDC], 2017; Guatteo et al., 2006).

Histopathology of the placenta, with modified Ziehl– Neelsen, Gimenez, Stamp, Giemsa or modified Koster stains; permit the observation of *C. burnetii* in inflammatory exudates (Guatteo et al., 2006; Sanchez et al., 2006). Due to similarities, *C. burnetii* can be confused with *Chlamydophila abortus* or *Brucella* spp., and thus, immunohistochemistry (IHC), using *C. burnetii* specific antibodies, or other more conclusive methods, should be used for definitive identification. Abortion induced by *C. burnetii* usually yields high numbers of bacteria for observation in trophoblasts of the allantochorion (Sanchez et al., 2006).

Histopathology, combined with serological testing, has been the diagnostic mainstay for Q fever for some years, as well as, the key methodology to differentiate between other causes of abortion in ruminants. Currently, direct detection and quantification by polymerase chain reaction (PCR) and serological ELISA (enzyme-linked immunosorbent assay) should be considered the methods of choice for clinical diagnosis, as PCR is still the most reliable tool for the diagnosis of infectious abortions and ELISA is the most sensitive method in detecting *C. burnetii* specific antibodies (Niemczuk, Szymańska-Czerwińska, Śmietanka, & Bocian, 2014; Sidi-Boumedine et al., 2010).

PCR detects *C. burnetii* DNA in a wide range of samples, such as placenta tissues, feces, vaginal mucus and milk. Primers and probes targeting the IS1111 element, which has multiple copies in the genome of *C. burnetii*, are more sensitive than primers and probes that target single copy genes, resulting in increased detection. Capability to detect and quantify *C. burnetii* DNA by real-time PCR has heightened diagnostic and study approaches. Individual vaginal discharge, milk and colostrum samples, or collective milk from a tank, can be used for analysis of bacterial shedding. Therefore, active monitoring systems may be implemented in regions that need to evaluate the prevalence of Q fever in their animal population, through PCR testing of bulk tank milk (BTM). Although vaginal swabs and birth products are indicated for abortion diagnosis, BTM samples are more appropriate to scrutinize the sanitary condition of dairy cattle and goat herds. This collective diagnostic approach to screen *C. burnetii* is deemed as more significant in relation to public health risk (EFSA Panel on Animal Health and Welfare (AHAW), 2010; Klee et al., 2006; Sidi-Boumedine et al., 2010).

A serological survey is the correct approach to evaluate prevalence. Serological assays are suitable for screening herds or flocks, but interpretation at the individual animal level is not possible. Indeed, a significant proportion of animals shedding *C. burnetii* bacteria, and even some aborted animals, are found to be seronegative, but the presence of specific anti-*C. burnetii* antibodies may provide evidence of a recent infection, as well as, of a past exposure (de Cremoux et al., 2012b; Guatteo, Beaudeau, Joly, & Seegers, 2007; Rousset et al., 2007; Rousset et al., 2009). Sampling should target a representative number of animals. Serological analyses may be carried out using enzyme-linked immunosorbent assay (ELISA), indirect immunofluorescence assay (IFA) or complement fixation test (CFT). Numerous studies have shown that relative sensitivity is lowest for the CFT, but on the contrary, it has high specificity for high levels of anti-*C. burnetii* antibodies, generated in aborted herds or flocks (Emery et al., 2014; Horigan, Bell, Pollard, Sayers, & Pritchard, 2011; Niemczuk et al., 2014; Rousset et al., 2007; Rousset et al., 2009).

The CFT is the most widely used test in veterinary laboratories, although commercially available ELISA tests for *C. burnetii* antibodies, in ruminants, are increasingly used. Compared to ELISA, the CFT lacks the sensitivity to detect *C. burnetii* specific antibodies in ruminant serum. IFA is the less reproducible test between operators and therefore between laboratories and research institutions. Although ELISA methods are not yet fully validated and harmonised, they are consistent and can be automated. Consequently, ELISA testing is recommended for routine serological screening of animals for Q fever and to date, is considered the most sensitive technique to detect *C. burnetii* specific antibodies (Horigan et al., 2011; Rousset et al., 2009).

Genotyping methods are very useful for epidemiological research, particularly to clarify links to the source of infection, understanding of epidemiological emerging factors, elucidating human outbreaks, and to a lesser extent, for evaluating control measures. Several typing methods have been used for the characterisation of *C. burnetii strains*, such as restriction endonuclease of genomic DNA, pulsed-field gel electrophoresis (PFGE), and sequence and/or restriction fragment length polymorphism (PCR-RFLP) analysis of *icd*, *com1* and *mucZ* genes. More recently, two PCR-based typing methods have been described, multi-locus variable number of tandem repeats analysis (MLVA) and multispacer sequence typing (MST) that permit the typing of *C. burnetii* without the need for isolation of the organism. To date, MLVA and MST are considered to be the most selective methods for *C. burnetii*, allowing the identification of up to 36 distinct genotypes. Additionally, databases have been established and their availability allows inter-laboratory comparisons to be made easily. This enables a better understanding of the propagation of *C. burnetii* isolates (linking outbreaks to their source) or to identify new emerging strains. Standardisation of MLVA is underway and should be available in the near future (World Organisation for Animal Health [OIE], 2015).

For specific laboratory research, it may be necessary to isolate the agent. For low contaminated inoculates of *C. burnetii*, direct isolation by inoculation of embryonated chicken eggs or cell culture is possible, being the latter a superior method (Samuel, & Hendrix, 2009).

Various other methods are or have been evaluated for analysis of *C. burnetii* in different samples, like *in-situ* hybridisation, DNA amplification, fluorescent *in-situ* hybridisation (FISH) and loop mediated isothermal amplification (LAMP) assays (Jensen et al., 2007; Samuel, & Hendrix, 2009).

Disease Control

In common with all zoonotic diseases, control of the disease in animals will influence the level of disease seen in man (Angelakis, & Raoult, 2010). In the case of a Q fever outbreak, sanitary and prophylactic measures should be applied at herd and human level, in order to limit disease transmission. It is mandatory to address the triad of human–animal–environmental aspects and to do an One Health approach in investigation and management of any outbreak (Bond et al., 2016).

Human and animal infections must be diagnosed early and treated immediately to prevent the development of chronic infections and secondary complications (Porter, Czaplicki, Mainil, Guattéo, & Saegerman, 2011). Balancing economic livestock interests and human health is particularly demanding when controlling zoonotic diseases outbreaks, including Q fever (van Asseldonk, Bontje, Backer, van Roermund, & Bergevoet, 2015).

According to the EFSA Panel on AHAW (2010), the choice of a Q fever control strategy will depend on the main objective of the control effort, that can be limited to avoiding the spreading of the disease or attempt the complete eradication of *C. burnetii* infection.

Therapeutic and prophylactic measures in small ruminants are intended to diminish abortion rates and bacterial shedding, thereby aiming to reduce environmental contamination (van den Brom et al., 2015).

In spite of the difficulty to determine susceptibility of *C. burnetii* to antibiotics, antibiotic treatment may be performed to reduce the number of abortions and the quantity of *C. burnetii* shed at parturition (Angelakis, & Raoult, 2010). In ruminants, antibiotic treatment generally consist in administering two injections of oxytetracycline (20 mg per kg body weight), during the last month of gestation, although this treatment does not totally suppress the abortions and the shedding of *C. burnetii* at lambing (Angelakis, & Raoult, 2010; Berri et al., 2007). Abortion in animals can be prevented with vaccination, and it is undoubted that a phase I vaccine must be used to control the disease and to reduce environmental contamination and therefore, the risk of transmission to humans, and might be considered a long-term control policy, especially in heavily infected herds (Angelakis, & Raoult, 2010; EFSA Panel on AHAW, 2010).

In goats, vaccination induces an overall decrease in shedding levels and the highest reduction is found in nulliparous animals (de Cremoux et al., 2012a). Thereby, before the very first pregnancy, the susceptible animals should be vaccinated (Bontje, Backer, Hogerwerf, Roest, & van Roermund, 2016; de Cremoux et al., 2012a).

The efficacy of the phase I vaccine was also studied in naturally infected cows (Guatteo, Seegers, Joly, & Beaudeau, 2008). When vaccinated while not pregnant, an initially non infected animal had a five times lower probability of becoming a shedder than an animal receiving a placebo (EFSA Panel on AHAW, 2010).

Besides antibiotic treatment and vaccination, other preventive measures can be adopted at the farm level, including the removal of risk material (placentas, aborted foetuses), manure management, culling of pregnant animals, identifying and culling of shedders, temporary breeding ban, control of animal movement between farms of differing infection status, appropriate tick control strategies, removing infected animals from herds or providing separate containment facilities in which to give birth, among others (Angelakis, & Raoult, 2010; EFSA Panel on AHAW, 2010).

In humans, regarding the clinical polymorphism of *C. burnetii* infection, there is no single management strategy. Recent studies have revealed that each situation requires specific treatment and follow-up. In case of primary infection, the main issues after diagnosis are screening for potential risk factors for complications and choice of a recommended regimen with doxycycline (200 mg/day) and hydroxychloroquine (600 mg/day), to prevent progression to persistent focalized infection (Eldin et al., 2017). Human Q fever may be prevented with a vaccine developed and commercialized in Australia, where it was used to immunize slaughterhouse personnel. This vaccine must not be administered to individuals having been in contact with *C. burnetii*, because this may lead to serious adverse reactions, such as sterile abscesses or systemic inflammatory syndrome (Parker, Barralet, & Bell, 2006; Schneeberger, Wintenberger, van der Hoek, & Stahl, 2014).

Q FEVER IN PORTUGAL

Q fever was identified for the first time in Portugal in 1948 (Fonseca, Pinto, Azevedo, & Lacerda, 1949a; Fonseca, Pinto, Azevedo, & Lacerda, 1949b). For many years it had been thought that acute Q fever merely expressed itself in Portugal as a pulmonary disease (Fonseca et al., 1949b), but in 1974, the first case with hepatic involvement was identified in the Infectious Diseases Department at Santa Maria's University Hospital (Mendes, Carmona, Malva, & Souza, 1989b). Several seroepidemiological studies have been conducted in Portugal confirming that the disease is endemic in the country (Filipe, Bacellar, & David de Morais, 1990; Mendes et al., 1989a; Parreira, 2008). Q fever is a notifiable disease in Portugal since January 1, 1999 and an average of 0.1 cases per 105 inhabitants per year have been reported (Direção-Geral da Saúde [DGS], 2011).

Unlike in other countries within Europe, where there is a clear trend towards a decrease in the number of human Q fever cases, in Portugal the numbers have been stable which has been reason for alert within Public Health stakeholders (Direção-Geral da Saúde [DGS], 2015; European Centre for Disease Prevention and Control [ECDC], 2014). Although no epidemics have been reported, it is believed that the disease is underdiagnosed and underreported (Palmela, Badura, & Valadas, 2012; Santos, Bacellar, & França, 2007a). For instance, a study performed by the Centre for Vectors and Infectious Diseases of the Ricardo Jorge National Health Institute (CEVDI/INSA) found serological confirmation of 32 cases between 2004 and 2005, as opposed to the 12 cases reported to the General Directorate of Health (DGS) countrywide for the same period (DGS, 2011; Santos et al., 2007a).

Sheep and goat traditional farming and has been widely present in Portugal and is part of the cultural and gastronomical background of the country. This close proximity to small ruminants may contribute to the endemicity of Q fever in Portugal (Alves et al., 2016). In a recent case series describing 7 cases of acute Q fever, admitted in a Portuguese University Hospital, between 2014 and 2015, Alves et al. (2016) have been able to retrieve detailed epidemiological data of all cases, mostly regarding contact or close proximity to sheep, cattle or goats, suggesting aerosol inhalation as the main route of transmission and a strong relationship between disease and occupational exposure (Alves et al., 2016). Risk for environmental exposure to Q fever has been previously pointed in a *Coxiella burnetii* prosthetic valve endocarditis of a 53-year-old patient with recurrent mechanical valve dehiscence on mitral position (Ferraz et al., 2016). This man had lived in a rural area with sheep and goats on the surroundings. Also recently, a study reported 2 rare manifestations of Q fever, namely splenic and hepatic abscesses and cerebral venous thrombosis, in a 47 and a 55-year-old man, both living on the country side and in contact with chicken and other farm animals (Gomes, Chaves, Gouveia, & Santos, 2014).

Nonetheless, a few studies also report disease in those exposed to companion animals. Q fever was detected in a 16-year-old female that presented to the emergency unit of a major Portuguese Hospital, complaining of severe retro-orbital headaches for the previous 6 days, with photophobia and vomiting for 2 days (Figueiredo, Candeias, & Brito, 2016). She used to visit her grandparents in a rural area, where they had 2 dogs. Interestingly, another very recent case report described a 60-year-old man who underwent kidney transplantation with a 34-year-old living donor renal allograft and underwent immunosuppressive therapy, and was only exposed to his cat (no other animal) (Godinho et al, 2015).

More recent attention has been given to Q fever in animals. In two studies, evidence for Q fever in aborted foetuses and in Zoo animals, using PCR technique with primers targeting *C. burnetii* genome (Clemente, Barahona, Andrade, & Botelho, 2009; Clemente, Fernandes, Barahona, Bernardino, & Botelho, 2008). In a later study, Cumbassá et al., (2015) sought evidence for *C. burnetii* infection in domestic, captive and wild animals, having found *C. burnetii* DNA in tissue of domestic, wild and zoo animals (Cumbassá et al, 2015). Simultaneously, a few serosurveys with wider sampling approaches, both in large and small ruminants, have shown *C. burnetii* circulation in Portugal. A 2013 cross-sectional study evaluated the exposure to *C. burnetii* in sheep and goats in the Centre of Portugal (Anastácio, Tavares, Carolino, Sidi-Boumedine, & da Silva, 2013). Results showed a global herd prevalence of 32.6%, higher in mixed herds (38.5%) and in sheep herds (37.5%) than in goat herds (28.8%). Global individual prevalence was estimated at 9.6% being higher in goats (10.4%) than in sheep (8.6%). Interestingly, authors have associated seropositivity to goats, older animals and larger herds. Another study from central Portugal studied bulk tank milk samples from cattle (n = 45) and small ruminant (n = 64) herds by both ELISA and PCR, showing an apparent seroprevalence of 45.9%, being higher in small ruminants (51.6%) than in cattle (37.8%). PCR analysis showed shedding of *C. burnetii* in 11.9% of bulk milk tank samples, being higher in cattle (20%) than in sheep and mixed herds (6.3%) (Anastácio et al., 2013). A study from the same year confirmed results of substantial endemicity of *C. burnetii* (Pimenta et al., 2015). Authors have studied bulk tank milk samples from 90 dairy farms and assayed using an ELISA kit, showing an apparent prevalence of 61.1% (Pimenta et al., 2015). Taken together, these serosurveys show a high level of exposure to *C. burnetii* in Portuguese small and large ruminant herds, proving the need to provide clearer understanding of Q fever epidemiology in Portugal, ideally by implementing monitoring programs on sentinel herds.

CONCLUSION

Coxiella burnetii infection can result in huge economic loss due to epizootic abortions, which are often associated with bacteria shedding in birth fluids and placentas, increasing the risk of infection to humans and animals. Important work has been made to prevent the spread of *C. burnetii* from small ruminants to humans, using either nonspecific and specific measures. However, these efforts have been hindered by the absence of effective veterinary interventions.

The knowledge of the epidemiology and the implementation of measures it seems to be urgent to an effective control, in animals which will have an important impact in the maintenance of human health. Consequently, it's imperative to determine the prevalence of *C. burnetii* infection in portuguese sheeps, evaluating simultaneously the prevalence in occupational portuguese workers, to determine and estimate the real circulation of *C. burnetii* among the risk population, trying, therefore to determine the major types of specific economical loss and the main sources of infection that occur in Portuguese professional workers.

REFERENCES

Abnave, P., Muracciole, X., & Ghigo, E. (2017). *Coxiella burnetii* Lipopolysaccharide: What Do We Know? *International Journal of Molecular Sciences*, *18*(12), 2509. doi:10.3390/ijms18122509 PMID:29168790

Agerholm, J. S. (2013). *Coxiella burnetii* associated reproductive disorders in domestic animals-a critical review. *Acta Veterinaria Scandinavica*, *55*(1), 13. doi:10.1186/1751-0147-55-13 PMID:23419216

Alves, J., Almeida, F., Duro, R., Ferraz, R., Silva, S., Sobrinho-Simões, J., & Sarmento, A. (2016). Presentation and diagnosis of acute Q fever in Portugal — A case series. *IDCases*, *7*, 34–37. doi:10.1016/j.idcr.2016.11.002 PMID:28070491

Anastácio, S., Tavares, N., Carolino, N., Sidi-Boumedine, K., & da Silva, G. J. (2013). Serological evidence of exposure to *Coxiella burnetii* in sheep and goats in central Portugal. *Veterinary Microbiology*, *167*(3-4), 500–505. doi:10.1016/j.vetmic.2013.08.004 PMID:24060100

Angelakis, E., & Raoult, D. (2010). Q fever. *Veterinary Microbiology*, *140*(3-4), 297–309. doi:10.1016/j.vetmic.2009.07.016 PMID:19875249

Arricau-Bouvery, N., & Rodolakis, A. (2005). Is Q fever an emerging or re-emerging zoonosis? *Veterinary Research*, *36*(3), 327–349. doi:10.1051/vetres:2005010 PMID:15845229

Baca, O., Klassen, D., & Aragon, A. (1993). Entry of *Coxiella burnetii* into host cells. *Acta Virologica. English Ed.*, *37*(2–3), 143–155. PMID:8105658

Bartelink, A. K., Stevens, H., van Kregten, E., Meijer, J. G., Beeres, M. P., & van Deuren, M. (2000). Acute and chronic Q fever; epidemiology, symptoms, diagnosis and therapy of infection caused by *Coxiella burnetii. Nederlands Tijdschrift voor Geneeskunde*, *144*(27), 1303–1306. PMID:10918908

Benson, W. W., Brock, D. W., & Mather, J. (1963). Serologic analysis of a penitentiary group using raw milk from a Q fever infected herd. *Public Health Reports*, *78*(8), 707–710. doi:10.2307/4591908 PMID:14049191

Berri, M., Rousset, E., Champion, J. L., Russo, P., & Rodolakis, A. (2007). Goats may experience reproductive failures and shed *Coxiella burnetii* at two successive parturitions after a Q fever infection. *Research in Veterinary Science*, *83*(1), 47–52. doi:10.1016/j.rvsc.2006.11.001 PMID:17187835

Berri, M., Souriau, A., Crosby, M., Crochet, D., Lechopier, P., & Rodolakis, A. (2001). Relationships between the shedding of *Coxiella burnetii*, clinical signs and serological responses of 34 sheep. *The Veterinary Record*, *148*(16), 502–505. doi:10.1136/vr.148.16.502 PMID:11345992

Berri, M., Souriau, A., Crosby, M., & Rodolakis, A. (2002). Shedding of *Coxiella burnetii* in ewes in two pregnancies following an episode of *Coxiella* abortion in a sheep flock. *Veterinary Microbiology*, *85*(1), 55–60. doi:10.1016/S0378-1135(01)00480-1 PMID:11792492

Blood, D. C., & Radostitis, O. M. (1989). *Veterinary Medicine* (7th ed.). London: Bailliere Tindall.

Bond, K. A., Vincent, G., Wilks, C. R., Franklin, L., Sutton, B., Stenos, J., ... Firestone, S. M. (2016). One Health approach to controlling a Q fever outbreak on an Australian goat farm. *Epidemiology and Infection*, *144*(6), 1129–1141. doi:10.1017/S0950268815002368 PMID:26493615

Bontje, D. M., Backer, J. A., Hogerwerf, L., Roest, H. I. J., & van Roermund, H. J. W. (2016). Analysis of Q fever in Dutch dairy goat herds and assessment of control measures by means of a transmission model. *Preventive Veterinary Medicine*, *123*, 71–89. doi:10.1016/j.prevetmed.2015.11.004 PMID:26708798

Capo, C., Lindberg, F. P., Meconi, S., Zaffran, Y., Tardei, G., Brown, E. J., ... Mege, J. L. (1999). Subversion of monocyte functions by *Coxiella burnetii*: Impairment of the cross-talk between αvβ3 integrin and CR3. *Journal of Immunology (Baltimore, Md.: 1950)*, *163*(11), 6078–6085. PMID:10570297

Capo, C., Moynault, A., Collette, Y., Olive, D., Brown, E. J., Raoult, D., & Mege, J.-L. (2003). *Coxiella burnetii* avoids macrophage phagocytosis by interfering with spatial distribution of complement receptor 3. *Journal of Immunology (Baltimore, Md.: 1950)*, *170*(8), 4217–4225. doi:10.4049/jimmunol.170.8.4217 PMID:12682255

Centers for Disease Control and Prevention (CDC). (2017). *Emergency preparedness and response: bioterrorism agents/diseases.* Q fever (Coxiella burnetii). Retrieved December, 15, 2017, from http://www.bt.cdc.gov/agent/agentlist-category.asp

Cerf, O., & Condron, R. (2006). *Coxiella burnetii* and milk pasteurization: An early application of the precautionary principle? *Epidemiology and Infection*, *134*(5), 946–951. doi:10.1017/S0950268806005978 PMID:16492321

Clemente, L., Barahona, M. J., Andrade, M. F., & Botelho, A. (2009). Diagnosis by PCR of *Coxiella burnetii* in aborted fetuses of domestic ruminants in Portugal. *The Veterinary Record*, *164*(12), 373–374. doi:10.1136/vr.164.12.373 PMID:19305010

Clemente, L., Fernandes, T. L., Barahona, M. J., Bernardino, R., & Botelho, A. (2008). Confirmation by PCR of *Coxiella burnetii* infection in animals at a zoo in Lisbon, Portugal. *The Veterinary Record*, *163*(7), 221–222. doi:10.1136/vr.163.7.221 PMID:18708658

Cleveland, K. O. (2017). Q Fever. *Medscape*. Retrieved December 15th, 2017 from https://emedicine.medscape.com/article/227156-overview

Cumbassá, A., Barahona, M. J., Cunha, M. V., Azórin, B., Fonseca, C., Rosalino, L. M., ... Botelho, A. (2015). *Coxiella burnetii* DNA detected in domestic ruminants and wildlife from Portugal. *Veterinary Microbiology*, *180*(1-2), 136–141. doi:10.1016/j.vetmic.2015.07.030 PMID:26345258

de Biase, D., Costagliola, A., Del Piero, F., Di Palo, R., & Coronati, D. Galiero, ... Paciello, O. (2018). *Coxiella burnetii* in Infertile Dairy Cattle with Chronic Endometritis. *Veterinary Pathology*. doi:10.1177/0300985818760376

de Cremoux, R., Rousset, E., Touratier, A., Audusseau, G., Nicollet, P., Ribaud, D., ... Le Pape, M. (2012a). Assessment of vaccination by a phase I *Coxiella burnetii*-inactivated vaccine in goat herds in clinical Q fever situation. *FEMS Immunology and Medical Microbiology*, *64*(1), 104–106. doi:10.1111/j.1574-695X.2011.00892.x PMID:22066485

de Cremoux, R., Rousset, E., Touratier, A., Audusseau, G., Nicollet, P., Ribaud, D., ... Le Pape, M. (2012b). *Coxiella burnetii* vaginal shedding and antibody responses in dairy goat herds in a context of clinical Q fever outbreaks. *FEMS Immunology and Medical Microbiology*, *64*(1), 120–122. doi:10.1111/j.1574-695X.2011.00893.x PMID:22066517

de Rooij, M. M., Borlée, F., Smit, L. A., de Bruin, A., Janse, I., Heederik, D. J., & Wouters, I. M. (2016). Detection of *Coxiella burnetii* in Ambient Air after a Large Q Fever Outbreak. *PLoS One*, *11*(3), e0151281. doi:10.1371/journal.pone.0151281 PMID:26991094

Direção-Geral da Saúde. (2011). *Doenças de Declaração Obrigatória, Direcção-Geral da Saúde, Lisboa, 2000-2004 e 2004 2008*. Retrieved 1, October, from http://www.dgs.pt

Direção-Geral da Saúde. (2015). *Doenças de Notificação Obrigatória (1999 a 2013)*. Available from http://www.dgs.pt

EFSA Panel on Animal Health and Welfare (AHAW). (2010). Scientific Opinion on Q Fever. *EFSA Journal*, *8*(5), 1595. doi:10.2903/j.efsa.2010.1595

Eldin, C., Mélenotte, C., Mediannikov, O., Ghigo, E., Million, M., Edouard, S., ... Raoult, D. (2017). From Q Fever to *Coxiella burnetii* Infection: A Paradigm Change. *Clinical Microbiology Reviews*, *30*(1), 115–190. doi:10.1128/CMR.00045-16 PMID:27856520

Emery, M. P., Ostlund, E. N., Aitichou, M., Ballin, J. D., McFarling, D., & McGonigle, L. (2014). *Coxiella burnetii* serology assays in goat abortion storm. *Journal of Veterinary Diagnostic Investigation*, *26*(1), 141–145. doi:10.1177/1040638713517233 PMID:24532695

European Centre for Disease Prevention and Control (ECDC). (2014). *Annual Epidemiological Report for 2014. Q fever*. Stockholm: ECDC.

Ferraz, R. V., Andrade, M., Silva, F., Andrade, P., Carvalho, C., Torres, J. P., ... Santos, L. (2016). Chronic Q fever: A missed prosthetic valve endocarditis possibly for years. *IDCases*, *6*, 55–57. doi:10.1016/j.idcr.2016.09.005 PMID:27713859

Figueiredo, C., Candeias, F., & Brito, M. J. (2016). Aseptic Meningitis Caused by *Coxiella burnetii*. *The Pediatric Infectious Disease Journal*, *35*(1), 115. doi:10.1097/INF.0000000000000935 PMID:26418239

Filipe, A. R., Bacellar, F., & David de Morais, J. A. (1990). Anticorpos contra *Rickettsieae* na população do sul de Portugal. *Revista Portuguesa de Doenças Infecciosas*, *13*(2), 85–89.

Fonseca, F., Pinto, M. R., Azevedo, J. F., & Lacerda, M. T. (1949a). Febre Q em Portugal. *Clínica Contemporânea*, *3*(21), 1159–1164.

Fonseca, F., Pinto, M. R., Azevedo, J. F., & Lacerda, M. T. (1949b). Febre Q em Portugal. *Clínica Contemporânea*, *3*(22), 1218–1227.

Fournier, P. E., Marrie, T. J., & Raoult, D. (1998). Diagnosis of Q Fever. *Journal of Clinical Microbiology*, *36*(7), 1823–1834. PMID:9650920

Gale, P., Kelly, L., Mearns, R., Duggan, J., & Snary, E. L. (2015). Q fever through consumption of unpasteurised milk and milk products - a risk profile and exposure assessment. *Journal of Applied Microbiology*, *118*(5), 1083–1095. doi:10.1111/jam.12778 PMID:25692216

Galiero, A., Fratini, F., Cammà, C., Di Domenico, M., Curini, V., Baronti, I., ... Cerri, D. (2016). Occurrence of *Coxiella burnetii* in goat and ewe unpasteurized cheeses: Screening and genotyping. *International Journal of Food Microbiology*, *237*, 47–54. doi:10.1016/j.ijfoodmicro.2016.08.008 PMID:27543815

Ghigo, E., Colombo, M. I., & Heinzen, R. A. (2012). The *Coxiella burnetii* parasitophorous vacuole. *Advances in Experimental Medicine and Biology*, *984*, 141–169. doi:10.1007/978-94-007-4315-1_8 PMID:22711631

Ghigo, E., Honstettre, A., Capo, C., Gorvel, J. P., Raoult, D., & Mege, J. L. (2004). Link between impaired maturation of phagosomes and defective *Coxiella burnetii* killing in patients with chronic Q fever. *The Journal of Infectious Diseases, 190*(10), 1767–7. doi:10.1086/425041 PMID:15499532

Godinho, I., Nogueira, E. L., Santos, C. M., Paulo, S. E., Fortes, A., Guerra, J. O., & Gomes da Costa, A. (2015). Chronic Q Fever in a renal transplant recipient: A case report. *Transplantation Proceedings, 47*(4), 1045–1047. doi:10.1016/j.transproceed.2015.03.022 PMID:26036515

Gomes, M. M., Chaves, A., Gouveia, A., & Santos, L. (2014). Two rare manifestations of Q fever: Splenic and hepatic abscesses and cerebral venous thrombosis, with literature review ma non troppo. *BMJ Case Reports, 2014*(feb05 1), bcr2013202843. doi:10.1136/bcr-2013-202843 PMID:24501338

Guatteo, R., Beaudeau, F., Berri, M., Rodolakis, A., Joly, A., & Seegers, H. (2006). Shedding routes of *Coxiella burnetii* in dairy cows: Implications for detection and control. *Veterinary Research, 37*(6), 827–833. doi:10.1051/vetres:2006038 PMID:16973121

Guatteo, R., Beaudeau, F., Joly, A., & Seegers, H. (2007). *Coxiella burnetii* shedding by dairy cows. *Veterinary Research, 38*(6), 849–860. doi:10.1051/vetres:2007038 PMID:17903418

Guatteo, R., Seegers, H., Joly, A., & Beaudeau, F. (2008). Prevention of *Coxiella burnetii* shedding in infected dairy herds using a phase I *C. burnetii* inactivated vaccine. *Vaccine, 26*(34), 4320–4328. doi:10.1016/j.vaccine.2008.06.023 PMID:18586060

Guidi, F., Petruzzelli, A., Ciarrocchi, F., Duranti, A., Valiani, A., Amagliani, G., & Blasi, G. (2017). Prevalence of *Coxiella burnetii* in cows' and ewes' bulk tank milk samples from selected dairy farms of Central Italy. *Italian Journal of Animal Science, 16*(4), 673–676. doi:10.1080/1828051X.2017.1321474

Hackstadt, T., & Williams, J. C. (1981). Biochemical stratagem for obligate parasitism of eukaryotic cells by *Coxiella burnetii. Proceedings of the National Academy of Sciences of the United States of America, 78*(5), 3240–3244. doi:10.1073/pnas.78.5.3240 PMID:6942430

Hatchette, T., Campbell, N., Hudson, R., Raoult, D., & Marrie, T. J. (2003). Natural history of Q fever in goats. *Vector Borne and Zoonotic Diseases (Larchmont, N.Y.), 3*(1), 11–15. doi:10.1089/153036603765627415 PMID:12804376

Horigan, M. W., Bell, M. M., Pollard, T. R., Sayers, A. R., & Pritchard, G. C. (2011). Q fever diagnosis in domestic ruminants: Comparison between complement fixation and commercial enzyme-linked immunosorbent assays. *Journal of Veterinary Diagnostic Investigation*, *23*(5), 924–931. doi:10.1177/1040638711416971 PMID:21908348

Jensen, T. K., Montgomery, D. L., Jaeger, P. T., Lindhardt, T., Agerholm, J. S., Bille-Hansen, V., & Boye, M. (2007). Application of fluorescent *in situ* hybridisation for demonstration of *Coxiella burnetii* in placentas from ruminant abortions. *APMIS: acta pathologica, microbiologica, et immunologica Scandinavica, 115*, 347–353.

Kazar, J. (2005). *Coxiella burnetii* Infection. *Annals of the New York Academy of Sciences*, *1063*(1), 105–114. doi:10.1196/annals.1355.018 PMID:16481501

Khalili, M., Sakhaee, E., & Babaei, H. (2011). Frequency of anti-*Coxiella burnetii* antibodies in cattle with reproductive disorders. *Comparative Clinical Pathology*, *21*(5), 917–919. doi:10.100700580-011-1199-2

Klee, S. R., Tyczka, J., Ellerbrok, H., Franz, T., Linke, S., Baljer, G., & Appel, B. (2006). Highly sensitive real-time PCR for specific detection and quantification of *Coxiella burnetii. BMC Microbiology*, *6*(1), 2. doi:10.1186/1471-2180-6-2 PMID:16423303

Klemmer, J., Njeru, J., Emam, A., El-Sayed, A., Moawad, A. A., Henning, K., ... El-Diasty, M. M. (2018). Q fever in Egypt: Epidemiological survey of *Coxiella burnetii* specific antibodies in cattle, buffaloes, sheep, goats and camels. *PLoS One*, *13*(2), e0192188. doi:10.1371/journal.pone.0192188 PMID:29466380

Koster, F. T., Williams, J. C., & Goodwin, J. S. (1985). Cellular immunity in Q fever: Modulation of responsiveness by a suppressor T cell-monocyte circuit. *Journal of Immunology (Baltimore, Md.: 1950)*, *135*(2), 1067–1072. PMID:2409135

Kovácová, E., & Kazár, J. (2002). Q fever still a query and underestimated infectious disease. *Acta Virologica. English Ed.*, *46*(4), 193–210. PMID:12693856

Lang, G. H. (1990). Coxiellosis (Q fever) in animals. In T. J. Marrie (Ed.), *Q Fever: The Disease* (Vol. 1, pp. 23–48). Boca Raton, FL: CRC Press.

Mangili, P., Amagliani, G., Micci, E., Brandi, G., Foglini, M., Cinti, B., ... Schiavano, G. F. (2016). A model for Coxiella burnetii monitoring in a sheep dairy farm. *JSM Biotechnology & Biomedical Engineering*, *3*, 1050.

Marrie, T. J., Stein, A., Janigan, D., & Raoult, D. (1996). Route of infection determines the clinical manifestations of acute Q fever. *The Journal of Infectious Diseases*, *173*(2), 484–487. doi:10.1093/infdis/173.2.484 PMID:8568318

Maurin, M., & Raoult, D. (1999). Q Fever. *Clinical Microbiology Reviews, 12*(4), 518–553. doi:10.1128/CMR.12.4.518 PMID:10515901

McGavin, M. D., & Zachary, J. F. (2007). *Pathologic basis of veterinary disease* (4th ed.). St. Louis, MO: Mosby.

Mendes, M. R., Carmona, M. H., & Malva, A. (1989). Estudo seroepidemiológico da febre Q numa população urbana e numa população de alto risco do Distrito de Lisboa. *Revista Portuguesa de Doenças Infecciosas, 12*(3), 159–162.

Mendes, M. R., Carmona, M. H., Malva, A., & Souza, R. D. (1989). Febre Q. Estudo retrospec-tivo (casuística do Serviço de Doenças Infecto-Contagiosas do Hospital de Santa Maria). *Revista Portuguesa de Doenças Infecciosas, 12*(3), 149–157.

Muskens, J., Wouda, W., von Bannisseht-Wijsmuller, T., & van Maanen, C. (2012). Prevalence of *Coxiella burnetii* infections in aborted fetuses and stillborn calves. *The Veterinary Record, 170*(10), 260. doi:10.1136/vr.100378 PMID:22186379

Niemczuk, K., Szymańska-Czerwińska, M., Śmietanka, K., & Bocian, Ł. (2014). Comparison of diagnostic potential of serological, molecular and cell culture methods for detection of Q fever in ruminants. *Veterinary Microbiology, 171*(1-2), 147–152. doi:10.1016/j.vetmic.2014.03.015 PMID:24725446

Palmela, C., Badura, R., & Valadas, E. (2012). Acute Q fever in Portugal. Epidemiological and clinical features of 32 hospitalized patients. *Germs, 2*(2), 43–59. doi:10.11599/germs.2012.1013 PMID:24432263

Parker, N. R., Barralet, J. H., & Bell, A. M. (2006). Q fever. *Lancet, 367*(9511), 679–688. doi:10.1016/S0140-6736(06)68266-4 PMID:16503466

Parreira, P. (2008). *Estudo da prevalência de anticorpos anti-Coxiella burnetii numa amostra de dadores de sangue de uma região portuguesa* (Master dissertation). Retrieved from Repositório da Universidade de Lisboa Faculdade de Medicina (FM), Dissertações e Mestrados: http://hdl.handle.net/10451/1035

Pellegrin, M., Delsol, G., Auvergnat, J. C., Familiades, J., Faure, H., Guiu, M., & Voigt, J. J. (1980). Granulomatous hepatitis in Q fever. *Human Pathology, 11*(1), 51–57. doi:10.1016/S0046-8177(80)80105-5 PMID:7364439

Pimenta, L., Alegria, N., Anastácio, S., Sidi-Boumedine, K., da Silva, G., Rabiço, Â., & Simões, J. (2015). Prevalence of *Coxiella burnetii* antibodies in Portuguese dairy cattle herds. *Tropical Animal Health and Production, 47*(1), 227–230. doi:10.100711250-014-0679-1 PMID:25339430

Porter, S. R., Czaplicki, G., Mainil, J., Guattéo, R., & Saegerman, C. (2011). Q Fever: Current State of Knowledge and Perspectives of Research of a Neglected Zoonosis. *International Journal of Microbiology, 248418*. doi:10.1155/2011/248418 PMID:22194752

Rodolakis, A. (2009). Q Fever in dairy animals. *Annals of the New York Academy of Sciences, 1166*(1), 90–93. doi:10.1111/j.1749-6632.2009.04511.x PMID:19538267

Roest, H. I., Post, J., van Gelderen, B., van Zijderveld, F. G., & Rebel, J. M. (2013). Q fever in pregnant goats: Humoral and cellular immune responses. *Veterinary Research*, *44*(1), 67. doi:10.1186/1297-9716-44-67 PMID:23915213

Roest, H.-J., van Gelderen, B., Dinkla, A., Frangoulidis, D., van Zijderveld, F., Rebel, J., & van Keulen, L. (2012). Q Fever in Pregnant Goats: Pathogenesis and Excretion of *Coxiella burnetii. PLoS One*, *7*(11), e48949. doi:10.1371/journal.pone.0048949 PMID:23152826

Rousset, E., Berri, M., Durand, B., Dufour, P., Prigent, M., Delcroix, T., ... Rodolakis, A. (2009). *Coxiella burnetii* Shedding Routes and Antibody Response after Outbreaks of Q Fever-Induced Abortion in Dairy Goat Herds. *Applied and Environmental Microbiology*, *75*(2), 428–433. doi:10.1128/AEM.00690-08 PMID:19011054

Rousset, E., Durand, B., Berri, M., Dufour, P., Prigent, M., Russo, P., ... Aubert, M. F. (2007). Comparative diagnostic potential of three serological tests for abortive Q fever in goat herds. *Veterinary Microbiology*, *124*(3-4), 286–297. doi:10.1016/j.vetmic.2007.04.033 PMID:17532581

Russell-Lodrigue, K. E., Andoh, M., Poels, M. W. J., Shive, H. R., Weeks, B. R., Zhang, G. Q., ... Samuel, J. E. (2009). *Coxiella burnetii* Isolates Cause Genogroup-Specific Virulence in Mouse and Guinea Pig Models of Acute Q Fever. *Infection and Immunity*, *77*(12), 5640–5650. doi:10.1128/IAI.00851-09 PMID:19786560

Russell-Lodrigue, K. E., Zhang, G. Q., McMurray, D. N., & Samuel, J. E. (2006). Clinical and Pathologic Changes in a Guinea Pig Aerosol Challenge Model of Acute Q Fever. *Infection and Immunity*, *74*(11), 6085–6091. doi:10.1128/IAI.00763-06 PMID:17057087

Samuel, J. E., & Hendrix, L. R. (2009). Laboratory maintenance of *Coxiella burnetii. Current Protocols in Microbiology, 6*(C.1), 1–16. doi:10.1002/9780471729259.mc06c01s15

Sanchez, J., Souriau, A., Buendia, A. J., Arricau-Bouvery, N., Martínez, C. M., Salinas, J., ... Navarro, J. A. (2006). Experimental *Coxiella burnetii* infection in pregnant goats: A histopathological and immunohistochemical study. *Journal of Comparative Pathology*, *135*(2-3), 108–115. doi:10.1016/j.jcpa.2006.06.003 PMID:16997003

Santos, A. S., Bacellar, F., & França, A. (2007a). Febre Q: Revisão de conceitos. *Revue de Médecine Interne*, *14*(2), 90–99.

Santos, A. S., de Sousa, R., Alves, F., Proença, P., Núncio, M. S., Dumler, J. S., & Bacellar, F. (2007b). Isolation of *Coxiella burnetii* from the blood of a patient with positive Anaplasma phagocytophilum serological results. *Clinical Microbiology and Infection*, *15*, 192–193. doi:10.1111/j.1469-0691.2008.02222.x PMID:19416284

Schneeberger, P. M., Wintenberger, C., van der Hoek, W., & Stahl, J. P. (2014). Q fever in the Netherlands - 2007–2010: What we learned from the largest outbreak ever. *Medecine et Maladies Infectieuses*, *44*(8), 339–353. doi:10.1016/j.medmal.2014.02.006 PMID:25108615

Shannon, J. G., & Heinzen, R. A. (2009). Adaptive Immunity to the Obligate Intracellular Pathogen *Coxiella burnetii. Immunologic Research*, *43*(1-3), 138–148. doi:10.100712026-008-8059-4 PMID:18813881

Siciliano, R., Barbosa Ribeiro, H., Furtado, R. H. M., Castelli, J., Sampaio, R., Santos, F., ... Strabelli, T. (2008). Endocardite por *Coxiella burnetii* (febre Q): Doença rara ou pouco diagnosticada? Relato dc caso. *Revista da Sociedade Brasileira de Medicina Tropical*, *41*(4), 409–412. doi:10.1590/S0037-86822008000400017 PMID:18853017

Sidi-Boumedine, K., Rousset, E., Henning, K., Ziller, M., Niemczuck, K., Roest, H. I. J., & Thiéry, R. (2010). *Development of harmonised schemes for the monitoring and reporting of Q-fever in animals in the European Union.* EFSA Scientific Report on Question No EFSA-Q-2009-00511. Retrieved 15, December, from https://efsa.onlinelibrary.wiley.com/doi/epdf/10.2903/sp.efsa.2010.EN-48

The Center for Food Security and Public Health (CFSPH). (2017). *Q fever*. Retrieved in April 24, 2018, from http://www.cfsph.iastate.edu/Factsheets/pdfs/q_fever.pdf

Tissot Dupont, H., Raoult, D., Brouqui, P., Janbon, F., Peyramond, D., Weiller, P. J., ... Poirier, R. (1992). Epidemiologic features and clinical presentation of acute Q fever in hospitalized patients: 323 French cases. *The American Journal of Medicine*, *93*(4), 427–434. doi:10.1016/0002-9343(92)90173-9 PMID:1415306 van Asseldonk, M. A. P. M., Bontje, D. M., Backer, J. A., van Roermund, H. J. W., & Bergevoet, R. H. M. (2015). Economic aspects of Q fever control in dairy goats. *Preventive Veterinary Medicine*, *121*(1-2), 115–122. doi:10.1016/j.prevetmed.2015.06.010 PMID:26164531

van den Brom, R., van Engelen, E., Roest, H. I., van der Hoek, W., & Vellema, P. (2015). *Coxiella burnetii* infections in sheep or goats: An opinionated review. *Veterinary Microbiology*, *181*(1-2), 119–129. doi:10.1016/j.vetmic.2015.07.011 PMID:26315774

van der Hoek, W., Dijkstra, F., Schimmer, B., Schneeberger, P. M., Vellema, P., Wijkmans, C., ... van Duynhoven, Y. (2010). Q fever in the Netherlands: An update on the epidemiology and control measures. *Eurosurveillance*, *15*(12), 19520. PMID:20350500

van Schaik, E. J., Chen, C., Mertens, K., Weber, M. M., & Samuel, J. E. (2013). Molecular pathogenesis of the obligate intracellular bacterium *Coxiella burnetii*. *Nature Reviews. Microbiology*, *11*(8), 561–573. doi:10.1038/nrmicro3049 PMID:23797173

Vanderburg, S., Rubach, M. P., Halliday, J. E., Cleaveland, S., Reddy, E. A., & Crump, J. A. (2014). Epidemiology of Coxiella burnetii infection in Africa: A OneHealth systematic review. *PLoS Neglected Tropical Diseases*, *8*(4), e2787. doi:10.1371/journal.pntd.0002787 PMID:24722554

Woldehiwet, Z. (2004). Q fever (coxiellosis): Epidemiology and pathogenesis. *Research in Veterinary Science*, *77*(2), 93–100. doi:10.1016/j.rvsc.2003.09.001 PMID:15196898

World Organisation for Animal Health (OIE). (2015). Manual of Diagnostic Tests and Vaccines for Terrestrial Animals 2015. *Terrestrial Manual*. Retrieved from http://www.oie.int/fileadmin/Home/eng/Health_standards/tahm/2.01.16_Q_FEVER.pdf

Wouda, W., & Dercksen, D. P. (2007). Abortion and stillbirth among dairy goats as a consequence of *Coxiella burnetii*. *Tijdschrift voor Diergeneeskunde*, *132*(23), 908–911. PMID:18085173

Compilation of References

(2005). Centers for Disease Control and Prevention Fatal rat-bite fever—Florida and Washington, 2003. *MMWR. Morbidity and Mortality Weekly Report*, *53*, 1198–1202. PMID:15635289

(2005). Centers for Disease Control and Prevention Outbreak of multidrug-resistant *Salmonella typhimurium* associated with rodents purchased at retail pet stores—United States, December 2003–October 2004. *MMWR. Morbidity and Mortality Weekly Report*, *54*, 429–433. PMID:15889011

(2005). Centers for Disease Control and Prevention Salmonellosis associated with pet turtles—Wisconsin and Wyoming, 2004. *MMWR. Morbidity and Mortality Weekly Report*, *54*, 223–226. PMID:15758895

Abnave, P., Muracciole, X., & Ghigo, E. (2017). *Coxiella burnetii* Lipopolysaccharide: What Do We Know? *International Journal of Molecular Sciences*, *18*(12), 2509. doi:10.3390/ijms18122509 PMID:29168790

Abu-Madi, M. A., Behnke, J. M., Boughattas, S., Al-Thani, A., Doiphode, S. H., & Deshmukh, A. (2016). Helminth infections among long-term-residents and settled immigrants in Qatar in the decade from 2005 to 2014: Temporal trends and varying prevalence among subjects from different regional origins. *Parasites & Vectors*, *9*(1), 153. doi:10.118613071-016-1433-5 PMID:26984202

Acha, P. N., & Szyfres, B. (2003). *Zoonoses and Communicable Diseases Common to Man and Animals* (Vol. 1-3). Washington, DC: Pan-American Health Organization.

Agerholm, J. S. (2013). *Coxiella burnetii* associated reproductive disorders in domestic animals-a critical review. *Acta Veterinaria Scandinavica*, *55*(1), 13. doi:10.1186/1751-0147-55-13 PMID:23419216

Agrawal, M. (2012). *Schistosomes and Schistosomiasis in South Asia*. New Delhi: Springer. doi:10.1007/978-81-322-0539-5

Ainsworth, G. C. (2003). Fungus Poisoning. In K. F. Kiple (Ed.), *The Cambridge historical dictionary of disease* (pp. 132–134). Cambridge, UK: Cambridge University Press.

Alho, A. M., Lima, C., Colella, V., Madeira de Carvalho, L., Otranto, D., & Cardoso, L. (2018). Awareness of zoonotic diseases and parasite control practices: A survey of dog and cat owners in Qatar. *Parasites & Vectors*, *11*(1), 133. doi:10.118613071-018-2720-0 PMID:29554937

Allen, H. A. (2015). Characterizing zoonotic disease detection in the United States: Who detects zoonotic disease outbreaks & how fast are they detected? *Journal of Infection and Public Health*, *8*(2), 194–201. doi:10.1016/j.jiph.2014.09.009 PMID:25488822

Allen-Scott, L. K., Buntain, B., Hatfield, J. M., Meisser, A., & Thomas, C. J. (2015). Academic institutions and one health: Building capacity for transdisciplinary research approaches to address complex health issues at the animal-human-ecosystem interface. *Acod Med.*, *90*(7), 866–871. doi:10.1097/ACM.0000000000000639 PMID:25650827

Alves, J., Almeida, F., Duro, R., Ferraz, R., Silva, S., Sobrinho-Simões, J., & Sarmento, A. (2016). Presentation and diagnosis of acute Q fever in Portugal — A case series. *IDCases*, *7*, 34–37. doi:10.1016/j.idcr.2016.11.002 PMID:28070491

Amábile-Cuevas, C. F. (2012). Antibiotic Resistance: From Darwin to Lederberg to Keynes. *Microbial Drug Resistance (Larchmont, N.Y.)*, *19*(2), 73–87. doi:10.1089/mdr.2012.0115 PMID:23046150

Anastácio, S., Tavares, N., Carolino, N., Sidi-Boumedine, K., & da Silva, G. J. (2013). Serological evidence of exposure to *Coxiella burnetii* in sheep and goats in central Portugal. *Veterinary Microbiology*, *167*(3-4), 500–505. doi:10.1016/j.vetmic.2013.08.004 PMID:24060100

Andersson, D. I., & Hughes, D. (2014). Microbiological effects of sublethal levels of antibiotics. *Nature Reviews. Microbiology*, *12*(7), 465–478. doi:10.1038/nrmicro3270 PMID:24861036

Angelakis, E., & Raoult, D. (2010). Q fever. *Veterinary Microbiology*, *140*(3-4), 297–309. doi:10.1016/j.vetmic.2009.07.016 PMID:19875249

Angen, Ø., Ståhl, M., Agerholm, J. S., Christoffersen, A. B., & Agger, J. F. (2011). Dynamics of relationship between the presence of Coxiella burnetii DNA, antibodies, and intrinsic variables in cow milk and bulk tank milk from Danish dairy cattle. *Journal of Dairy Science*, *94*(12), 5750–5759. doi:10.3168/jds.2011-4197 PMID:22118065

Anonymous. (2011). *Compassion in World Farming. Antibiotics in Farm Animal Production*. Public Health and Animal Welfare. Compassion in World Farming. Retrieved from http://www.fao.org/fileadmin/user_upload/animalwelfare/antibiotics in animal farming.pdf

Arricau-Bouvery, N., & Rodolakis, A. (2005). Is Q fever an emerging or re-emerging zoonosis? *Veterinary Research*, *36*(3), 327–349. doi:10.1051/vetres:2005010 PMID:15845229

Asante, M. (2000). *The Egyptian philosophers: Ancient African voices from Imhotep to Akhenaten*. Chicago, IL: African American Images.

Asnis, D. S., Conetta, R., Teizeira, A. A., Waldman, G., & Sampson, B. A. (2000). The West Nile outbreak of 1999 in New York: The Flushing Hospital experience. *Clinical Infectious Diseases*, *30*(3), 413–418. doi:10.1086/313737 PMID:10722421

Astobiza, I., Ruiz-Fons, F., Pinero, A., Barandika, J. F., Hurtado, A., & García-Perez, A. L. (2012). Estimation of *Coxiella burnetii* prevalence in dairy cattle in intensive systems by serological and molecular analyses of bulk-tank milk samples. *Journal of Dairy Science*, *95*(4), 1632–1638. doi:10.3168/jds.2011-4721 PMID:22459811

Atlas, R. M. (2013). One Health: Its Origins and Future. In J.S. Mackenzie, M. Jeggo, P. Daszak, & J.A. Richt (Eds.), The Concept and Examples of a One Health Approach = One Health: The Human-Animal-Environment Interfaces in Emerging Infectious Diseases, vol. 1 = Current Topics in Microbiology and Immunologie (pp. 1-13). Berlin, Germany: Springer. doi:10.1007/82_2012_223

Aubry-Damon, H., Grenet, K., Sall-Ndiaye, P., Che, D., Cordeiro, E., Bougnoux, M. E., ... Andremont, A. (2004). Antimicrobial resistance in commensal flora of pig farmers. *Emerging Infectious Diseases*, *10*(5), 873–879. doi:10.3201/eid1005.030735 PMID:15200822

Aucken, H. M., & Pitt, T. L. (1993). Lipopolysaccharide profile typing as a technique for comparative typing of gram-negative bacteria. *Journal of Clinical Microbiology*, *31*(5), 1286–1289. PMID:7684751

Baca, O. G., & Paretsky, D. (1983). Q fever and *Coxiella burnetii*: A model for host-parasite interactions. *Microbiological Reviews*, *47*(2), 127–149. PMID:6348504

Baca, O., Klassen, D., & Aragon, A. (1993). Entry of *Coxiella burnetii* into host cells. *Acta Virologica. English Ed.*, *37*(2–3), 143–155. PMID:8105658

Barber, M., & Rozwadowska-Dowzenko, M. (1948). Infection by penicillin-resistant *Staphylococci*. *Lancet*, *2*(6530), 641–644. doi:10.1016/S0140-6736(48)92166-7 PMID:18890505

Barbour, A.G. (1998). Fall and rise of Lyme disease and other Ixodes tick-borne infections in North America and Europe. *Br Med Bull.*, *54*, 647-58.

Bardosh, K., & Thys, S. (2012). *Socio-cultural research on neglected zoonoses in Africa: a literature review analysis*. Poster presented at the Ecohealth conference, Kunming, India.

Barger, G. (1931). *Ergot and Ergotism. A monograph based on the Dohme lectures delivered in Johns Hopkins University, Baltimore*. London, UK: Gurney & Jackson. Retrieved from http://ergotism.info/en/1931_barger_ergotism.htm

Bartelink, A.K., Stevens, H., van Kregten, E., Meijer, J.G., Beeres, M.P., & van Deuren, M. (2000). Acute and chronic Q fever; epidemiology, symptoms, diagnosis and therapy of infection caused by Coxiella burnetii. *Ned Tijdschr Geneeskd*, *144*(27), 1303-6.

Bartelink, A. K., Stevens, H., van Kregten, E., Meijer, J. G., Beeres, M. P., & van Deuren, M. (2000). Acute and chronic Q fever; epidemiology, symptoms, diagnosis and therapy of infection caused by *Coxiella burnetii*. *Nederlands Tijdschrift voor Geneeskunde*, *144*(27), 1303–1306. PMID:10918908

Bartelink, A. K., & van Kregten, E. (1995). *Streptococcus suis* as threat to pig-farmers and abattoir workers. *Lancet*, *346*(8991-8992), 1707. doi:10.1016/S0140-6736(95)92874-X PMID:8551847

Bartlett, P. C., & Judge, L. J. (1997). The role of epidemiology in public health. *Revue Scientifique et Technique OIE*, *16*(2), 331–336. doi:10.20506/rst.16.2.1020 PMID:9501345

Bauer, V. H. (1973). *Das Antoniusfeuer in Kunst und Medizin*. Berlin: Springer Verlag. doi:10.1007/978-3-642-65768-9

Beare, P. A., Jeffrey, B. M., Long, C. M., Martens, C. M., & Heinzen, R. A. (2018). Genetic mechanisms of *Coxiella burnetii* lipopolysaccharide phase variation. *PLoS Pathogens*, *14*(3), e1006922. doi:10.1371/journal.ppat.1006922 PMID:29481553

Béchir, M., Schelling, E., Wyss, K., Daugla, D. M., Daoud, S., Tanner, M., & Zinsstag, J. (2004). Approche novatrice des vaccinations en santé publique et en médecine vétérinaire chez les pasteurs nomades au Tchad: Expériences et coûts. *Medecine Tropicale*, *64*(5), 497–502. PMID:15771021

Beetz, A., Uvnas-Moberg, K., Henri, J., & Kotrschal, K. (2012). Psychological and psycho-physiological effects of human-animal interactions: The possible role of oxytocin. *Frontiers in Psychology*, *3*. doi:10.3389/fpsyg.2012.00234

Bennett, S., Woods, T., Liyanage, W. M., & Smith, D. L. (1991). A simplified general method for cluster-sample surveys of health in developing countries. *World Health Statistics Quarterly*, *44*, 98–106. PMID:1949887

Benson, W. W., Brock, D. W., & Mather, J. (1963). Serologic analysis of a penitentiary group using raw milk from a Q fever infected herd. *Public Health Reports*, *78*(8), 707–710. doi:10.2307/4591908 PMID:14049191

Berger, S. (2009). *Bakterien in Krieg und Frieden. Eine Geschichte der medizinischen Bakteriologie in Deutschland, 1890-1933*. Göttingen, Germany: Wallstein.

Bergey, D. H., Krieg, N. R., & Holt, J. G. (1984). *Bergey's manual of systematic bacteriology*. Baltimore, MD: Williams & Wilkins.

Berón, W., Gutierrez, M. G., Rabinovitch, M., & Colombo, M. I. (2002). *Coxiella burnetii* Localizes in a Rab7-Labeled Compartment with Autophagic Characteristics. *Infection and Immunity*, *70*(10), 5816–5821. doi:10.1128/IAI.70.10.5816-5821.2002 PMID:12228312

Berri, M., Rousset, E., Champion, J. L., Russo, P., & Rodolakis, A. (2007). Goats may experience reproductive failures and shed *Coxiella burnetii* at two successive parturitions after a Q fever infection. *Research in Veterinary Science*, *83*(1), 47–52. doi:10.1016/j.rvsc.2006.11.001 PMID:17187835

Berri, M., Souriau, A., Crosby, M., Crochet, D., Lechopier, P., & Rodolakis, A. (2001). Relationships between the shedding of *Coxiella burnetii*, clinical signs and serological responses of 34 sheep. *The Veterinary Record*, *148*(16), 502–505. doi:10.1136/vr.148.16.502 PMID:11345992

Berri, M., Souriau, A., Crosby, M., & Rodolakis, A. (2002). Shedding of *Coxiella burnetii* in ewes in two pregnancies following an episode of *Coxiella* abortion in a sheep flock. *Veterinary Microbiology*, *85*(1), 55–60. doi:10.1016/S0378-1135(01)00480-1 PMID:11792492

Bewley, K. R. (2013). Animal Models of Q Fever (*Coxiella burnetii*). *Comparative Medicine*, *63*(6), 469–476. PMID:24326221

Bhat, A. H., Ganguly, B., Tiwari, A. K., & Das, A. K. (2017). *Canine Pravovirus ns1 gene and hicken Anemia vp3 gene induce partial oncolysis of Canine Transmissible Venereal Tumor*. Scientific Reports 7. Retrieved from https://www.nature.com/articles/s41598-017-15734-6

Blood, D. C., & Radostitis, O. M. (1989). *Veterinary Medicine* (7th ed.). London: Bailliere Tindall.

Boden, K., Wolf, K., Hermann, B., & Frangoulidis, D. (2015). First isolation of *Coxiella burnetii* from clinical material by cell-free medium (ACCM2). *European Journal of Clinical Microbiology & Infectious Diseases*, *34*(5), 1017–1022. doi:10.100710096-015-2321-1 PMID:25876216

Bond, K. A., Vincent, G., Wilks, C. R., Franklin, L., Sutton, B., Stenos, J., ... Firestone, S. M. (2016). One Health approach to controlling a Q fever outbreak on an Australian goat farm. *Epidemiology and Infection*, *144*(6), 1129–1141. doi:10.1017/S0950268815002368 PMID:26493615

Bonfoh, B., Kasymbekov, J., Durr, S., Toktobaev, N., Doherr, M. G., Schueth, T., ... Schelling, E. (2012). Representative seroprevalences of brucellosis in humans and livestock in Kyrgyzstan. *EcoHealth*, *9*(2), 132–138. doi:10.100710393-011-0722-x PMID:22143553

Bonfoh, B., Wasem, A., Traoré, A. N., Fané, A., Spillmann, H., Simbé, C. F., ... Zinsstag, J. (2003). Microbiological quality of cows' milk taken at different intervals from the udder to the selling point in Bamako (Mali). *Food Control*, *14*(7), 495–500. doi:10.1016/S0956-7135(02)00109-3

Bontje, D. M., Backer, J. A., Hogerwerf, L., Roest, H. I. J., & van Roermund, H. J. W. (2016). Analysis of Q fever in Dutch dairy goat herds and assessment of control measures by means of a transmission model. *Preventive Veterinary Medicine*, *123*, 71–89. doi:10.1016/j.prevetmed.2015.11.004 PMID:26708798

Brennan, R. E., Russell, K., Zhang, G., & Samuel, J. E. (2004). Both Inducible Nitric Oxide Synthase and NADPH Oxidase Contribute to the Control of Virulent Phase I *Coxiella burnetii* Infections. *Infection and Immunity*, *72*(11), 6666–6675. doi:10.1128/IAI.72.11.6666-6675.2004 PMID:15501800

Bresalier, M., Cassidy, A., & Woods, A. (2015). One Health in History. In J. Zinsstag, E. Schelling, D. Waltner-Toews, M. Whittacker, & M. Tanner (Eds.), *One Health. The Theory and Practice of Integrated Health Approaches* (pp. 1–15). Wallingford, UK: CABI. doi:10.1079/9781780643410.0001

Bruchhausen, W. (2006). Medizin zwischen den Welten. Geschichte und Gegenwart des medizinischen Pluralismus im südöstlichen Tansania. Göttingen, Germany: v&r unipress/Bonn University Press.

Burnet, F. M., & Freeman, M. (1937). Experimental studies on the virus of Q fever. *The Medical Journal of Australia*, *2*, 299–302.

Burnham, G., Lafta, R., Doocy, S., & Roberts, L. (2006). Mortality after the 2003 invasion of Iraq: A cross-sectional cluster sample survey. *Lancet*, *368*(9545), 1421–1428. doi:10.1016/S0140-6736(06)69491-9 PMID:17055943

Byers, K. B., & Harding, A. L. (2006). Epidemiology of laboratory associated infections. In Biological Safety Principles and Practices (pp. 53–77). American Society of Microbiology.

Canadian Integrated Program for Antimicrobial Resistance Surveillance (CIPARS). (2007) *Salmonella Heidelberg ceftiofur-related resistance in human and retail chicken isolates*. Available at: http://www.phac-aspc. gc.ca/cipars-picra/heidelberg/heidelberg-eng.php

Capo, C., Lindberg, F. P., Meconi, S., Zaffran, Y., Tardei, G., Brown, E. J., ... Mege, J. L. (1999). Subversion of monocyte functions by *Coxiella burnetii*: Impairment of the cross-talk between αvβ3 integrin and CR3. *Journal of Immunology (Baltimore, Md.: 1950)*, *163*(11), 6078–6085. PMID:10570297

Capo, C., Moynault, A., Collette, Y., Olive, D., Brown, E. J., Raoult, D., & Mege, J.-L. (2003). *Coxiella burnetii* avoids macrophage phagocytosis by interfering with spatial distribution of complement receptor 3. *Journal of Immunology (Baltimore, Md.: 1950)*, *170*(8), 4217–4225. doi:10.4049/jimmunol.170.8.4217 PMID:12682255

Carmichael, A. (1993). Bubonic Plague. In K. F. Kiple (Ed.), *The Cambridge world history of human disease* (pp. 628–631). Cambridge, UK: Cambridge University Press. doi:10.1017/CHOL9780521332866.083

Cassidy, A. (2016). One Medicine? Advocating (Inter)disciplinarity at the Interfaces of Animal Health, Human Health, and the Environment. In S. Frickel, M. Albert, & B. Prainsack (Eds.), *Investigating Interdisciplinary Collaboration. Theory and Practice across Disciplines* (pp. 213–236). New Brunswick, NJ: Rutgers University Press.

Centers for Disease Control and Prevention (CDC). (2017). *Emergency preparedness and response: bioterrorism agents/diseases.* Q fever (Coxiella burnetii). Retrieved December, 15, 2017, from http://www.bt.cdc.gov/agent/agentlist-category.asp

Centers for Disease Control and Prevention Update. (2003). multistate outbreak of monkeypox—Illinois, Indiana, Kansas, Missouri, Ohio, and Wisconsin, 2003. *MMWR. Morbidity and Mortality Weekly Report*, *52*, 642–646. PMID:12855947

Cerf, O., & Condron, R. (2006). *Coxiella burnetii* and milk pasteurization: An early application of the precautionary principle? *Epidemiology and Infection*, *134*(5), 946–951. doi:10.1017/S0950268806005978 PMID:16492321

Chandler, M., & Day, M. (2017). Obesity and associated co-morbidities in people and companion animals: A One Health Prespective. *Journal of Comparative Pathology*, *156*(4), 296–309. doi:10.1016/j.jcpa.2017.03.006 PMID:28460795

Chaumartin, H. (1946). *Le mal des ardents et le feu Saint-Antoine. Etude historique médicale, hagiographique et légendaire*. Vienne, France: Imprimerie Ternet-Martin.

Chen, W., Fang, T., Zhou, X., Zhang, D., Shi, X., & Shi, C. (2016). IncHI2 plasmids Are predominant in antibiotic resistant *Salmonella* Isolates. *Frontiers in Microbiology*, *7*, 1566. doi:10.3389/fmicb.2016.01566 PMID:27746775

Cherniack, E. P., & Chernuack, A. R. (2014). The benefits of pets and animal assisted therapy to the health of older individuals. *Current Gerontology and Geriatrics Research*, *2014*, 623203. doi:10.1155/2014/623203 PMID:25477957

Chevalier, V., de la Rocque, S., Baldet, T., Vial, L., & Roger, F. (2004). Epidemiological processes involved in the emergence of vector-borne diseases: West Nile fever, Rift Valley fever, Japanese encephalitis and Crimean-Congo haemorrhagic fever. *Rev sci tech Off Int Epiz, 23*(2), 535-555.

Chien, Y.-J. (2013). How did international agencies perceive the avian influenza problem? The adoption and manufacture of the 'One World, One Health' framework. *Sociology of Health & Illness*, *35*(2), 213–226. doi:10.1111/j.1467-9566.2012.01534.x PMID:23095003

Chmielewski, T., & Tylewska-Wierzbanowska, S. (2012). Q Fever at the Turn of the Century. *Polish Journal of Microbiology*, *61*(2), 81–93. PMID:23163207

Cipolla, Bonizzi, & Zecconi. (2011). *From "One Health" to "One Communication": The Contribution of Communication in Veterinary Medicine to Public Health Report of an informal expert consultation*. Academic Press.

Cleaveland, S., Fevre, E. M., Kaare, M., & Coleman, P. G. (2002). Estimating human rabies mortality in the United Republic of Tanzania from dog bite injuries. *Bulletin of the World Health Organization*, *80*, 304–310. PMID:12075367

Cleaveland, S., Laurenson, M. K., & Taylor, L. H. (2001). Diseases of humans and their domestic mammals: Pathogen characteristics, host range and the risk of emergence. *Philosophical Transactions of the Royal Society of London. Series B, Biological Sciences*, *356*(1411), 991–999. doi:10.1098/rstb.2001.0889 PMID:11516377

Clemente, L., Barahona, M. J., Andrade, M. F., & Botelho, A. (2009). Diagnosis by PCR of *Coxiella burnetii* in aborted fetuses of domestic ruminants in Portugal. *The Veterinary Record*, *164*(12), 373–374. doi:10.1136/vr.164.12.373 PMID:19305010

Clemente, L., Fernandes, T. L., Barahona, M. J., Bernardino, R., & Botelho, A. (2008). Confirmation by PCR of *Coxiella burnetii* infection in animals at a zoo in Lisbon, Portugal. *The Veterinary Record*, *163*(7), 221–222. doi:10.1136/vr.163.7.221 PMID:18708658

Cleveland, K. O. (2017). Q Fever. *Medscape*. Retrieved December 15th, 2017 from https://emedicine.medscape.com/article/227156-overview

Clifford, D. L., Kazwala, R. R., Sadiki, H., Roug, A., Muse, E. A., Coppolillo, P. C., & Mazet, J. A. (2013). Tuberculosis infection in wildlife from the Ruaha ecosystem Tanzania: Implications for wildlife, domestic animals, and human health. *Epidemiology and Infection*, *141*(07), 1371–1381. doi:10.1017/S0950268813000836 PMID:23601163

Coelho, A. C., & García Díez, J. (2015). Biological Risks and Laboratory-Acquired Infections: A Reality That Cannot be Ignored in Health Biotechnology. *Frontiers in Bioengineering and Biotechnology*, *3*, 56. doi:10.3389/fbioe.2015.00056 PMID:25973418

Coetzee, J., Corcoran, C., Prentice, E., Moodley, M., Mendelson, M., Poirel, L., ... Brink, A. J. (2016). Emergence of plasmid-mediated colistin resistance (MCR-1) among *Escherichia coli* isolated from South African patients. *South African Medical Journal*, *106*(5), 449–450. doi:10.7196/SAMJ.2016.v106i5.10710 PMID:27138657

Colville, J. L., & Berryhill, D. L. (2007). *Handbook of Zoonoses: Identification and Prevention*. St. Louis, MO: Mosby, Inc.

Cook, R. A., Karesh, W. B., & Osofsky, S. A. (Eds.). (2004). *The Manhattan Principles on 'One World One Health*. New York, NY: Wildlife Conservation Society.

Costa, D., Poeta, P., Saenz, Y., Vinue, L., Rojo-Bezares, B., Jouini, A., ... Torres, C. (2007). Detection of *Escherichia coli* harbouring extended-spectrum β-lactamases of the CTX-M, TEM and SHV classes in faecal samples of wild animals in Portugal. *The Journal of Antimicrobial Chemotherapy*, *59*, 1311–1312. PMID:17023496

Coughlin, S. S. (2006). Ethical issues in epidemiologic research and public health practice. *Emerging Themes in Epidemiology*, *3*(1), 16. doi:10.1186/1742-7622-3-16 PMID:17018147

Courtenay, M., Sweeney, J., Zielinska, P., Brown, B. S., & La Ragione, R. (2015). One Health: An opportunity For an inter-professional approach to health care. *Journal of Interprofessional Care*, *29*(6), 641–642. doi:10.3109/13561820.2015.1041584 PMID:26652637

Courvalin, P. (2008). Predictable and unpredictable evolution of antibiotic resistance. *Journal of Internal Medicine*, *264*(1), 4–16. doi:10.1111/j.1365-2796.2008.01940.x PMID:18397243

Cox, H. R. (1941). Cultivation of rickettsiae of the rocky mountain spotted fever, typhus and Q fever groups in the embryonic tissues of developing chicks. *Science*, *94*(2444), 399–403. doi:10.1126cience.94.2444.399 PMID:17798222

Craddock, S. (2014). Precarious connections: Making therapeutic production happen for malaria and tuberculosis. *Social Science & Medicine*, *129*, 36–43. doi:10.1016/j.socscimed.2014.07.039 PMID:25142906

Craddock, S., & Hinchliffe, S. (2015). One world, one health? Social science engagements with the one health agenda. *Social Science & Medicine, 129*, 1–4. doi:10.1016/j.socscimed.2014.11.016 PMID:25434985

Cumbassá, A., Barahona, M. J., Cunha, M. V., Azórin, B., Fonseca, C., Rosalino, L. M., ... Botelho, A. (2015). *Coxiella burnetii* DNA detected in domestic ruminants and wildlife from Portugal. *Veterinary Microbiology, 180*(1-2), 136–141. doi:10.1016/j.vetmic.2015.07.030 PMID:26345258

da Costa, P. M., Loureiro, L., & Matos, A. J. F. (2013). Transfer of multi-drug resistant bacteria between intermingled ecological niches: The interface between humans, animals and the environment. *International Journal of Environmental Research and Public Health, 10*(1), 278–294. doi:10.3390/ijerph10010278 PMID:23343983

Danta-Torres, F., Chomel, B., & Otranto, D. (2012). Ticks and tick-borne diseases: A One Health perspective. *Trends in Parasitology, 28*(10), 437–446. doi:10.1016/j.pt.2012.07.003 PMID:22902521

Das, U. (2004). *Health and Environment: Challenges and Strategics*. Compendium of 6th Assoc. of Public Health Veterinarians conference, Nimpith, Sunderbans, India.

Das, U. (2006). *Community participation and rural health care with reference to role of professional organizations*. Compendium of 7th Association of Public Health Veterinarians Conference, Bhubaneswar, India.

Das, U. (2015a). *Therapeutic Veterinary Public Health—A new concept in Human Health Care*. Brochure of 14th World Congress on Public Health, Kolkata, India. Abs. No. 797, 75.

Das, U. (2015b). *Utilization of dog in Therapeutic Veterinary Public Health—The Subject of Tomorrow*. Compendium of 12th Convention of Indian Society for Advancement of Canine Practice, Allahabad, India.

Das, U. (2015c). Genesis of 'Veterinary Public Health'and Route to 'One Health'. *Intas Polivet, 16*, 182–186.

Das, U. (2017). *Shaping Veterinary Public Health in New Dimension. In Veterinary Public Health: One Health 1st edition* (pp. 213–217). New Delhi, India: New Delhi Publishers.

Das, U., & Das, A. K. (2000). Review of canine transmissible venereal sarcoma. *Veterinary Research Communications*, *24*(8), 545–556. doi:10.1023/A:1006491918910 PMID:11305746

Das, U., & Mukherjee, B. (2006). Pet therapy—A new concept in human health care. *Intas Polivet*, *7*, 198–199.

Daszak, P. (2000). Emerging infectious diseases of wildlife— Threats to biodiversity and human health. *Science*, *287*(5452), 443–449. doi:10.1126cience.287.5452.443 PMID:10642539

Davies, G., Cox, H., Parker, R., & Dyer, R. (1938). A Filter-Passing Infectious Agent Isolated from Ticks. *Public Health Reports (1896-1970)*, *53*(52), 2259-2282. doi:10.2307/4582746

Davin-Regli, A., & Pagès, J. M. (2012). Cross-resistance between biocides and antimicrobials: An emerging question. *Revue Scientifique et Technique (International Office of Epizootics)*, *31*, 89–104. PMID:22849270

de Biase, D., Costagliola, A., Del Piero, F., Di Palo, R., & Coronati, D. Galiero, ... Paciello, O. (2018). *Coxiella burnetii* in Infertile Dairy Cattle with Chronic Endometritis. *Veterinary Pathology*. doi:10.1177/0300985818760376

De Craemer, W. (1983). A cross-cultural perspective on personhood. *The Milbank Memorial Fund Quarterly. Health and Society*, *61*(1), 19–34. doi:10.2307/3349814 PMID:6552386

de Cremoux, R., Rousset, E., Touratier, A., Audusseau, G., Nicollet, P., Ribaud, D., ... Le Pape, M. (2012a). Assessment of vaccination by a phase I *Coxiella burnetii*-inactivated vaccine in goat herds in clinical Q fever situation. *FEMS Immunology and Medical Microbiology*, *64*(1), 104–106. doi:10.1111/j.1574-695X.2011.00892.x PMID:22066485

de Cremoux, R., Rousset, E., Touratier, A., Audusseau, G., Nicollet, P., Ribaud, D., ... Le Pape, M. (2012b). *Coxiella burnetii* vaginal shedding and antibody responses in dairy goat herds in a context of clinical Q fever outbreaks. *FEMS Immunology and Medical Microbiology*, *64*(1), 120–122. doi:10.1111/j.1574-695X.2011.00893.x PMID:22066517

De Rooij, M. M. T., Borlée, F., Smit, L. A. M., de Bruin, A., Janse, I., Heederik, D. J. J., & Wouters, I. M. (2016). Detection of *Coxiella burnetii* in Ambient Air after a Large Q Fever Outbreak. *PLoS One*, *11*(3), e0151281. doi:10.1371/journal.pone.0151281 PMID:26991094

Dean, A. S., Bonfoh, B., Kulo, A. E., Boukaya, G. A., Amidou, M., Hattendorf, J., ... Schelling, E. (2013). Epidemiology of brucellosis and Q Fever in linked human and animal populations in northern Togo. *PLoS One*, 8.

Dean, A. S., Schelling, E., Bonfoh, B., Kulo, A. E., Boukaya, G. A., & Pilo, P. (2014). Deletion in the gene Bru-Ab2_0168 of Brucella abortus strains: Diagnostic challenges. *Clinical Microbiology and Infection*, *20*, 550–553.

Derrick, E. H. (1937). "Q" Fever, new fever entity: Clinical features, diagnosis and laboratory investigation. *The Medical Journal of Australia*, *2*, 281–299.

Diguimbaye-Djaibé, C., Hilty, M., Ngandolo, R., Mahamat, H. H., Pfyffer, G. E., Baggi, F., … Zinsstag, J. (2006). Mycobacterium bovis isolates from tuberculous lesions in Chadian zebu carcasses. *Emerging Infectious Diseases*, *12*(5), 769–771. Available at http://www.cdc.gov/ncidod/eid/vol12no05/pdfs/05-0691.pdf

Diop, C. (1974). *The African Origin of Civilization: Myth or Reality*. Chicago, IL: Lawrence Hill & Co.

Direção-Geral da Saúde. (2011). *Doenças de Declaração Obrigatória, Direcção-Geral da Saúde, Lisboa, 2000-2004 e 2004-2008*. Retrieved 1, October, from http://www.dgs.pt

Direção-Geral da Saúde. (2015). *Doenças de Notificação Obrigatória (1999 a 2013)*. Available from http://www.dgs.pt

Dutil, L. R., Irwin, R., Finley, L. K., Ng, B., Avery, P., Boerlin, A. M., ... Pillai, D. R. (2010). Ceftiofur resistance in *Salmonella enterica* serovar Heidelberg from chicken meat and humans, Canada. *Emerging Infectious Diseases*, *16*(1), 48–54. doi:10.3201/eid1601.090729 PMID:20031042

Dzidic, S., Suskovic, J., & Kos, B. (2008). Antibiotic resistance mechanisms in bacteria: Biochemical and genetic aspects. *Food Technology and Biotechnology*, *46*(1), 11–21.

Economou, V., & Gousia, P. (2015). Agriculture and food animals as a source of antimicrobial-resistant bacteria. *Infection and Drug Resistance*, *8*, 49–61. doi:10.2147/IDR.S55778 PMID:25878509

EFSA Panel on Animal Health and Welfare (AHAW). (2010). Scientific Opinion on Q Fever. *EFSA Journal*, *8*(5), 1595. doi:10.2903/j.efsa.2010.1595

El Sherbini, A., Kabbash, I., Schelling, E., El Shennawy, S., Shalapy, N., Elnaby, G. H., ... Eisa, A. (2007). Seroprevalences and local variation of human and livestock brucellosis in two villages in Gharbia Governorate, Egypt. *Transactions of the Royal Society of Tropical Medicine and Hygiene*, *101*(9), 923–928. doi:10.1016/j.trstmh.2007.04.020 PMID:17604066

Eldin, C., Mélenotte, C., Mediannikov, O., Ghigo, E., Million, M., Edouard, S., ... Raoult, D. (2017). From Q Fever to *Coxiella burnetii* Infection: A Paradigm Change. *Clinical Microbiology Reviews*, *30*(1), 115–190. doi:10.1128/CMR.00045-16 PMID:27856520

Elliot, K. (2011). *Is a little pollution good for you?* New York, NY: Oxford University Press. doi:10.1093/acprof:oso/9780199755622.001.0001

Elmer, P. (2004). *The healing arts: Health, disease and society in Europe, 1500-1800*. Manchester, UK: Manchester University Press.

Emery, M. P., Ostlund, E. N., Aitichou, M., Ballin, J. D., McFarling, D., & McGonigle, L. (2014). *Coxiella burnetii* serology assays in goat abortion storm. *Journal of Veterinary Diagnostic Investigation*, *26*(1), 141–145. doi:10.1177/1040638713517233 PMID:24532695

Enserink, M. (2010). Infectious diseases. Questions abound in Q-fever explosion in the Netherlands. *Science*, *327*, 266–267. PMID:20075230

Erickson, H. L. (2007). Philosophy and theory of holism. *The Nursing Clinics of North America*, *42*(2), 139–163. doi:10.1016/j.cnur.2007.03.001 PMID:17544676

European Centre for Disease Prevention and Control (ECDC). (2014). *Annual Epidemiological Report for 2014. Q fever*. Stockholm: ECDC.

Executive Board. (1951). *EB7.R78 Joint WHO/FAO Expert Group on Zoonoses: Report on First Session*. Geneva, Switzerland: WHO.

Executive Board. (1970). *EB45.R4 Socio-economic Consequences of the Zoonoses*. Geneva, Switzerland: WHO.

Executive Board. (1971). *EB47.R44 Socio-economic Consequences of the Zoonoses*. Geneva, Switzerland: WHO.

Executive Board. (1972). *EB49.R11 Socio-economic Consequences of the Zoonoses*. Geneva, Switzerland: WHO.

Faes, C., Aerts, M., Litiere, S., Meroc, E., Van der Stede, Y., & Mintiens, K. (2011). Estimating herd prevalence on the basis of aggregate testing of animals. *Journal of the Royal Statistical Society. Series A, (Statistics in Society)*, *174*(1), 155–174. doi:10.1111/j.1467-985X.2010.00652.x

FAO, OIE, & WHO. (2010). *The FAO-OIE-WHO Collaboration: Sharing Responsibilities and Coordinating Global Activities at the Animal–Human–Ecosystems Interfaces. A Tripartite Concept Note*. Available from http://www.fao.org/docrep/012/ak736e/ak736e00.pdf

FAO, OIE, & WHO. (2012). High-Level Technical Meeting to Address Health Risks at the Human-Animal-Ecosystems Interfaces. Mexico City, Mexico 15-17 November 2011. Authors.

FAO, OIE, WHO, UNSIC, UNICEF, & WB. (2008). *Contributing to One World, One Health: A Strategic Framework for Reducing Risks of Infectious Diseases at the Animal–Human–Ecosystems Interface*. Authors.

FAO. (2016). *Drivers, dynamics and epidemiology of antimicrobial resistance in animal production*. Rome, Italy: FAO.

Far Eastern Rural Hygiene Conference. (1937). *Current Science*, *6*(2), 70-72.

Fenollar, F., Thuny, F., Xeridat, B., Lepidi, H., & Raoult, D. (2006). Endocarditis after acute Q fever in patients with previously undiagnosed valvulopathies. *Clinical Infectious Diseases*, *42*(6), 818–821. doi:10.1086/500402 PMID:16477559

Fernández-Aguilar, X., Cabezón, Ó., Colom-Cadena, A., Lavín, S., & López-Olvera, J. R. (2016). Serological survey of *Coxiella burnetii* at the wildlife–livestock interface in the Eastern Pyrenees, Spain. *Acta Veterinaria Scandinavica*, *58*(1), 26. doi:10.118613028-016-0209-4 PMID:27121001

Ferraz, R. V., Andrade, M., Silva, F., Andrade, P., Carvalho, C., Torres, J. P., ... Santos, L. (2016). Chronic Q fever: A missed prosthetic valve endocarditis possibly for years. *IDCases*, *6*, 55–57. doi:10.1016/j.idcr.2016.09.005 PMID:27713859

Figueiredo, C., Candeias, F., & Brito, M. J. (2016). Aseptic Meningitis Caused by *Coxiella burnetii*. *The Pediatric Infectious Disease Journal*, *35*(1), 115. doi:10.1097/INF.0000000000000935 PMID:26418239

Filipe, A. R., Bacellar, F., & David de Morais, J. A. (1990). Anticorpos contra *Rickettsieae* na população do sul de Portugal. *Revista Portuguesa de Doenças Infecciosas*, *13*(2), 85–89.

Firdessa, R., Berg, S., Hailu, E., Schelling, E., Gumi, B., Erenso, G., ... Aseffa, A. (2013). Mycobacterial lineages causing pulmonary and extrapulmonary tuberculosis, Ethiopia. *Emerging Infectious Diseases*, *19*(3), 460–463. doi:10.3201/eid1903.120256 PMID:23622814

Fischer, J., Rodriguez, I., Schmoger, S., Friese, A., Roesler, U., Helmuth, R., & Guerra, B. (2013). *Salmonella enterica* subsp. *enterica* producing VIM-1 carbapenemase isolated from livestock farms. *The Journal of Antimicrobial Chemotherapy*, *68*(2), 478–480. doi:10.1093/jac/dks393 PMID:23034713

Foltz, R. C. (2005). Islam, Animals, and Vegetarianism. In *The Encyclopeadia of Religion and Nature* (pp. 873–875). London: Continuum.

Fonseca, F., Pinto, M. R., Azevedo, J. F., & Lacerda, M. T. (1949a). Febre Q em Portugal. *Clínica Contemporânea*, *3*(21), 1159–1164.

Forde, M., Morrison, K., Dewailly, E., Badrie, N., & Robertson, L. (2011). Strengthening integrated research and capacity development within the Caribbean region. *BMC International Health and Human Rights*, *11*(Suppl. 2), S7. doi:10.1186/1472-698X-11-S2-S7 PMID:22166013

Founou, L. L., Founou, R. C., & Essack, S. Y. (2016). Antibiotic resistance in the food chain: A developing country-perspective. *Frontiers in Microbiology*, *7*, 1881. doi:10.3389/fmicb.2016.01881 PMID:27933044

Fournier, P. E., Marrie, T. J., & Raoult, D. (1998). Diagnosis of Q Fever. *Journal of Clinical Microbiology*, *36*(7), 1823–1834. PMID:9650920

Frankson, R., Hueston, W., Christian, K., Olson, D., Lee, M., Valeri, L., ... Rubin, C. (2016). One Health core competency domains. *Frontiers in Public Health*, *4*, 192. doi:10.3389/fpubh.2016.00192 PMID:27679794

French, W. (2005). Francis of Assisi. In *The Encyclopeadia of Religion and Nature* (pp. 670–672). London: Continuum.

Gale, P., Kelly, L., Mearns, R., Duggan, J., & Snary, E. L. (2015). Q fever through consumption of unpasteurised milk and milk products - a risk profile and exposure assessment. *Journal of Applied Microbiology*, *118*(5), 1083–1095. doi:10.1111/jam.12778 PMID:25692216

Galiero, A., Fratini, F., Cammà, C., Di Domenico, M., Curini, V., Baronti, I., ... Cerri, D. (2016). Occurrence of *Coxiella burnetii* in goat and ewe unpasteurized cheeses: Screening and genotyping. *International Journal of Food Microbiology*, *237*, 47–54. doi:10.1016/j.ijfoodmicro.2016.08.008 PMID:27543815

Ganguly, B., Das, U., & Das, A. K. (2016). Canine Transmissible Venereal Tumour: A Review. *Veterinary and Comparative Oncology, 14*(1), 1–12. doi:10.1111/vco.12060 PMID:23981098

Garrity, G. M., Bell, J. A., & Lilburn, T. (2015). Coxiellaceae fam. nov. In W. B. Whitman, F. Rainey, P. Kämpfer, M. Trujillo, J. Chun, P. DeVos, B. Hedlund & S. Dedysh (Eds.), Bergey's Manual of Systematics of Archaea and Bacteria. Wiley. doi:10.1002/9781118960608.fbm00223

Ghigo, E., Capo, C., Tung, C. H., Raoult, D., Gorvel, J. P., & Mege, J. L. (2002). *Coxiella burnetii* Survival in THP-1 Monocytes Involves the Impairment of Phagosome Maturation: IFN-γ Mediates its Restoration and Bacterial Killing. *Journal of Immunology (Baltimore, Md.: 1950), 169*(8), 4488–4495. doi:10.4049/jimmunol.169.8.4488 PMID:12370385

Ghigo, E., Colombo, M. I., & Heinzen, R. A. (2012). The *Coxiella burnetii* parasitophorous vacuole. *Advances in Experimental Medicine and Biology, 984*, 141–169. doi:10.1007/978-94-007-4315-1_8 PMID:22711631

Ghigo, E., Honstettre, A., Capo, C., Gorvel, J. P., Raoult, D., & Mege, J. L. (2004). Link between impaired maturation of phagosomes and defective *Coxiella burnetii* killing in patients with chronic Q fever. *The Journal of Infectious Diseases, 190*(10), 1767–7. doi:10.1086/425041 PMID:15499532

Gibbs, S. E. J., & Gibbs, E. P. G. (2012). The Historical, Present, and Future Role of Veterinarians in One Health. In J.S. Mackenzie, M. Jeggo, P. Daszak, & J.A. Richt (Eds.), The Concept and Examples of a One Health Approach = One Health: The Human-Animal-Environment Interfaces in Emerging Infectious Diseases, vol. 1 = Current Topics in Microbiology and Immunologie (pp. 31-47). Berlin, Germany: Springer. doi:10.1007/82_2012_259

Gibbs, E. (2014). The evolution of One Health: A decade of progress and challenges for the future. *The Veterinary Record, 174*(4), 85–91. doi:10.1136/vr.g143 PMID:24464377

Gilbertson, D. (1993). Trichinosis. In K. F. Kiple (Ed.), *The Cambridge world history of human disease* (pp. 1055–1058). Cambridge, UK: Cambridge University Press. doi:10.1017/CHOL9780521332866.207

Githeko, A. K., Lindsay, S. W., Confalonieri, U. E., & Patz, J. A. (2000). Climate change and vector-borne diseases: A regional analysis. *Bulletin of the World Health Organization, 78*(9), 1136–1147. PMID:11019462

Godinho, I., Nogueira, E. L., Santos, C. M., Paulo, S. E., Fortes, A., Guerra, J. O., & Gomes da Costa, A. (2015). Chronic Q Fever in a renal transplant recipient: A case report. *Transplantation Proceedings*, *47*(4), 1045–1047. doi:10.1016/j.transproceed.2015.03.022 PMID:26036515

Gomes, M. M., Chaves, A., Gouveia, A., & Santos, L. (2014). Two rare manifestations of Q fever: Splenic and hepatic abscesses and cerebral venous thrombosis, with literature review ma non troppo. *BMJ Case Reports*, *2014*(feb05 1), bcr2013202843. doi:10.1136/bcr-2013-202843 PMID:24501338

Gonjalo, J. D., Wolpaw, D. R., Lehman, E., & Chuang, C. H. (2014). Palint-centered interprofessional collaborative care: Factors associated with bedside interprofessional rounds. *Journal of General Internal Medicine*, *29*(7), 1040–1047. doi:10.100711606-014-2817-x PMID:24615186

Grace, D., Gilbert, J., Lapar, M. L., Unger, F., Fevre, S., Nguyen-Viet, H., & Schelling, E. (2011). Zoonotic emerging infectious disease in selected countries in southeast Asia: Insights from ecohealth. *EcoHealth*, *8*(1), 55–62. doi:10.100710393-010-0357-3 PMID:21174223

Gradmann, C. (2010). Robert Koch and the invention of the carrier state: Tropical medicine, veterinary infections and epidemiology around 1900. *Studies in History and Philosophy of Biological and Biomedical Sciences*, *41*(3), 232–240. doi:10.1016/j.shpsc.2010.04.012 PMID:20934644

Grant, S., & Olsen, C. W. (1995). Preventing zoonotic diseases in immunocompromised persons: The role of physicians and veterinarians. *Emerging Infectious Diseases*, *5*(1), 159–163. doi:10.3201/eid0501.990121 PMID:10081686

Grubbs, B., Artese, A., Schmitt, K., Cormier, E., & Panton, L. (2016). A pilot study to assess the feasibility of group exercise and animal assisted therapy in older adults. *Journal of Aging and Physical Activity*, *24*(2), 322–331. doi:10.1123/japa.2015-0107 PMID:26439234

Gsell, O. (1993). Leptospirosis. In K. F. Kiple (Ed.), *The Cambridge world history of human disease* (pp. 840–842). Cambridge, UK: Cambridge University Press. doi:10.1017/CHOL9780521332866.143

Guan, Y., Chen, H., Li, K., Riley, S., Leung, G., Webster, R., ... Yuen, K. (2007). A model to control the epidemic of H5N1 influenza at the source. *BMC Infectious Diseases*, *7*(1), 132. doi:10.1186/1471-2334-7-132 PMID:17999754

Guatteo, R., Beaudeau, F., Berri, M., Rodolakis, A., Joly, A., & Seegers, H. (2006). Shedding routes of *Coxiella burnetii* in dairy cows: Implications for detection and control. *Veterinary Research, 37*(6), 827–833. doi:10.1051/vetres:2006038 PMID:16973121

Guatteo, R., Beaudeau, F., Joly, A., & Seegers, H. (2007). *Coxiella burnetii* shedding by dairy cows. *Veterinary Research, 38*(6), 849–860. doi:10.1051/vetres:2007038 PMID:17903418

Guatteo, R., Seegers, H., Joly, A., & Beaudeau, F. (2008). Prevention of *Coxiella burnetii* shedding in infected dairy herds using a phase I *C. burnetii* inactivated vaccine. *Vaccine, 26*(34), 4320–4328. doi:10.1016/j.vaccine.2008.06.023 PMID:18586060

Guatteo, R., Seegers, H., Taurel, A. F., Joly, A., & Beaudeau, F. (2011). Prevalence of *Coxiella burnetii* infection in domestic ruminants: A critical review. *Veterinary Microbiology, 149*(1-2), 1–16. doi:10.1016/j.vetmic.2010.10.007 PMID:21115308

Guidi, F., Petruzzelli, A., Ciarrocchi, F., Duranti, A., Valiani, A., Amagliani, G., & Blasi, G. (2017). Prevalence of *Coxiella burnetii* in cows' and ewes' bulk tank milk samples from selected dairy farms of Central Italy. *Italian Journal of Animal Science, 16*(4), 673–676. doi:10.1080/1828051X.2017.1321474

Gumi, B., Schelling, E., Berg, S., Firdessa, R., Erenso, G., Mekonnen, W., ... Zinsstag, J. (2012). Zoonotic transmission of tuberculosis between pastoralists and their livestock in South-East Ethiopia. *EcoHealth, 9*(2), 139–149. doi:10.100710393-012-0754-x PMID:22526748

Hackstadt, T., & Williams, J. C. (1981). Biochemical stratagem for obligate parasitism of eukaryotic cells by *Coxiella burnetii. Proceedings of the National Academy of Sciences of the United States of America, 78*(5), 3240–3244. doi:10.1073/pnas.78.5.3240 PMID:6942430

Haller, J. S. Jr. (2003). Ergotism. In K. F. Kiple (Ed.), *The Cambridge historical dictionary of disease* (pp. 120–121). Cambridge, UK: Cambridge University Press.

Hamburg, M. A., & Lederberg, J. C. (2003). *Microbial threats to health.* Washington, DC: National Academy Press.

Hamilton, W., Ryder, D., Cooper, H. Jr, Williams, D., & Weinberg, A. (2015). Enviornmental Health: A survey of Texas primary care physicians. *Texas Medicine, 101*, 62–70. PMID:17094519

Hanczaruk, M., Cutler, S. J., Toman, R., & Frangoulidis, D. (2012). Coxiella burnetii: Q Fever. In BSL3 and BSL4 Agents. In M. C. Elschner, S. J. Cutler, M. Weidmann, & P. Butaye (Eds.), Epidemiology, Microbiology and Practical Guidelines (pp. 57-69). Weinheim: Wiley-Blackwell. doi:10.1002/9783527645114.ch19

Handbuch der speciellen Pathologie und Therapie der chronischen Krankheiten nach den Erfahrungen der bewährtesten Ärzte unserer Zeit systematisch dargestellt. (1841). (Vol. 1-3). Berlin: Veit.

Harbottle, H., White, D. G., McDermott, P. F., Walker, R. D., & Zhao, S. (2006). Comparison of Multilocus sequence typing, Pulse Field Electrophoresis and antimicrobial susceptibility for characterization of Salmonella enterica serovar Newport isolates. *Journal of Clinical Microbiology*, *44*(7), 2449–2457. doi:10.1128/JCM.00019-06 PMID:16825363

Hatchette, T., Campbell, N., Hudson, R., Raoult, D., & Marrie, T. J. (2003). Natural history of Q fever in goats. *Vector Borne and Zoonotic Diseases (Larchmont, N.Y.)*, *3*(1), 11–15. doi:10.1089/153036603765627415 PMID:12804376

Hechemy, K. E. (2012). History and Prospects of *Coxiella burnetii* Research. In R. Toman, R. Heinzen, J. Samuel, & J. L. Mege (Eds.), *Coxiella burnetii: Recent Advances and New Perspectives in Research of the Q Fever Bacterium. Advances in Experimental Medicine and Biology* (Vol. 984). Dordrecht: Springer. doi:10.1007/978-94-007-4315-1_1

Heinzen, R. A., Scidmore, M. A., Rockey, D. D., & Hackstadt, T. (1996). Differential interaction with endocytic and exocytic pathways distinguish parasitophorous vacuoles of *Coxiella burnetii* and Chlamydia trachomatis. *Infection and Immunity*, *64*(3), 796–809. PMID:8641784

Heppell, C. W., Egan, J. R., & Hall, I. (2017). A human time dose response model for Q fever. *Epidemics*, *21*, 30–38. doi:10.1016/j.epidem.2017.06.001 PMID:28666604

Highland, C. (2001). *Meditations of John Muir*. Berkeley, CA: Wilderness Press.

Hill, A. B. (1965). The environment and disease: Association or causation? *Proceedings of the Royal Society of Medicine*, *58*, 295–300. PMID:14283879

Hinchliffe, S. (2015). More than one world, more than one health: Re-configuring interspecies health. *Social Science & Medicine*, *129*, 28–35. doi:10.1016/j.socscimed.2014.07.007 PMID:25022470

Hoover, T. A., Culp, D. W., Vodkin, M. H., Williams, J. C., & Thompson, H. A. (2002). Chromosomal DNA Deletions Explain Phenotypic Characteristics of Two Antigenic Variants, Phase II and RSA 514 (Crazy), of the *Coxiella burnetii* Nine Mile Strain. *Infection and Immunity*, *70*(12), 6726–6733. doi:10.1128/IAI.70.12.6726-2733.2002 PMID:12438347

Horigan, M. W., Bell, M. M., Pollard, T. R., Sayers, A. R., & Pritchard, G. C. (2011). Q fever diagnosis in domestic ruminants: Comparison between complement fixation and commercial enzyme-linked immunosorbent assays. *Journal of Veterinary Diagnostic Investigation*, *23*(5), 924–931. doi:10.1177/1040638711416971 PMID:21908348

Horton, R., & Lo, S. (2015). Planetary health: A new science for exceptional action. *Lancet*, *386*(10007), 1921–1922. doi:10.1016/S0140-6736(15)61038-8 PMID:26188746

Hotta, A., Kawamura, M., To, H., Andoh, M., Yamaguchi, T., Fukushi, H., & Hirai, K. (2002). Phase Variation Analysis of *Coxiella burnetii* during Serial Passage in Cell Culture by Use of Monoclonal Antibodies. *Infection and Immunity*, *70*(8), 4747–4749. doi:10.1128/IAI.70.8.4747-4749.2002 PMID:12117996

Howe, D., & Mallavia, L. P. (2000). *Coxiella burnetii* Exhibits Morphological Change and Delays Phagolysosomal Fusion after Internalization by J774A.1 Cells. *Infection and Immunity*, *68*(7), 3815–3821. doi:10.1128/IAI.68.7.3815-3821.2000 PMID:10858189

Ikuenobe, P. (2006). *Philosophical perspectives on communalism and morality in African traditions*. Oxford, UK: Lexington Books.

Imran, S., Alam, K., & Beaumont, N. (2014). Reinterpreting the definition of sustainable development for a more ecocentric reorientation. *Sustainable Development*, *22*(2), 134–144. doi:10.1002d.537

Ingwe, R., Ebegbulem, J. & Ikeji, C. (2010). Ecocentric and anthropocentric policies and crises in climate/environment, finance and economy: Implications of the emerging green policy of the Obama administration for Africa's sustainable development. *African Journal of Political Science and International Relations*, *4*(1), 1-12.

Intergovernmental Panel on Climate Change (IPCC) – Climate Change. (2007). Synthesis report - Summary for policymakers. Available: http://www.ipcc.ch/pdf/assessment-report/ar4/syr/ ar4_syr_spm.pdf

International Live Stock Research Institute. (2012). Mapping of poverty and likely zoonoses hot spot. Zoonoses Project 4. Report to Deptt. of International Development. Author.

International Risk Governance Council. (2005). *White Paper on Risk Governance. Towards an Integrative Approach*. IRGC. Retrieved from http://www.irgc.org/IMG/pdf/IRGC_WP_No_1_Risk_Governance__reprinted_version_.pdf

Iyioke, I. V. (2016). *Re-conceptualizing responsibility in clinical trials: An insight with the African notion of self* (Unpublished doctoral dissertation). Michigan State University, East Lansing, MI.

Jensen, T. K., Montgomery, D. L., Jaeger, P. T., Lindhardt, T., Agerholm, J. S., Bille-Hansen, V., & Boye, M. (2007). Application of fluorescent *in situ* hybridisation for demonstration of *Coxiella burnetii* in placentas from ruminant abortions. *APMIS: acta pathologica, microbiologica, et immunologica Scandinavica, 115*, 347–353.

Jessup, D. A., Miller, M. A., Johnson, K., Conrad, P. A., Tinkar, M. T., Estes, J., & Mazet, J. A. (2007). Seaotters in a dirty ocean. *Journal of the American Veterinary Medical Association, 23*, 1648–1652.

Jiang, & Young, & Hardee. (2008). Population, Urbanization, And The Environment. *World Watch, 21*(5), 34–39.

Jiménez-Arribas, G., Léautaud, V., & Amábile-Cuevas, C. F. (2001). Regulatory locus soxRS partially protects *Escherichia coli* against ozone. *FEMS Microbiology Letters, 195*(2), 175–177. doi:10.1016/S0378-1097(01)00007-6 PMID:11179648

Joakim Larsson, D. G. (2014). Antibiotics in the environment. *Upsala Journal of Medical Sciences, 119*(2), 108–112. doi:10.3109/03009734.2014.896438 PMID:24646081

Joakim Larsson, D. G., & Fick, J. (2009). Transparency throughout the production chain – a way to reduce pollution from the manufacturing of pharmaceuticals. *Regulatory Toxicology and Pharmacology, 53*(3), 161–163. doi:10.1016/j.yrtph.2009.01.008 PMID:19545507

Johnston, C. (2013). Lessons from medical ethics. In C. M. Wathes, S. A. Corr, S. A. May, S. P. McCulloch, & M. C. Whiting (Eds.), *Veterinary & Animal Ethics*. Oxford, UK: Blackwell Publishing Ltd.

Joint WHO/FAO Expert Committee on Zoonoses. (1959). *Second Report = WHO Technical Report Series, 169, FAO agricultural studies, 47*. Author.

Joint WHO/FAO Expert Group on Zoonoses. (1951). *Report on the first session = WHO Technical Report Series, 40*. Author.

Jonas, O., & Warford, L. (2014). *Global Program for Avian Influenza Control and Human Pandemic Preparedness and Response. Project Accomplishments.* Washington, DC: The World Bank.

Jones, K. E., Patel, N. G., Levy, M. A., Storeygard, A., Balk, D., Gittleman, J. L., & Daszak, P. (2008). Global trends in emerging infectious diseases. *Nature*, *451*(7181), 990–993. doi:10.1038/nature06536 PMID:18288193

Jones, R. M., Nicas, M., Hubbard, A. E., & Reingold, A. L. (2006). The infectious dose of *Coxiella burnetii* (Q Fever). *Applied Biosafety: Journal of the American Biological Safety Association*, *11*(1), 32–41. doi:10.1177/153567600601100106

Kaeberlein, M. (2016). The biology of aging: Citizen scientists and their pets as a bridge between research on model organisms and human subjects. *Veterinary Pathology*, *53*(2), 291–298. doi:10.1177/0300985815591082 PMID:26077786

Kahn, L. H. (2006). Confronting Zoonoses, Linking Human and Veterinary Medicine. *Emerging Infectious Diseases*, *12*(4), 556–561. doi:10.3201/eid1204.050956 PMID:16704801

Kahn, L. H., Kaplan, B., Monath, T. P., & Steele, J. H. (2008). Teaching "One Medicine One Health". *The American Journal of Medicine*, *121*, 169–170.

Kahn, L. H., Kaplan, B., & Steele, J. H. (2007). Confronting zoonoses through closer collaboration between medicine and veterinary medicine (as 'one medicine'). *Veterinaria Italiana*, *43*, 5–19. PMID:20411497

Kaindi, D. W., Schelling, E., Wangoh, J. M., Imungi, J. K., Farah, Z., & Meile, L. (2012). Towards one health disease surveillance: The Southern African Centre for Infectious Disease Surveillance approach. *The Onderstepoort Journal of Veterinary Research*, *79*, 454. PMID:23327374

Kant, I. (2004). Animals may be Used. In A. Linzey & P. B. Clarke (Eds.), *Animal Rights: A Historical Anthology* (pp. 78–79). New York, NY: Columbia University Press.

Kant, I. (2004). Duties to Animals are Indirect. In A. Linzey & P. B. Clarke (Eds.), *Animal Rights: A Historical Anthology* (pp. 126–127). New York, NY: Columbia University Press.

Kaphagawani, D. (2004). African conception of a person: A critical survey. In K. Wiredu (Ed.), *A Companion to African Philosophy* (pp. 332–342). Blackwell Publishing; doi:10.1002/9780470997154.ch26

Karesh, W. B., & Robert, A. (2005). Wildlife Trade and Global Disease Emergence. *Emerging Infectious Diseases, 11*(7), 1000–1002. doi:10.3201/eid1107.050194 PMID:16022772

Kazar, J. (2005). *Coxiella burnetii* Infection. *Annals of the New York Academy of Sciences, 1063*(1), 105–114. doi:10.1196/annals.1355.018 PMID:16481501

Kelbessa, W. (2005). The utility of ethical dialogue for marginalized voices in Africa. In Proceedings of Sharpening policy tools for marginalized managers of natural resources. Addis Ababa University.

Kelbessa, W. (2011). *Indigenous and Modern environmental ethics: A study of the indigenous Oromo environmental ethic and modern issues of environment and development*. Washington, DC: Cultural Heritage and Contemporary Change, Series II.

Kelbessa, W. (2011). Indigenous Environmental Philosophy. In J. Garfield & W. Edelglass (Eds.), *The Oxford Handbook of World Philosophy* (pp. 574–581). Oxford, UK: Oxford University Press. doi:10.1093/oxfordhb/9780195328998.003.004

Kelly, A. M., Ferguson, J. D., Galligan, D. T., Salman, M. Osburn, B. I. (2013), One health, food security, and veterinary medicine. *Journal of the American Veterinary Medical Association, 242*(6), 739-743. doi:10.2460/javma.242.6.739

Keusch, G. T. (2009). Sustaining Global Surveillance and Response to Emerging Zoonotic Diseases. Academic Press.

Keusch, G., Pappaioanou, M., Scott, K., Tsai, P., & Gonzalez, M. (2009). *Sustaining global surveillance and response to emerging zoonotic diseases*. Washington, DC: National Academy Press.

Khalili, M., Sakhaee, E., & Babaei, H. (2012). Frequency of anti-*Coxiella burnetii* antibodies in cattle with reproductive disorders. *Comparative Clinical Pathology, 21*(5), 917–919. doi:10.100700580-011-1199-2

Khavkin, T., & Tabibzadeh, S. S. (1988). Histologic, immunofluorescence, and electron microscopic study of infectious process in mouse lung after intranasal challenge with *Coxiella burnetii. Infection and Immunity, 56*(7), 1792–1799. PMID:3290107

Kim, S. G., Kim, E. H., Lafferty, C. J., & Dubovi, E. (2005). *Coxiella burnetii* in Bulk Tank Milk Samples, United States. *Emerging Infectious Diseases*, *11*(4), 619–621. doi:10.3201/eid1104.041036 PMID:15829205

King, L. (2008). One World, One Health. *Proceedings of the 2008 World Veterinary Congress*, 10-16.

Klee, S. R., Tyczka, J., Ellerbrok, H., Franz, T., Linke, S., Baljer, G., & Appel, B. (2006). Highly sensitive real-time PCR for specific detection and quantification of *Coxiella burnetii*. *BMC Microbiology*, *6*(1), 2. doi:10.1186/1471-2180-6-2 PMID:16423303

Klemmer, J., Njeru, J., Emam, A., El-Sayed, A., Moawad, A. A., Henning, K., ... El-Diasty, M. M. (2018). Q fever in Egypt: Epidemiological survey of *Coxiella burnetii* specific antibodies in cattle, buffaloes, sheep, goats and camels. *PLoS One*, *13*(2), e0192188. doi:10.1371/journal.pone.0192188 PMID:29466380

Korte, G. (2016, December 13). Obama signs $6.3 billion law for cancer research, drug treatment. *USA Today*.

Koster, F. T., Williams, J. C., & Goodwin, J. S. (1985). Cellular immunity in Q fever: Modulation of responsiveness by a suppressor T cell-monocyte circuit. *Journal of Immunology (Baltimore, Md.: 1950)*, *135*(2), 1067–1072. PMID:2409135

Kovácová, E., & Kazár, J. (2002). Q fever still a query and underestimated infectious disease. *Acta Virologica. English Ed.*, *46*(4), 193–210. PMID:12693856

Kozajda, A., & Bródka, K., & SzadkowskaStańczyk, I. (2013). Factors influencing biosafety level and LAI among the staff of medical laboratories. *Medycyna Pracy*, *64*(4), 473–486. PMID:24502112

Krauss, H., Weber, A., Appel, M., Enders, B., Graevenitz, A. v., Isenberg, H. D., … Zahner, H. (2004). Zoonosen. Von Tier zu Mensch übertragbare Infektionskrankheiten (3rd ed.). Köln, Germany: Deutscher Ärzte-Verlag.

Krauße, G., & Zandhof, K. J. (1990). Institut für Hygiene und Technologie der Lebensmittel tierischen Ursprungs. In A. von den Driesch (Ed.), 200 Jahre tierärztliche Lehre und Forschung in München (pp. 83-96). Stuttgart, Germany: Schattauer.

Krönke, F. (2001). *Perception of Ill-health in a FulBe Pastoralist Community and Its Implications on Health Interventions in Chad* (Doctoral dissertation). Available from http://pages.unibas.ch/diss/2002/ DissB_6478.htm

Kuroiwa, Y., Oyanagi, R., Fuse, S., Mori, T., Ueno, H., & Tsutsumi, H. (2007). Persistent hepatitis and repeated wheezing in an infant. *The Pediatric Infectious Disease Journal*, *26*(8), 763–769. doi:10.1097/INF.0b013e3180f60bfe PMID:17848898

Landers, T. F., Cohen, B., Wittum, T. E., & Larson, E. L. (2012). A Review of Antibiotic Use in Food Animals: Perspective, Policy, and Potential. *Public Health Reports*, *127*(1), 4–22. doi:10.1177/003335491212700103 PMID:22298919

Lang, G. H. (1990). Coxiellosis (Q fever) in animals. In T. J. Marrie (Ed.), *Q Fever: The Disease* (Vol. 1, pp. 23–48). Boca Raton, FL: CRC Press.

Leonard, E., Pearl, D., Finley, R., Janecko, N., Reid-Smith, R., Peregrine, A., & Weese, J. (2012). Comparison of antimicrobial resistance patterns of *Salmonella* spp. and *Escherichia coli* recovered from pet dogs from volunteer households in Ontario (2005–2006). *The Journal of Antimicrobial Chemotherapy*, *67*(1), 174–181. doi:10.1093/jac/dkr430 PMID:22016151

Leopold, W. (1949). *A Sand County Almanac*. Oxford, UK: Oxford University Press.

Lerner, H., & Berg, C. (2017). A Comparison of Three Holistic Approaches to Health: One Health, EcoHealth, and Planetary Health. *Frontiers in Veterinary Science*, *4*(163). doi:10.3389/fvets.2017.00163 PMID:29085825

Levine, G. N., Allen, K., Braun, L. T., Christian, H. E., Friedmann, E., Taubert, K. A., ... Lange, R. A. (2013). Pet ownership and cardiovascular Risk: A scientific statement from the American Heart Association. *Circulation*, *127*(23), 2353–2363. doi:10.1161/CIR.0b013e31829201e1 PMID:23661721

Levin, J. (1839). *Vergleichende Darstellung der von den Hausthieren auf Menschen übertragbaren Krankheiten*. Berlin: Schroeder.

Levy, S. B., & Marshall, B. (2004). Antibacterial resistance worldwide: Causes, challenges and responses. *Nature Medicine*, *10*(12), 122–129. doi:10.1038/nm1145 PMID:15577930

Lewis, H. B. (2008). One world, one health, one medicine: From the perspective of companion animal practice. *Proceedings of the 2008 World Veterinary Congress*, 10-16.

Lindahl & Grace. (2015). Article. *Infection Ecology and Epidemiology, 5*. doi:10.3402/iee.v5.30048

Lindberg, R., Jarnheimer, P., Olsen, B., Johansson, M., & Tysklind, M. (2004). Determination of antibiotic substances in hospital sewage water using solid phase extraction and liquid chromatography/ mass spectrometry and group analogue internal standards. *Chemosphere*, *57*(10), 1479–1488. doi:10.1016/j.chemosphere.2004.09.015 PMID:15519392

Lindberg, R., Wennberg, P., Johansson, M., Tysklind, M., & Andersson, B. (2005). Screening of human antibiotic substances and determination of weekly mass flows in five sewage treatment plants in Sweden. *Environmental Science & Technology*, *39*(10), 3421–3429. doi:10.1021/es048143z PMID:15952345

Liu, Y. y., Wang, Y., Walsh, T., Yi, L., Zhang, R., Spencer, J., ... Shen, J. (2016). Emergence of plasmid-mediated colistin resistance mechanism MCR-1 in animals and human beings in China: A microbiological and molecular biological study. *The Lancet Infectious Diseases*, *16*(2), 161–168. doi:10.1016/S1473-3099(15)00424-7 PMID:26603172

Loutan, L., Bierens de Haan, D., & Subilia, L. (1997). The health of asylum seekers: From communicable disease screening to post-traumatic disorders. *Bulletin de la Société de Pathologie Exotique*, *90*(4), 233–237. PMID:9479457

Lyons, M. (1992). *The Colonial Disease: A Social History of Sleeping Sickness in Northern Zaire, 1900-1940*. Cambridge, UK: Cambridge University Press. doi:10.1017/CBO9780511583704

Macpherson, C. N. (2005). Human behaviour and the epidemiology of parasitic zoonoses. *International Journal for Parasitology*, *35*(11-12), 1319–1331. doi:10.1016/j.ijpara.2005.06.004 PMID:16102769

Maltezou, H. C., & Raoult, D. (2002). Q fever in children. *The Lancet Infectious Diseases*, *2*(11), 686–691. doi:10.1016/S1473-3099(02)00440-1 PMID:12409049

Mangili, P., Amagliani, G., Micci, E., Brandi, G., Foglini, M., Cinti, B., ... Schiavano, G. F. (2016). A model for *Coxiella burnetii* monitoring in a sheep dairy farm. *JSM Biotechnology & Biomedical Engineering*, *3*, 1050.

Marfin, A. A., Peterson, L. R., Eidson, M., Miller, J., Hadler, J., Farello, C., & ... . (2000). Widespread West Nile virus activity, eastern United States. *Emerging Infectious Diseases*, *7*(4), 730–735. doi:10.3201/eid0704.017423 PMID:11585539

Marietta, D. (1995). *For People and the Planet: Holism and Humanism in Environmental ethics*. Philadelphia, PA: Temple University Press.

Mariner, J. C., Pfeiffer, D. U., Costard, S., Knopf, L., Zingeser, J., Chibeu, D., & Mehta, P. (2011). *Surveillance for the Present and the Future. Challenges of Animal Health Information Systems and Surveillance for Animal Diseases and Zoonoses*. FAO.

Marrie, T. J., Stein, A., Janigan, D., & Raoult, D. (1996). Route of infection determines the clinical manifestations of acute Q fever. *The Journal of Infectious Diseases*, *173*(2), 484–487. doi:10.1093/infdis/173.2.484 PMID:8568318

Marshall, B. M., & Levy, S. B. (2011). Food animals and antimicrobials: Impacts on human health. *Clinical Microbiology Reviews*, *24*(4), 718–733. doi:10.1128/CMR.00002-11 PMID:21976606

Martinez, J. L., & Baquero, F. (2009). *Antibiotics and the Evolution of Antibiotic Resistance*. Available online at http://onlinelibrary.wiley.com/doi/10.1002/9780470015902.a0021782/full

Matchak, R. L. (2015). Pet ownership and physical health. *Current Opinion in Psychiatry*, *28*(5), 386–392. doi:10.1097/YCO.0000000000000183 PMID:26164613

Mathew, A. G., Cissell, R., & Liamthong, S. (2007). Antibiotic resistance in bacteria associated with food animals: A United States perspective of livestock production. *Foodborne Pathogens and Disease*, *4*(2), 115–133. doi:10.1089/fpd.2006.0066 PMID:17600481

Matolino, B. (2011). The (mal) function of "it" in Ifeanyi Menkiti's normative account of person. *African Studies Quarterly*, *12*(4), 23–37.

Maurin, M., Benoliel, A. M., Bongrand, P., & Raoult, D. (1992). Phagolysosomes of *Coxiella burnetii*-infected cell lines maintain an acidic pH during persistent infection. *Infection and Immunity*, *60*(12), 5013–5016. PMID:1452331

Maurin, M., & Raoult, D. (1999). Q Fever. *Clinical Microbiology Reviews*, *12*(4), 518–553. doi:10.1128/CMR.12.4.518 PMID:10515901

Mayr, A., & Mahnel, H. (1990). Institut für Medizinische Mikrobiologie, Infektions- und Seuchenmedizin. In A. von den Driesch (Ed.), 200 Jahre tierärztliche Lehre und Forschung in München (pp. 169-179). Stuttgart, Germany: Schattauer.

Mazet, J. A., Clifford, D. L., Coppolillo, P. B., Deolalikar, A. B., Erickson, J. D., & Kazwala, R. R. (2009). A 'one health' approach to address emerging zoonoses: The HALI project in Tanzania. *PLoS Medicine*, 6.

Mbiti, J. (1970). *African Religions and Philosophy*. New York, NY: Praeger Publishers.

McDade, J. E. (1990). Historical aspects of Q fever. In T. J. Marrie (Ed.), Q Fever: The Disease (pp. 6-15). Boca Raton, FL: CRC Press.

McGann, P., Snesrud, E., Maybank, R., Corey, B., Ong, A. C., Clifford, R., ... Schaecher, K. E. (2016). *Escherichia coli* harboring *mcr-1* and *bla*CTX-M on a novel IncF plasmid: First report of mcr-1 in the USA. *Antimicrobial Agents and Chemotherapy*, *60*(7), 4420–4421. doi:10.1128/AAC.01103-16 PMID:27230792

McGavin, M. D., & Zachary, J. F. (2007). *Pathologic basis of veterinary disease* (4th ed.). St. Louis, MO: Mosby.

McMichael, A.J. (2002). Population, environment, disease, and survival: past patterns, uncertain futures. *Lancet, 359*, 1145-8.

Mendes, M. R., Carmona, M. H., & Malva, A. (1989). Estudo seroepidemiológico da febre Q numa população urbana e numa população de alto risco do Distrito de Lisboa. *Revista Portuguesa de Doenças Infecciosas*, *12*(3), 159–162.

Mendes, M. R., Carmona, M. H., Malva, A., & Souza, R. D. (1989). Febre Q. Estudo retrospec-tivo (casuística do Serviço de Doenças Infecto-Contagiosas do Hospital de Santa Maria). *Revista Portuguesa de Doenças Infecciosas*, *12*(3), 149–157.

Menkiti, I. (2004). On the normative conception of a person. In K. Wiredu (Ed.), *A companion to African philosophy* (pp. 324–331). New York, NY: Blackwell Publishing.

Meredith, A. L., Cleaveland, S. C., Denwood, M. J., Brown, J. K., & Shaw, D. J. (2015). *Coxiella burnetii* (Q-Fever) Seroprevalence in Prey and Predators in the United Kingdom: Evaluation of Infection in Wild Rodents, Foxes and Domestic Cats Using a Modified ELISA. *Transboundary and Emerging Diseases*, *62*(6), 639–649. doi:10.1111/tbed.12211 PMID:24479951

Messenger, A. M., Barnes, A. N., & Gray, G. C. (2014). Reverse zoonotic disease transmission (zooanthroponosis): A systematic review of seldom-documented human biological threats to animals. *PLoS One*, *9*(2), e89055. doi:10.1371/journal.pone.0089055 PMID:24586500

Michelle, A. R. (1993). *The Advancement of Veterinary Science: Vol. 3: History of the Healing Professions: Parallels between Veterinary and Medical History*. CAB International.

Miller, A. L., Wang, Y., Mooseker, M. S., & Koleske, A. J. (2004). The Abl-related gene (Arg) requires its F-actin–microtubule cross-linking activity to regulate lamellipodial dynamics during fibroblast adhesion. *The Journal of Cell Biology, 165*(3), 407–420. doi:10.1083/jcb.200308055 PMID:15138293

Miller, L., & Hurley, K. (2009). *Infectious Disease Management in Animal Shelters*. John Wiley and Sons.

Million, M., & Raoult, D. (2013). 66 - Q Fever. In A. J. Magill, D. R. Hill, T. Solomon, & E. T. Ryan (Eds.), *Hunter's Tropical Medicine and Emerging Infectious Disease* (9th ed.; pp. 558–560). London: W.B. Saunders; doi:10.1016/B978-1-4160-4390-4.00066-7

Mill, J. S. (2004). Duties to Animals are Direct. In A. Linzey & P. B. Clarke (Eds.), *Animal Rights: A Historical Anthology* (pp. 138–140). New York, NY: Columbia University Press.

Mizuno, S., Fujinaga, T., Tajima, M., Otomo, K., & Koike, T. (1989). Role of lymphocytes in dogs experimentally re-challenged with canine transmissible sarcoma. *Jpn. J.Vet. Sci., 51*(1), 86–95. doi:10.1292/jvms1939.51.86 PMID:2927041

Montavon, A., Jean-Richard, V., Bechir, M., Daugla, D. M., Abdoulaye, M., Bongo Naré, R. N., ... Zinsstag, J. (2013). Health of mobile pastoralists in the Sahel - assessment of 15 years of research and development. *Tropical Medicine & International Health, 18*(9), 1044–1052. doi:10.1111/tmi.12147 PMID:23834073

Mori, M., & Roest, H.J. (2018). Farming, Q fever and public health: agricultural practices and beyond. *Arch Public Health., 6*, 76. doi:. doi:10.118613690-017-0248-y

Mori, M., Boarbi, M., Michel, P., Bakinahe, R., Rits, K., Wattiau, P., & Fretin, D. (2013). In Vitro and In Vivo Infectious Potential of *Coxiella burnetii*: A Study on Belgian Livestock Isolates. *PLoS One, 8*(6), e67622. doi:10.1371/journal.pone.0067622 PMID:23840751

Mor, S. M., Robbins, A. H., Jarvin, I., Kaufman, G. E., & Lindenmayer, J. M. (2013). Curriculum asset mapping for One Health education. *Journal of Veterinary Medical Education, 40*(4), 363–369. doi:10.3138/jvme.0313-0525R PMID:24072190

Morse, S. S., Mazet, J. A. K., Woolhouse, M., Parrish, C. R., Carroll, D., Karesh, W. B., ... Daszak, P. (2012). Parediction and prevention of the next pandemic zoonosis. *Lancet, 380*(9857), 1956–1965. doi:10.1016/S0140-6736(12)61684-5 PMID:23200504

Munita, J. M., & Arias, C. A. (2016). Mechanisms of antibiotic resistance. *Microbiology Spectrum, 4*(2). doi:10.1128/microbiolspec.VMBF-0016-2015 PMID:27227291

Muskens, J., Wouda, W., von Bannisseht-Wijsmuller, T., & van Maanen, C. (2012). Prevalence of *Coxiella burnetii* infections in aborted fetuses and stillborn calves. *The Veterinary Record, 170*(10), 260. doi:10.1136/vr.100378 PMID:22186379

Mutsaers, I. (2015). One-health approach as counter-measure against "autoimmune" responses in biosecurity. *Social Science & Medicine, 129*, 123–130. doi:10.1016/j.socscimed.2014.09.042 PMID:25446776

Naicker, P. R. (2011). The impact of climate change and other factors on zoonotic diseases. *Archives of Clinical Microbiology, 2*(4).

Narayan, K. G. (2011). Veterinary Public Health—A route to One Health. *Proceedings of the 9th Conference of Association of Public Health Veterinarians, Challenges and strategies for Veterinary Public Health in India*, 1-6.

Narayanan, V. (2005). Hinduism. In *The Encyclopeadia of Religion and Nature* (pp. 763–777). London: Continuum.

Nasi, R., Brown, D., Wilkie, D., Bennett, E., Tutin, C., Van Tol, G., & Christophersen, T. (2008). Conservation and use of wildlife-based resources: the bushmeat crisis. In CBD Technical Series no. 33. Secretariat of the Convention on Biological Diversity and Center for International Forestry Research (pp. 1–50). CIFOR.

Nass, S. J., & Gorby, H. (2015). The role of clinical studies for pets with naturally occurring tumors in Transational Cancer Res: Workshop Summary. National Academic Press.

National Action Plan on Antimicrobial Resistance (NAP-AMR). (2017). Government of India.

Natterson, H. B., & Bowlers, K. Z. (2012). *The astonishing connection between human and animal health*. New York: A.A. Knopf.

Nelson, M. (2010). *Teaching holism in environmental ethics* (Unpublished pedagogical paper). Michigan State University, East Lansing, MI.

Niehaus, I. (2002). Bodies, heat, and taboos: Conceptualizing modern personhood in the South African Lowveld. *Ethnology, 41*(3), 189. doi:10.2307/4153025

Niemczuk, K., Szymańska-Czerwińska, M., Śmietanka, K., & Bocian, Ł. (2014). Comparison of diagnostic potential of serological, molecular and cell culture methods for detection of Q fever in ruminants. *Veterinary Microbiology, 171*(1-2), 147–152. doi:10.1016/j.vetmic.2014.03.015 PMID:24725446

Nutter, F. W. (1999). Understanding the interrelationships between botanical, human, and veterinary epidemiology: The Ys and Rs of it all. *Ecosystem Health*, *5*(3), 131–140. doi:10.1046/j.1526-0992.1999.09922.x

Omran, A. R. (1971). The epidemiologic transition. A theory of the epidemiology of population change. *The Milbank Quarterly*, *49*(4), 509–538. doi:10.2307/3349375 PMID:5155251

Omsland, A., Cockrell, D. C., Howe, D., Fischer, E. R., Virtaneva, K., Sturdevant, D. E., & Heinzen, R. A. (2009). Host cell-free growth of the Q fever bacterium *Coxiella burnetii*. *Proceedings of the National Academy of Sciences of the United States of America*, *106*(11), 4430–4434. doi:10.1073/pnas.0812074106 PMID:19246385

Osei Sekyere, J. (2014). Antibiotic Types and Handling Practices in Disease Management among Pig Farms in Ashanti Region, Ghana. *Journal of Veterinary Medicine*, 8. PMID:26464936

Ostfeld, R.S., & Holt, R.D. (2004). Are predators good for your health? Evaluating evidence for top-down regulation of zoonotic disease reservoirs. *Front Ecol Environ.*, 2, 13-20.

Oyston, P. C., & Davies, C. (2011). Q fever: The neglected biothreat agent. *Journal of Medical Microbiology*, *60*(1), 9–21. doi:10.1099/jmm.0.024778-0 PMID:21030501

Packard, R. M. (2007). *The making of a tropical disease. A short history of malaria*. Baltimore, MD: Johns Hopkins University Press.

Pagel, S. W., & Gautier, P. (2012). Use of Antimicrobial Agents in Livestock. *Revue Scientifique et Technique (International Office of Epizootics)*, *31*(1), 145–188. doi:10.20506/rst.31.1.2106 PMID:22849274

Palmela, C., Badura, R., & Valadas, E. (2012). Acute Q fever in Portugal. Epidemiological and clinical features of 32 hospitalized patients. *Germs*, *2*(2), 43–59. doi:10.11599/germs.2012.1013 PMID:24432263

Paloni, M., & Khanna, C. (2008). Translation of new cancer treatments from pet dogs to humans. *Nature Reviews. Cancer*, *8*(2), 147–156. doi:10.1038/nrc2273 PMID:18202698

Parker, N. R., Barralet, J. H., & Bell, A. M. (2006). Q fever. *Lancet*, *367*(9511), 679–688. doi:10.1016/S0140-6736(06)68266-4 PMID:16503466

Parkes, M. W., Charron, D. F., & Sanchez, A. (2012). Better together: field-building networks at the frontiers of ecohealth research. In D. F. Charron (Ed.), *Ecohealth Research in Practice: Innovative Applications of an Ecosystem Approach to Health.* Ottawa: Springer and International Development Research Centre. doi:10.1007/978-1-4614-0517-7_21

Parreira, P. (2008). *Estudo da prevalência de anticorpos anti-Coxiella burnetii numa amostra de dadores de sangue de uma região portuguesa* (Master dissertation). Retrieved from Repositório da Universidade de Lisboa Faculdade de Medicina (FM), Dissertações e Mestrados: http://hdl.handle.net/10451/1035

Pastorino, B., de Lamballerie, X., & Charrel, R. (2017). Biosafety and Biosecurity in European Containment Level 3 Laboratories: Focus on French Recent Progress and Essential Requirements. *Frontiers in Public Health, 5*, 121. doi:10.3389/fpubh.2017.00121 PMID:28620600

Patterson, D. (2003). Rabies. In K. F. Kiple (Ed.), *The Cambridge historical dictionary of disease* (pp. 270–275). Cambridge, UK: Cambridge University Press.

Patz, Graczyk, Geller, & Vittor. (2000). Effects of environmental change on emerging parasitic diseases. *Int J Parasitol., 30*, 1395-406.

Patz, J. A., Confalonieri, U. E. C., Amerasinghe, F. P., Chua, K. B., Daszak, P., & Hyatt, A. D. (2005). Human health: ecosystem regulation of infectious diseases. In Millennium ecosystem assessment. Condition and Trends Working Group. Ecosystems and human well-being: current state and trends. Vol. 1: Findings of the Condition and Trends Working Group. Washington, DC: Island Press.

Paul, N., Moodley, A., Ghibaudo, G., & Guardabassi, L. (2011). Carriage of methicillin-resistant *Staphylococcus pseudintermedius* in small animal veterinarians: Indirect evidence of zoonotic transmission. *Zoonoses and Public Health, 58*(8), 533–539. doi:10.1111/j.1863-2378.2011.01398.x PMID:21824350

Paulson, J. A., & Zaoutis, T. E. (2015). Council on Environmental Health, Committee on Infectious Diseases. Non therapeutic use of antimicrobial agents in animal agriculture: Implications for pediatrics. *Pediatrics, 136*, 1670–1677. doi:10.1542/peds.2015-3630

Pavlovsky, E. N. (1966). *Natural nidality of transmissible diseases.* Urbana, IL: University of Illinois Press. doi:10.1097/00000441-196611000-00067

Pellegrin, M., Delsol, G., Auvergnat, J. C., Familiades, J., Faure, H., Guiu, M., & Voigt, J. J. (1980). Granulomatous hepatitis in Q fever. *Human Pathology*, *11*(1), 51–57. doi:10.1016/S0046-8177(80)80105-5 PMID:7364439

Pemberton, N., & Worboys, M. (2007). *Mad dogs and Englishmen. Rabies in Britain, 1830-2000*. Basingstoke, UK: Palgrave Macmillan.

Philip, C. (1948). Comments on the Name of the Q Fever Organism. *Public Health Reports (1896-1970)*, *63*(2), 58-58. doi:10.2307/4586402

Pierce, J., & Jameton, A. (2004). *The ethics of environmentally responsible health care*. Oxford, UK: Oxford University Press, Inc. doi:10.1016/j.scitotenv.2004.03.034

Pike, R. M. (1976). Laboratory associated infections: Summary and analysis of 3921 cases. *Health Laboratory Science*, *13*(2), 105–114. PMID:946794

Pimenta, L., Alegria, N., Anastácio, S., Sidi-Boumedine, K., da Silva, G., Rabiço, Â., & Simões, J. (2015). Prevalence of *Coxiella burnetii* antibodies in Portuguese dairy cattle herds. *Tropical Animal Health and Production*, *47*(1), 227–230. doi:10.100711250-014-0679-1 PMID:25339430

Pinto, L., Radhouani, H., Coelho, C., Martins da Costa, P., Simões, R., Brandão, R. M. L., ... Poeta, P. (2010). Genetic detection of extended-spectrum β-lactamases *Escherichia coli* in birds of prey from Serra da Estrela Natural Reserve of Portugal. *Applied and Environmental Microbiology*, *76*, 4118–4120. doi:10.1128/AEM.02761-09 PMID:20418435

Piot, C. (1999). *Remotely global: Village modernity in West Africa*. Chicago, IL: The University of Chicago Press.

Polley, L. (2005). Navigating parasite webs and parasite flow: Emerging and re-emerging parasitic zoonoses of wildlife origin. *International Journal for Parasitology*, *35*(11-12), 1279–1294. doi:10.1016/j.ijpara.2005.07.003 PMID:16168994

Porter, S. R., Czaplicki, G., Mainil, J., Guattéo, R., & Saegerman, C. (2011). Q Fever: Current State of Knowledge and Perspectives of Research of a Neglected Zoonosis. *International Journal of Microbiology*, *248418*. doi:10.1155/2011/248418 PMID:22194752

Porter, V. R. (1999). Fragmented ethics and 'Bridges Bioethics.'. *The Hastings Center Report*, *29*(1), 38–40. doi:10.2307/3528538 PMID:10052010

Porter, V. R., & Whitehouse, P. J. (1998). Deep and global bioethics for a livable world. *Scientist (Philadelphia, Pa.)*, *12*(1), 9.

Potter, V. R. (1971). *Bioethics: Bridge to the future*. Englewood Cliffs, NJ: Prentice-Hall, Inc.

Potter, V. R. (1988). *Global bioethics: Building on the Leopold legacy*. East Lansing, MI: Michigan State University Press.

Potter, V. R. (1990). Getting to the Year 3000: Can global bioethics overcome evolution's fatal flaw? *Perspectives in Biology and Medicine*, *8*(2), 185–186. doi:10.1080/10590509009373376 PMID:11642811

Potter, V. R., & Potter, L. (1995). Global bioethics: Converting sustainable development to global survival. *Medicine and Global Survival*, *2*(3), 9–17. PMID:14627015

Press Information Bureau Government of India. (2007). *'Vision and Road Map' released at the conclusion of the three-day International Ministerial Conference on Avian and Pandemic Influenza*. Retrieved on 14 August from https://www.cdc.gov/onehealth/pdf/delhi/vision_roadmap.pdf

Price, L. B., Stegger, M., Hasman, H., Aziz, M., Larsen, J., Andersen, P. S., … Aarestrup, F.M. (2012). *Staphylococcus aureus* CC398: host adaptation and emergence of methicillin resistance in livestock. *MBio, 3*, 305–311. doi: .00305-11 doi:10.1128/mBio

Quigley, D. (2006). A review of improved ethical practices in environmental and public health research: Case examples from Native communities. *Ethical Practices in Environmental and Public Health*, *33*(2), 130-147. doi:. doi:10.1023/A:1021132602330

Rabinowitz, P. M., Kock, R., Kachani, M., Kunkel, R., Thomas, J., Gilbert, J., ... Rubin, C. (2013). Toward proof of concept of a one health approach to disease prediction and control. *Emerging Infectious Diseases*, *19*(12). doi:10.3201/eid1912.130265 PMID:24295136

Randolph, S.E. (2008). Dynamics of tick-borne disease systems: minor role of recent climate change. *Rev sci tech Off Int Epiz, 27*(2), 367-381.

Randolph, T. F., Schelling, E., Grace, D., Nicholson, C. F., Leroy, J. L., Cole, D. C., ... Ruel, M. (2007). Invited review: Role of livestock in human nutrition and health for poverty reduction in developing countries. *Journal of Animal Science*, *85*(11), 2788–2800. doi:10.2527/jas.2007-0467 PMID:17911229

Raoult, D., Brouqui, P., Marchou, B., & Gastaut, J. A. (1992). Acute and chronic Q fever in patients with cancer. *Clinical Infectious Diseases*, *14*(1), 127–130. doi:10.1093/clinids/14.1.127 PMID:1571416

Raoult, D., Marrie, T., & Mege, J. (2005). Natural history and pathophysiology of Q fever. *The Lancet Infectious Diseases*, *5*(4), 219–226. doi:10.1016/S1473-3099(05)70052-9 PMID:15792739

Raoult, D., Vestris, G., & Enea, M. (1990). Isolation of 16 strains of *Coxiella burnetii* from patients by using a sensitive centrifugation cell culture system and establishment of the strains in HEL cells. *Journal of Clinical Microbiology*, *28*(11), 2482–2484. PMID:2254424

Reimer, L. G. (1993). Q fever. *Clinical Microbiology Reviews*, *6*(3), 193–198. doi:10.1128/CMR.6.3.193 PMID:8358703

Robinson, T. P., Bu, D. P., Carrique-Mas, J., Fevre, E. M., Gilbert, M., Grace, D., ... Woolhouse, M. E. J. (2016). Antibiotic resistance is the quintessential one health issue. *Transactions of the Royal Society of Tropical Medicine and Hygiene*, *110*(7), 377–380. doi:10.1093/trstmh/trw048 PMID:27475987

Rodolakis, A. (2009). Q Fever in dairy animals. *Annals of the New York Academy of Sciences*, *1166*(1), 90–93. doi:10.1111/j.1749-6632.2009.04511.x PMID:19538267

Roest, H. I., Post, J., van Gelderen, B., van Zijderveld, F. G., & Rebel, J. M. (2013). Q fever in pregnant goats: Humoral and cellular immune responses. *Veterinary Research*, *44*(1), 67. doi:10.1186/1297-9716-44-67 PMID:23915213

Roest, H.-J., van Gelderen, B., Dinkla, A., Frangoulidis, D., van Zijderveld, F., Rebel, J., & van Keulen, L. (2012). Q Fever in Pregnant Goats: Pathogenesis and Excretion of *Coxiella burnetii*. *PLoS One*, *7*(11), e48949. doi:10.1371/journal.pone.0048949 PMID:23152826

Romano, P. S., Gutierrez, M. G., Beron, W., Rabinovitch, M., & Colombo, M. I. (2007). The autophagic pathway is actively modulated by phase II *Coxiella burnetii* to efficiently replicate in the host cell. *Cellular Microbiology*, *9*(4), 891–909. doi:10.1111/j.1462-5822.2006.00838.x PMID:17087732

Rousset, E., Berri, M., Durand, B., Dufour, P., Prigent, M., Delcroix, T., ... Rodolakis, A. (2009). *Coxiella burnetii* Shedding Routes and Antibody Response after Outbreaks of Q Fever-Induced Abortion in Dairy Goat Herds. *Applied and Environmental Microbiology*, *75*(2), 428–433. doi:10.1128/AEM.00690-08 PMID:19011054

Rousset, E., Durand, B., Berri, M., Dufour, P., Prigent, M., Russo, P., ... Aubert, M. F. (2007). Comparative diagnostic potential of three serological tests for abortive Q fever in goat herds. *Veterinary Microbiology*, *124*(3-4), 286–297. doi:10.1016/j.vetmic.2007.04.033 PMID:17532581

Russell-Lodrigue, K. E., Andoh, M., Poels, M. W. J., Shive, H. R., Weeks, B. R., Zhang, G. Q., ... Samuel, J. E. (2009). *Coxiella burnetii* Isolates Cause Genogroup-Specific Virulence in Mouse and Guinea Pig Models of Acute Q Fever. *Infection and Immunity, 77*(12), 5640–5650. doi:10.1128/IAI.00851-09 PMID:19786560

Russell-Lodrigue, K. E., Zhang, G. Q., McMurray, D. N., & Samuel, J. E. (2006). Clinical and Pathologic Changes in a Guinea Pig Aerosol Challenge Model of Acute Q Fever. *Infection and Immunity, 74*(11), 6085–6091. doi:10.1128/IAI.00763-06 PMID:17057087

Samuel, J. E., & Hendrix, L. R. (2009). Laboratory maintenance of *Coxiella burnetii. Current Protocols in Microbiology, 6*(C.1), 1–16. doi:10.1002/9780471729259.mc06c01s15

Sanchez, J., Souriau, A., Buendia, A. J., Arricau-Bouvery, N., Martínez, C. M., Salinas, J., ... Navarro, J. A. (2006). Experimental *Coxiella burnetii* infection in pregnant goats: A histopathological and immunohistochemical study. *Journal of Comparative Pathology, 135*(2-3), 108–115. doi:10.1016/j.jcpa.2006.06.003 PMID:16997003

Sandoz, K. M., Sturdevant, D. E., Hansen, B., & Heinzen, R. A. (2014). Developmental transitions of *Coxiella burnetii* grown in axenic media. *Journal of Microbiological Methods, 96*, 104–110. doi:10.1016/j.mimet.2013.11.010 PMID:24286928

Santos, A. S., Bacellar, F., & França, A. (2007a). Febre Q: Revisão de conceitos. *Revue de Médecine Interne, 14*(2), 90–99.

Santos, A. S., de Sousa, R., Alves, F., Proença, P., Núncio, M. S., Dumler, J. S., & Bacellar, F. (2007b). Isolation of *Coxiella burnetii* from the blood of a patient with positive Anaplasma phagocytophilum serological results. *Clinical Microbiology and Infection, 15*, 192–193. doi:10.1111/j.1469-0691.2008.02222.x PMID:19416284

Satterthwaite, D., McGranahan, G., & Tacoli, C. (2010). Urbanization and its implications for food and farming. *Philos Trans R Soc B Biol Sci., 365*, 2809-20.

Saunders, L. Z. (2000). Virchow's Contributions to Veterinary Medicine: Celebrated Then, Forgotten Now. *Veterinary Pathology, 37*(3), 199–207. doi:10.1354/vp.37-3-199 PMID:10810984

Schelling, E. (2002). *Human and animal health in nomadic pastoralist of Chad: Zoonoses, morbidity and health services* (Doctoral dissertation). Available from https://edoc.unibas.ch/57/1/DissB_6478.pdf

Schelling, E., Bechir, M., Ahmed, M. A., Wyss, K., Randolph, T. F., & Zinsstag, J. (2007). Human and animal vaccination delivery to remote nomadic families, Chad. *Emerging Infectious Diseases*, *13*(3), 373–379. doi:10.3201/eid1303.060391 PMID:17552089

Schelling, E., Daoud, S., Daugla, D. M., Diallo, P., Tanner, M., & Zinsstag, J. (2005). Morbidity and nutrition patterns of three nomadic pastoralist communities of Chad. *Acta Tropica*, *95*(1), 16–25. doi:10.1016/j.actatropica.2005.03.006 PMID:15866506

Schelling, E., Diguimbaye, C., Daoud, S., Nicolet, J., Boerlin, P., Tanner, M., & Zinsstag, J. (2003). Brucellosis and Q-fever seroprevalences of nomadic pastoralists and their livestock in Chad. *Preventive Veterinary Medicine*, *61*(4), 279–293. doi:10.1016/j.prevetmed.2003.08.004 PMID:14623412

Schelling, E., & Kimani, T. (2007). *Human and animal health response capacity and costs: a rapid appraisal of the 2007 Rift Valley fever outbreak in Kenya*. International Livestock Research Institute.

Schmidt, K., Dressel, K. M., Niedrig, M., Mertens, M., Schüle, S. A., & Groschup, M. H. (2013). Public Health and Vector-Borne Diseases – A New Concept for Risk Governance. *Zoonoses and Public Health*, *2013*(Mar), 11. doi:10.1111/zph.12045 PMID:23480672

Schmithausen, L. (2005). Buddhism. In *The Encyclopeadia of Religion and Nature* (pp. 232–236). London: Continuum.

Schneeberger, P. M., Wintenberger, C., van der Hoek, W., & Stahl, J. P. (2014). Q fever in the Netherlands - 2007–2010: What we learned from the largest outbreak ever. *Medecine et Maladies Infectieuses*, *44*(8), 339–353. doi:10.1016/j.medmal.2014.02.006 PMID:25108615

Schwabe, C. W. (1978). *Cattle, Priests, and Progress in Medicine*. Minneapolis, MN: University of Minnesota Press.

Schwabe, C. W. (1984). *Veterinary medicine and human health* (3rd ed.). Baltimore, MD: Williams and Wilkins.

Schwartz, S. & Bilsky, W. (1987). Towards a universal psychological structure of human values. *Journal of Personality and Social Psychology*, (53), 550-562.

Schweitzer, A. (2004). Duties to Life. In A. Linzey & P. B. Clarke (Eds.), *Animal Rights: A Historical Anthology* (pp. 152–153). New York, NY: Columbia University Press.

Scott, G. H., Williams, J. C., & Stephenson, E. H. (1987). Animal models in Q fever: Pathological responses of inbred mice to phase I *Coxiella burnetii. Microbiology, 133*(3), 691–700. doi:10.1099/00221287-133-3-691 PMID:3655728

Scott, H. H. (1942). *A History of Tropical Medicine* (Vol. 1-2). London, UK: Arnold.

Scott, S., & Duncan, C. J. (2001). *Biology of Plagues. Evidence from Historical Populations*. Cambridge, UK: Cambridge University Press. doi:10.1017/CBO9780511542527

Seshadri, R., Paulsen, I. T., Eisen, J. A., Read, T. D., Nelson, K. E., & Nelson, W. C. (2003). Complete genome sequence of the Q-fever pathogen *Coxiella burnetii. Proceedings of the National Academy of Sciences of the United States of America, 100*(9), 5455–5460. doi:10.1073/pnas.0931379100

Shaffer, L. E. (2008). Role of surveillance in disease prevention and control: Cross species surveillance contribution to one medicine. *Proceedings of Annual Meeting of American Veterinary Medical Association.*

Shannon, J. G., & Heinzen, R. A. (2008). Infection of human monocyte-derived macrophages with *Coxiella burnetii. Methods in Molecular Biology (Clifton, N.J.), 431*, 189–200. PMID:18287757

Shannon, J. G., & Heinzen, R. A. (2009). Adaptive Immunity to the Obligate Intracellular Pathogen *Coxiella burnetii. Immunologic Research, 43*(1-3), 138–148. doi:10.100712026-008-8059-4 PMID:18813881

Shannon, J. G., Howe, D., & Heinzen, R. A. (2005). Virulent *Coxiella burnetii* does not activate human dendritic cells: Role of lipopolysaccharide as a shielding molecule. *Proceedings of the National Academy of Sciences of the United States of America, 102*(24), 8722–8727. doi:10.1073/pnas.0501863102 PMID:15939879

Shomaker, T. S., Green, E. M., & Yandow, S. M. (2013). Prespective: One Health: a compelling convergence. *Academic Medicine, 90*, 866–871. PMID:23165268

Shortridge, K. F., Peiris, J. S. M., & Guan, Y. (2003). The next influenza pandemic: Lessons from Hong Kong. *Journal of Applied Microbiology, 94*(s1), 70S–79S. doi:10.1046/j.1365-2672.94.s1.8.x PMID:12675938

Shrestha, K., Acharya, K. P., & Shrestha, S. (2018). One health: The interface between veterinary and human health. *International Journal of One Health, 4*, 8–14. doi:10.14202/IJOH.2018.8-14

Shrestha, R. K., Stoller, J. K., Honari, G., Procop, G. W., & Gordon, S. M. (2004). Pneumonia due to *Cryptococcus neoformans* in a patient receiving infliximab: Possible zoonotic transmission from a pet cockatiel. *Respiratory Care*, *49*, 606–608. PMID:15165294

Siciliano, R., Barbosa Ribeiro, H., Furtado, R. H. M., Castelli, J., Sampaio, R., Santos, F., ... Strabelli, T. (2008). Endocardite por *Coxiella burnetii* (febre Q): Doença rara ou pouco diagnosticada? Relato de caso. *Revista da Sociedade Brasileira de Medicina Tropical*, *41*(4), 409–412. doi:10.1590/S0037-86822008000400017 PMID:18853017

Sidi-Boumedine, K., Rousset, E., Henning, K., Ziller, M., Niemczuck, K., Roest, H. I. J., & Thiéry, R. (2010). *Development of harmonised schemes for the monitoring and reporting of Q-fever in animals in the European Union.* EFSA Scientific Report on Question No EFSA-Q-2009-00511. Retrieved 15, December, from https://efsa.onlinelibrary.wiley.com/doi/epdf/10.2903/sp.efsa.2010.EN-48

Singer, P. (2004). All Animals are Equal. In A. Linzey & P. B. Clarke (Eds.), *Animal Rights: A Historical Anthology* (pp. 138–140). New York, NY: Columbia University Press.

Skultety, L., Hajduch, M., Flores-Ramirez, G., Miernyk, J. A., Ciampor, F., Toman, R., & Sekeyova, Z. (2011). Proteomic comparison of virulent phase I and avirulent phase II of *Coxiella burnetii*, the causative agent of Q fever. *Journal of Proteomics*, *74*(10), 1974–1984. doi:10.1016/j.jprot.2011.05.017 PMID:21616182

Slifkoa, Huw, Smith, & Rose. (2000). Emerging parasite zoonoses associated with water and food. *International Journal for Parasitology*, 1379-1393.

St Aquinas, T. (2004). Animals are not Rational Creatures. In A. Linzey & P. B. Clarke (Eds.), *Animal Rights: A Historical Anthology* (pp. 7–11). New York, NY: Columbia University Press.

Stefanovska, J. (2014). *Report to EDENext projet from WG16: Public Health and Vector-Borne Diseases. A New Concept for Risk Governance*. (Unpublished)

Stein, M. (2008), Zoonosen. Fragile Barriere zwischen den Arten. *Research*Eu. Magazin des europäischen Forschungsraums, Sonderausgabe Oktober ‚Mensch sein Tier sein‘*, 34.

Stein, A., Louveau, C., Lepidi, H., Ricci, F., Baylac, P., Davoust, B., & Raoult, D. (2005). Q Fever Pneumonia: Virulence of *Coxiella burnetii* Pathovars in a Murine Model of Aerosol Infection. *Infection and Immunity*, *73*(4), 2469–2477. doi:10.1128/IAI.73.4.2469-2477.2005 PMID:15784593

Stein, A., Saunders, N. A., Taylor, A. G., & Raoult, D. (1993). Phylogenic homogeneity of *Coxiella burnetii* strains as determinated by 16S ribosomal RNA sequencing. *FEMS Microbiology Letters, 113*(3), 339–344. doi:10.1111/j.1574-6968.1993.tb06537.x PMID:7505761

Stokstad, E. L. R., & Jukes, T. H. (1950). Further observations on the "animal protein factor." *Proceedings of the Society for Experimental Biology and Medicine, 73*(*3*), 523–528. 10.3181/00379727-73-17731

Tangwa, G. B. (2004). Some African Reflections on Biomedical and Environmental Ethics. In K. Wiredu (Ed.), *A Companion to African philosophy* (pp. 387–395). Oxford, UK: Blackwell Publishers.

Taylor, L. H., Latham, S. M., & Woolhouse, M. E. J. (2001). Risk factors for human disease emergence. *Philosophical Transactions of the Royal Society of London. Series B, Biological Sciences, 356*(1411), 983–989. doi:10.1098/rstb.2001.0888 PMID:11516376

Tempels, P., Rubbens, A., & King, C. (1959). *Bantu philosophy*. Paris: Présence Africaine.

The Center for Food Security and Public Health (CFSPH). (2017). *Q fever*. Retrieved in April 24, 2018, from http://www.cfsph.iastate.edu/Factsheets/pdfs/q_fever.pdf

The Internet Encyclopedia of Philosophy. (n.d.). *Bioethics*. Retrieved June 26, 2014, from http://www.iep.utm.edu/bioethic/#SH2a

The World Organisation for Animal Health (OIE). (2012). Manual of Diagnostic Tests and Vaccines for Terrestrial Animals. *Terrestrial Manual*. Retrieved from http://www.oie.int/fileadmin/Home/eng/Health_standards/tahm/2.01.16_Q_FEVER.pdf

Tirado, F., Gomez, A., & Rocamora, V. (2015). The global condition of epidemics: Panoramas in A (H1N1) influenza and their consequences for One World One Health program. *Social Science & Medicine, 129*, 113–122. doi:10.1016/j.socscimed.2014.09.003 PMID:25218795

Tissot Dupont, H., Raoult, D., Brouqui, P., Janbon, F., Peyramond, D., Weiller, P. J., ... Poirier, R. (1992). Epidemiologic features and clinical presentation of acute Q fever in hospitalized patients: 323 French cases. *The American Journal of Medicine, 93*(4), 427–434. doi:10.1016/0002-9343(92)90173-9 PMID:1415306

Toole, M. J., & Waldman, R. J. (1997). The public health aspects of complex emergencies and refugee situations. *Annual Review of Public Health, 18*(1), 283–312. doi:10.1146/annurev.publhealth.18.1.283 PMID:9143721

Tucker, M. E. (2005). Confucianism. In *The Encyclopeadia of Religion and Nature* (pp. 407–411). London: Continuum.

Tujulin, E., Lilliehöök, B., Macellaro, A., Sjöstedt, A., & Norlander, L. (1999). Early cytokine induction in mouse P388D1 macrophages infected by *Coxiella burnetii. Veterinary Immunology and Immunopathology*, *68*(2-4), 159–168. doi:10.1016/S0165-2427(99)00023-9 PMID:10438316

UNHCR. (2017). *Global trends: Forced displacements in 2017*. UNHCR.

United Nations Department of Economics and Social Affairs. (2003). *World Population Prospects*. United Nations.

United Nations, Department of Economic and Social Affairs, Population Division. (2015). *World Population Prospects: The 2015 Revision, Key Findings and Advance Tables*. Working Paper No. ESA/P/WP.241.

United Nations. (1975). *Report of the World Food Conference in Rome, 5-16 November 1974*. New York, NY: United Nations.

UNSCN. (2010). *Progress in Nutrition. 6th report on the world nutrition situation*. Geneva, Switzerland: UNSCN.

UNSCN. (2014). *Nutrition and the Post-2015 Sustainable Development Goals. A Technical Note*. Geneva, Switzerland: UNSCN.

UNSCN. (2017a). *Global Governance for Nutrition and the role of UNSCN*. Discussion Paper. Geneva, Switzerland: UNSCN.

UNSCN. (2017b). *By 2030, end all forms of malnutrition and leave no one behind*. Discussion Paper. Geneva, Switzerland: UNSCN.

UNSCN. (2017c). *Sustainable Diets for Healthy People and a Healthy Planet*. Discussion Paper. Geneva, Switzerland: UNSCN.

US General Accounting Office West Nile virus outbreak. (2000). *Lessons for public health preparedness*. Washington, DC: The Office. GAO/HEHS-00-180.

Vadovic, P., Slaba, K., Fodorova, M., Skultety, L., & Toman, R. (2005). Structural and Functional Characterization of the Glycan Antigens Involved in Immunobiology of Q Fever. *Annals of the New York Academy of Sciences*, *1063*(1), 149–153. doi:10.1196/annals.1355.023 PMID:16481506 van Asseldonk, M. A. P. M., Bontje, D. M., Backer, J. A., van Roermund, H. J. W., & Bergevoet, R. H. M. (2015). Economic aspects of Q fever control in dairy goats. *Preventive Veterinary Medicine*, *121*(1-2), 115–122. doi:10.1016/j.prevetmed.2015.06.010 PMID:26164531

Van Boeckel, T. P., Brower, C., Gilbert, M., Grenfell, B. T., Levin, S., Robinson, T. P., ... Laxminarayan, R. (2015). Global Trends in Antimicrobial Use in Food Animals. *Proceedings of the National Academy of Sciences of the United States of America*, *112*(18), 5649–5654. doi:10.1073/pnas.1503141112 PMID:25792457

Van den Brom, R., van Engelen, E., Luttikholt, S., Moll, L., van Maanen, K., & Vellema, P. (2012). *Coxiella burnetii* in bulk tank milk samples from dairy goat and dairy sheep farms in The Netherlands in 2008. *The Veterinary Record*, *170*(12), 310. doi:10.1136/vr.100304 PMID:22351793

Van den Brom, R., van Engelen, E., Roest, H. I., Van der Hoek, W., & Vellema, P. (2015). *Coxiella burnetii* infections in sheep or goats: An opinionated review. *Veterinary Microbiology*, *181*(1-2), 119–129. doi:10.1016/j.vetmic.2015.07.011 PMID:26315774

Van der Hoek, W., Dijkstra, F., Schimmer, B., Schneeberger, P. M., Vellema, P., Wijkmans, C., ... van Duynhoven, Y. (2010). Q fever in the Netherlands: An update on the epidemiology and control measures. *Eurosurveillance*, *25*(12), 19520. doi:10.2807/ese.15.12.19520-en PMID:20350500

van Loenhout, J. A., Paget, W. J., Vercoulen, J. H., Wijkmans, C. J., Hautvast, J. L. A., & van der Velden, K. (2012). Assessing the long-term health impact of Q-fever in the Netherlands: A prospective cohort study started in 2007 on the largest documented Q-fever outbreak to date. *BMC Infectious Diseases*, *12*(1), 280. doi:10.1186/1471 2334-12-280 PMID:23110336

van Schaik, E. J., Chen, C., Mertens, K., Weber, M. M., & Samuel, J. E. (2013). Molecular pathogenesis of the obligate intracellular bacterium *Coxiella burnetii*. *Nature Reviews. Microbiology*, *11*(8), 561–573. doi:10.1038/nrmicro3049 PMID:23797173

van Vlissingen, M. (2001). Professional ethics in veterinary science – considering the consequences as a tool for problem solving. *Veterinary Sciences for Tomorrow*, *1*, 1–8.

Vanderburg, S., Rubach, M. P., Halliday, J. E., Cleaveland, S., Reddy, E. A., & Crump, J. A. (2014). Epidemiology of Coxiella burnetii infection in Africa: A OneHealth systematic review. *PLoS Neglected Tropical Diseases*, *8*(4), e2787. doi:10.1371/journal.pntd.0002787 PMID:24722554

Vandersmissen, A. (2010). *'One Health': From a Classical Concept to a Modern Dynamics for Global Co-operation*. Paper presented at Operationalizing 'One Health': A Policy Perspective -Taking Stock and Shaping an Implementation Roadmap, Stone Mountain, GA. Retrieved 14 August 2018 from https://www.cdc.gov/onehealth/pdf/atlanta/alain_vandersmissen.pdf

Veldman, K., Cavaco, L. M., Mevius, D., Battisti, A., Franco, A., Botteldoorn, N., ... Aarestrup, S. (2011). International collaborative study on the occurrence of plasmid mediated quinolone resistance in *Salmonella enterica* and *Escherichia coli* isolated from animals, humans, food and the environment in 13 European countries. *The Journal of Antimicrobial Chemotherapy*, *66*(6), 1278–1286. doi:10.1093/jac/dkr084 PMID:21393198

Verbrugghe, E., Boyen, F., Gaastra, W., Bekhuis, L., Leyman, B., Van Parys, A., ... Pasmans, F. (2012). The complex interplay between stress and bacterial infections in animals. *Veterinary Microbiology*, *155*(2-4), 115–127. doi:10.1016/j.vetmic.2011.09.012 PMID:21963418

Verharen, C. C. (1995). Afrocentrism and Acentrism: A marriage of science and philosophy. *Journal of Black Studies*, *26*(1), 62–76. doi:10.1177/002193479502600105

Verharen, C. C. (2006). Philosophy against empire: An ancient Egyptian renaissance. *Journal of Black Studies*, *36*(6), 958–973. doi:10.1177/0021934705286128

Vermeulen, V. (2010). Forschung an Tieren. In *Forschungsethik. Eine Einführung* (pp. 82–97). Stuttgart: J. B. Metzler.

Vincent, G. A., Graves, S. R., Robsond, J. M., Nguyen, C., Hussain-Yusuf, H., Islama, A., ... Stenos, J. (2015). Isolation of *Coxiella burnetii* from serum of patients with acute Q fever. *Journal of Microbiological Methods*, *119*, 74–78. doi:10.1016/j.mimet.2015.10.008 PMID:26462766

Virchow, R. (1855). Infectionen durch contagiöse Thiergifte. In *Intoxicationen, Zoonosen und Syphilis = Handbuch der speciellen Pathologie und Therapie, 2(1)*. Erlangen: Enke.

Virchow, R. (1864). *Darstellung der Lehre von den Trichinen mit Rücksicht auf die dadurch gebotenen Vorsichtsmaaßregeln für Laien und Ärzte*. Berlin, Germany: Reimer.

Vohl, D. E., & Heinzen, R. A. (2007). Microreview: Lounging in a lysosome: the intracellular lifestyle of *Coxiella burnetii*. *Cellular Microbiology*, *9*(4), 829–840. doi:10.1111/j.1462-5822.2007.00901.x PMID:17381428

von Braun, J., Ruel, M. T., & Gillespie, S. (2010). Bridging the gap: Linking agriculture and health to achieve the Millenium Development Goals. In P. Pintrup-Andersen (Ed.), *The African Food System and its Interaction with Human Health and Nutrition* (pp. 279–303). Ithaca, NY: Cornell University Press.

von Engelhardt, D. (1984). Kausalität und Konditionalität in der modernen Medizin. In H. Schipperges (Ed.), *Pathogenese. Grundzüge und Perspektiven einer Theoretischen Pathologie*. Berlin, Germany: Springer.

VWB/VSF Canada. (2010). *One Health for One World: A Compendium of Case Studies*. Available at: https:// www.vetswithoutborders.ca/images/pdfs/OHOW%20 Compendium%20Case%20Studies.pdf

Wagner, E. (Ed.). (1874). *Handbuch der allgemeinen Pathologie*. Leipzig, Germany: Otto Wigand.

Weiss, R. (2003, April 7). African's Apes are imperiled, Researchers Warn. *Washington Post*.

Wendt, A., Kreienbrock, L., & Campe, A. (2014). Zoonotic Disease Surveillance – Inventory of Systems Integrating Human and Animal Disease Information. *Zoonoses and Public Health*, n/a. doi:10.1111/zph.12120 PMID:24712724

Whitehouse, P. J. (1999). The ecomedical disconnection syndrome. *The Hastings Center Report*, *29*(1), 41–44. doi:10.2307/3528539 PMID:10052011

WHO, EU, ILRI, DBL, FAO, OIE, & AU. (2009). *Integrated Control of Neglected Zoonotic Diseases in Africa / Applying the 'One Health' Concept*. Available at: http://whqlibdoc. who.int/hq/2008/WHO_HTM_NTD_NZD_2008.1_eng.pdf

Wilkie, D. S., & Carpenter, J. F. (1999). Bushmeat hunting in the Congo Basin: An assessment of impacts and options for mitigation. *Biodiversity and Conservation*, *8*(7), 927–955. doi:10.1023/A:1008877309871

Wilkinson, L. (1981). Glanders: Medicine and veterinary medicine in common pursuit of a contagious disease. *Medical History, 25*(04), 363–384. doi:10.1017/S0025727300034876 PMID:7038356

Wilkinson, L. (1988). Understanding the Nature of Rabies: An Historical Perspective. In J. B. Campbell & K. M. Charlton (Eds.), *Rabies = Developments in Veterinary Virology, 7* (pp. 1–23). Boston, MA: Springer. doi:10.1007/978-1-4613-1755-5_1

Wilkinson, L. (1992). *Animals and disease. An introduction to the history of comparative medicine*. Cambridge, UK: Cambridge University Press.

Wilkinson, L. (1992). *Animals and Disease. An introduction to the history of comparative medicine*. Cambridge, UK: Cambridge University Press.

Wilkinson, L. (1993). Anthrax. In K. F. Kiple (Ed.), *The Cambridge world history of human disease* (pp. 582–584). Cambridge, UK: Cambridge University Press. doi:10.1017/CHOL9780521332866.070

Wilson, I. G. (2004). Airborne *Campylobacter infection* in a poultry worker: Case report and review of the literature. *Communicable Disease and Public Health, 7*, 349–353. PMID:15779805

Winau, R. (1887). *Medizin in Berlin*. Berlin, Germany: Walter de Gruyter.

Winkler, M. S., Krieger, G. R., Divall, M. J., Singer, B. H., & Utzinger, J. (2012). Health impact assessment of industrial development projects: A spatio-temporal visualization. *Geospatial Health, 6*(2), 299–301. doi:10.4081/gh.2012.148 PMID:22639132

Wiredu, K. (2004). Introduction: African philosophy in our time. In K. Wiredu (Ed.), *A Companion to African Philosophy* (pp. 1–28). Blackwell Publishing.

Woldehiwet, Z. (2004). Q fever (coxiellosis): Epidemiology and pathogenesis. *Research in Veterinary Science, 77*(2), 93–100. doi:10.1016/j.rvsc.2003.09.001 PMID:15196898

Wolf, M. (2015, March). Is there really such a thing as "one health"? Thinking about a more than human world from the perspective of cultural anthropology. *Social Science & Medicine, 129*, 5–11. doi:10.1016/j.socscimed.2014.06.018 PMID:24961737

Woolhouse, M. E. J. (2008). Epidemiology: Emerging diseases go global. *Nature, 451*(7181), 898–899. doi:10.1038/451898a PMID:18288175

Woolhouse, M., Ward, M., van Bunnik, B., & Farrar, J. (2015). Antimicrobial resistance in humans, livestock and the wider environment. *Philosophical Transactions of the Royal Society of London. Series B, Biological Sciences*, *370*(1670), 20140083. doi:10.1098/rstb.2014.0083 PMID:25918441

Woolridge, M. (2012). Evidence for the circulation of antimicrobial-resistant strains and genes in nature and especially between humans and animals. *Revue Scientifique et Technique (International Office of Epizootics)*, *31*, 231–247. PMID:22849279

World Bank Group. (2018). *Operational Framework for strengthening human, animal and environmental public health systems at their interface = Report number 122980-GLB*. Washington, DC: World Bank.

World Bank. (1986). *Poverty and Hunger: Issues and Options for Food Security in Developing Countries*. Washington, DC: World Bank.

World Bank. (2010a). People, Pathogens, and Our Planet: Vol. 1. *Towards a One Health Approach for Controlling Zoonotic Diseases*. Washington, DC: The World Bank.

World Bank. (2010b). People, Pathogens and Our Planet: Vol. 2. *The Economics of One Health*. Washington, DC: The World Bank.

World Health Assembly. (1954). *WHA7-TD-8 Report of technical discussions at the Seventh World Health Assembly*. Author.

World Health Assembly. (1969). *WHA22.35 Socio-economic Consequences of the Zoonoses*. Author.

World Health Organization, International Agency for Research on Cancer. (2013, October 17). *Press Release, No. 221*. WHO.

World Health Organization. (1975). The Veterinary contributions to public health practice. Report of a joint FAO/WHO Expert Committee on Veterinary Public Health. Geneva, WHO. *Technical Report Series (World Health Organization)*, *573*, 79.

World Health Organization. (2002). *Future trends in veterinary public health*. Report of a Joint FAO, WHO & OIE Expert Committee on Veterinary Public Health, Geneva, WHO Tech Rep. Ser., 907, p-85.

World Health Organization. (2006). *Global Early Warning and Response System for Major Animal Diseases including Zoonoses (GLEWS)*. Final version adopted by WHO, FAO & OIE tripartite. 2006:1-26.

World Health Organization. (2006). The Control of Neglected Zoonotic Diseases: A Route to Poverty Alleviation: Report of a Joint WHO/DFID-AHP. Meeting with the participation of FAO and OIE = WHO/SDE/FOS/2006.1, Geneva, Switzerland.

World Health Organization. (2014). *Antimicrobial resistance: global report on surveillance*. WHO.

World Health Organization. (2014). Guidance framework for testing of genetically modified mosquitoes. A health information product by the WHO-executed UNICEF/UNDP/World Bank/World Health Organizations Special Program for Research and Training in Tropical Diseases. Geneva, Switzerland: WHO.

World Health Report. (2007). *A Safer Future: Global Public Health Security*. Geneva, Switzerland: WHO.

World Organisation for Animal Health (OIE). (2015). Manual of Diagnostic Tests and Vaccines for Terrestrial Animals 2015. *Terrestrial Manual.* Retrieved from http://www.oie.int/fileadmin/Home/eng/Health_standards/tahm/2.01.16_Q_FEVER.pdf

Wouda, W., & Dercksen, D. P. (2007). Abortion and stillbirth among dairy goats as a consequence of *Coxiella burnetii. Tijdschrift voor Diergeneeskunde*, *132*(23), 908–911. PMID:18085173

Wurtz, N., Papa, A., Hukic, M., Di Caro, A., Leparc-Goffart, I., Leroy, E., ... Raoult, D. (2016). Survey of laboratory acquired infections around the world in biosafety level 3 and 4 laboratories. *European Journal of Clinical Microbiology & Infectious Diseases*, *35*(8), 1247–1258. doi:10.100710096-016-2657-1 PMID:27234593

Wydra, K. (2012). The One Health Concept in a development context. In M. Kappas, U. Groß, & D. Kelleher (Eds.), *Global Health - A challenge for interdisciplinary research*. Göttingen, Germany: Universitätsverlag.

Ziman, J. (1998). Why must scientists become more ethically sensitive than they used to be? *Science*, *282*(5395), 1813–1814. doi:10.1126cience.282.5395.1813 PMID:11645122

Zinkernagel, R. M., & Doherty, P. C. (1974). Immunological surveillance against altered self components by sensitized T lymphocytes in lymphocytic choriomeningitis. *Nature*, 251.

Zinsstag, J., Schelling, E., Waltner-Toews, D., & Tanner, M. (2011). *From "one medicine" to "one health" and systemic approaches to health and well-being*. Academic Press.

Zinsstag, J. (2012). Convergence of Ecohealth and One Health. *EcoHealth*, *9*(4), 371–373. doi:10.100710393-013-0812-z PMID:23392841

Zinsstag, J., Mackenzie, J. S., Jeggo, M., Heymann, D. L., Patz, J. A., & Daszak, P. (2012). Mainstreaming one health. *EcoHealth*, *9*(2), 107–110. doi:10.100710393-012-0772-8 PMID:22777051

Zinsstag, J., Schelling, E., Daoud, S., Schierle, J., Hofmann, P., Diguimbaye, C., ... Tanner, M. (2002). Serum retinol of Chadian nomadic pastoralist women in relation to their livestocks' milk retinol and beta-carotene content. *International Journal for Vitamin and Nutrition Research*, *72*(4), 221–228. doi:10.1024/0300-9831.72.4.221 PMID:12214559

Zinsstag, J., Schelling, E., Roth, F., Bonfoh, B., de Savigny, D., & Tanner, M. (2007). Human benefits of animal interventions for zoonosis control. *Emerging Infectious Diseases*, *13*(4), 527–531. doi:10.3201/eid1304.060381 PMID:17553265

Zinsstag, J., Schelling, E., Waltner-Toews, D., & Tanner, M. (2011, September 1). From "one medicine" to "one health" and systemic approaches to health and well-being. *Preventive Veterinary Medicine*, *101*(3-4), 148–156. doi:10.1016/j.prevetmed.2010.07.003 PMID:20832879

Zinsstag, J., Schelling, E., Waltner-Toews, D., Whittaker, M., & Tanner, M. (2015). Preface. In J. Zinsstag, E. Schelling, D. Waltner-Toews, M. Whittacker, & M. Tanner (Eds.), *One Health. The Theory and Practice of Integrated Health Approaches* (pp. xv–xvi). Wallingford, UK: CABI. doi:10.1079/9781780643410.0000

Zinsstag, J., Waltner-Toews, D., & Tanner, M. (2015). Theoretical Issues of One Health. In J. Zinsstag, E. Schelling, D. Waltner-Toews, M. Whittacker, & M. Tanner (Eds.), *One Health. The Theory and Practice of Integrated Health Approaches* (pp. 16–25). Wallingford, UK: CABI. doi:10.1079/9781780643410.0016

Related References

To continue our tradition of advancing information science and technology research, we have compiled a list of recommended IGI Global readings. These references will provide additional information and guidance to further enrich your knowledge and assist you with your own research and future publications.

Abu Seman, S. A., & Ramayah, T. (2017). Are We Ready to App?: A Study on mHealth Apps, Its Future, and Trends in Malaysia Context. In J. Pelet (Ed.), *Mobile Platforms, Design, and Apps for Social Commerce* (pp. 69–83). Hershey, PA: IGI Global. doi:10.4018/978-1-5225-2469-4.ch005

Aggarwal, S., & Azad, V. (2017). A Hybrid System Based on FMM and MLP to Diagnose Heart Disease. In S. Bhattacharyya, S. De, I. Pan, & P. Dutta (Eds.), *Intelligent Multidimensional Data Clustering and Analysis* (pp. 293–325). Hershey, PA: IGI Global. doi:10.4018/978-1-5225-1776-4.ch011

Akaichi, J., & Mhadhbi, L. (2016). A Clinical Decision Support System: Ontology-Driven Approach for Effective Emergency Management. In J. Moon & M. Galea (Eds.), *Improving Health Management through Clinical Decision Support Systems* (pp. 270–294). Hershey, PA: IGI Global. doi:10.4018/978-1-4666-9432-3.ch013

Akerkar, R. (2016). Towards an Intelligent Integrated Approach for Clinical Decision Support. In A. Aggarwal (Ed.), *Managing Big Data Integration in the Public Sector* (pp. 187–205). Hershey, PA: IGI Global. doi:10.4018/978-1-4666-9649-5.ch011

Al-Busaidi, S. S. (2018). Interdisciplinary Relationships Between Medicine and Social Sciences. In M. Al-Suqri, A. Al-Kindi, S. AlKindi, & N. Saleem (Eds.), *Promoting Interdisciplinarity in Knowledge Generation and Problem Solving* (pp. 124–137). Hershey, PA: IGI Global. doi:10.4018/978-1-5225-3878-3.ch009

Al Kareh, T., & Thoumy, M. (2018). The Impact of Health Information Digitization on the Physiotherapist-Patient Relationship: A Pilot Study of the Lebanese Community. *International Journal of Healthcare Information Systems and Informatics, 13*(2), 29–53. doi:10.4018/IJHISI.2018040103

Alenzuela, R. (2017). Research, Leadership, and Resource-Sharing Initiatives: The Role of Local Library Consortia in Access to Medical Information. In S. Ram (Ed.), *Library and Information Services for Bioinformatics Education and Research* (pp. 199–211). Hershey, PA: IGI Global. doi:10.4018/978-1-5225-1871-6.ch012

Ameri, H., Alizadeh, S., & Noughabi, E. A. (2017). Application of Data Mining Techniques in Clinical Decision Making: A Literature Review and Classification. In E. Noughabi, B. Raahemi, A. Albadvi, & B. Far (Eds.), *Handbook of Research on Data Science for Effective Healthcare Practice and Administration* (pp. 257–295). Hershey, PA: IGI Global. doi:10.4018/978-1-5225-2515-8.ch012

Anand, S. (2017). Medical Image Enhancement Using Edge Information-Based Methods. In B. Singh (Ed.), *Computational Tools and Techniques for Biomedical Signal Processing* (pp. 123–148). Hershey, PA: IGI Global. doi:10.4018/978-1-5225-0660-7.ch006

Angjellari-Dajci, F., Sapienza, C., Lawless, W. F., & Kavanagh, K. (2016). Human Capital Accumulation in Medical Simulated Learning Environments: A Framework for Economic Evaluation. In M. Russ (Ed.), *Quantitative Multidisciplinary Approaches in Human Capital and Asset Management* (pp. 65–88). Hershey, PA: IGI Global. doi:10.4018/978-1-4666-9652-5.ch004

Anil, M., Ayyildiz-Tamis, D., Tasdemir, S., Sendemir-Urkmez, A., & Gulce-Iz, S. (2016). Bioinspired Materials and Biocompatibility. In M. Bououdina (Ed.), *Emerging Research on Bioinspired Materials Engineering* (pp. 294–322). Hershey, PA: IGI Global. doi:10.4018/978-1-4666-9811-6.ch011

Anton, J. L., Soriano, J. V., Martinez, M. I., & Garcia, F. B. (2018). Comprehensive E-Learning Appraisal System. In M. Khosrow-Pour, D.B.A. (Ed.), Encyclopedia of Information Science and Technology, Fourth Edition (pp. 5787-5799). Hershey, PA: IGI Global. doi:10.4018/978-1-5225-2255-3.ch503

Arabi, M. (2016). Redesigning the Organizational Structure to Reach Efficiency: The Case of Ministry of Health and Medical Education of Iran. In R. Gholipour & K. Rouzbehani (Eds.), *Social, Economic, and Political Perspectives on Public Health Policy-Making* (pp. 257–294). Hershey, PA: IGI Global. doi:10.4018/978-1-4666-9944-1.ch012

Assis-Hassid, S., Heart, T., Reychav, I., & Pliskin, J. S. (2016). Modelling Factors Affecting Patient-Doctor-Computer Communication in Primary Care. *International Journal of Reliable and Quality E-Healthcare*, *5*(1), 1–17. doi:10.4018/IJRQEH.2016010101

Atzori, B., Hoffman, H. G., Vagnoli, L., Messeri, A., & Grotto, R. L. (2018). Virtual Reality as Distraction Technique for Pain Management in Children and Adolescents. In M. Khosrow-Pour, D.B.A. (Ed.), Encyclopedia of Information Science and Technology, Fourth Edition (pp. 5955-5965). Hershey, PA: IGI Global. doi:10.4018/978-1-5225-2255-3.ch518

Audibert, M., Mathonnat, J., Pélissier, A., & Huang, X. X. (2018). The Impact of the New Rural Cooperative Medical Scheme on Township Hospitals' Utilization and Income Structure in Weifang Prefecture, China. In I. Management Association (Ed.), Health Economics and Healthcare Reform: Breakthroughs in Research and Practice (pp. 109-121). Hershey, PA: IGI Global. doi:10.4018/978-1-5225-3168-5.ch007

Ayyachamy, S. (2016). Analysis and Comparison of Developed 2D Medical Image Database Design using Registration Scheme, Retrieval Scheme, and Bag-of-Visual-Words. In N. Dey & A. Ashour (Eds.), *Classification and Clustering in Biomedical Signal Processing* (pp. 149–168). Hershey, PA: IGI Global. doi:10.4018/978-1-5225-0140-4.ch007

Babalola, A. C. (2016). Literacy and Decision Making on Health Issues among Married Women in Southwest Nigeria. In V. Wang (Ed.), *Handbook of Research on Advancing Health Education through Technology* (pp. 191–212). Hershey, PA: IGI Global. doi:10.4018/978-1-4666-9494-1.ch009

Babu, A., & Ayyappan, S. (2017). A Methodological Evaluation of Crypto-Watermarking System for Medical Images. In C. Bhatt & S. Peddoju (Eds.), *Cloud Computing Systems and Applications in Healthcare* (pp. 189–217). Hershey, PA: IGI Global. doi:10.4018/978-1-5225-1002-4.ch010

Bakke, A. (2017). Ethos in E-Health: From Informational to Interactive Websites. In M. Folk & S. Apostel (Eds.), *Establishing and Evaluating Digital Ethos and Online Credibility* (pp. 85–103). Hershey, PA: IGI Global. doi:10.4018/978-1-5225-1072-7.ch005

Bali, S. (2018). Enhancing the Reach of Health Care Through Telemedicine: Status and New Possibilities in Developing Countries. In U. Pandey & V. Indrakanti (Eds.), *Open and Distance Learning Initiatives for Sustainable Development* (pp. 339–354). Hershey, PA: IGI Global. doi:10.4018/978-1-5225-2621-6.ch019

Barrett, T. E. (2018). Essentials for Education and Training for Tomorrow's Physicians. In C. Smith (Ed.), *Exploring the Pressures of Medical Education From a Mental Health and Wellness Perspective* (pp. 230–252). Hershey, PA: IGI Global. doi:10.4018/978-1-5225-2811-1.ch010

Barrett, T. J. (2016). Knowledge in Action: Fostering Health Education through Technology. In V. Wang (Ed.), *Handbook of Research on Advancing Health Education through Technology* (pp. 39–62). Hershey, PA: IGI Global. doi:10.4018/978-1-4666-9494-1.ch003

Berrahal, S., & Boudriga, N. (2017). The Risks of Wearable Technologies to Individuals and Organizations. In A. Marrington, D. Kerr, & J. Gammack (Eds.), *Managing Security Issues and the Hidden Dangers of Wearable Technologies* (pp. 18–46). Hershey, PA: IGI Global. doi:10.4018/978-1-5225-1016-1.ch002

Bhagat, A. P., & Atique, M. (2016). Medical Image Mining Using Fuzzy Connectedness Image Segmentation: Efficient Retrieval of Patients' Stored Images. In W. Karâa & N. Dey (Eds.), *Biomedical Image Analysis and Mining Techniques for Improved Health Outcomes* (pp. 184–209). Hershey, PA: IGI Global. doi:10.4018/978-1-4666-8811-7.ch009

Bhargava, P. (2018). Blended Learning: An Effective Application to Clinical Teaching. In S. Tang & C. Lim (Eds.), *Preparing the Next Generation of Teachers for 21st Century Education* (pp. 302–320). Hershey, PA: IGI Global. doi:10.4018/978-1-5225-4080-9.ch018

Binh, N. T., & Tuyet, V. T. (2016). The Combination of Adaptive Filters to Improve the Quality of Medical Images in New Wavelet Domain. In N. Dey & A. Ashour (Eds.), *Classification and Clustering in Biomedical Signal Processing* (pp. 46–76). Hershey, PA: IGI Global. doi:10.4018/978-1-5225-0140-4.ch003

Bird, J. L. (2017). Writing Healing Narratives. In V. Bryan & J. Bird (Eds.), *Healthcare Community Synergism between Patients, Practitioners, and Researchers* (pp. 1–28). Hershey, PA: IGI Global. doi:10.4018/978-1-5225-0640-9.ch001

Bottrighi, A., Leonardi, G., Piovesan, L., & Terenziani, P. (2016). Knowledge-Based Support to the Treatment of Exceptions in Computer Interpretable Clinical Guidelines. *International Journal of Knowledge-Based Organizations*, *6*(3), 1–27. doi:10.4018/IJKBO.2016070101

Bougoulias, K., Kouris, I., Prasinos, M., Giokas, K., & Koutsouris, D. (2017). Ob/Gyn EMR Software: A Solution for Obstetricians and Gynecologists. In A. Moumtzoglou (Ed.), *Design, Development, and Integration of Reliable Electronic Healthcare Platforms* (pp. 101–111). Hershey, PA: IGI Global. doi:10.4018/978-1-5225-1724-5.ch006

Bouslimi, R., Ayadi, M. G., & Akaichi, J. (2018). Medical Image Retrieval in Healthcare Social Networks. *International Journal of Healthcare Information Systems and Informatics, 13*(2), 13–28. doi:10.4018/IJHISI.2018040102

Bouzaabia, O., Bouzaabia, R., & Mejri, K. (2017). Role of Internet in the Development of Medical Tourism Service in Tunisia. In A. Capatina & E. Rancati (Eds.), *Key Challenges and Opportunities in Web Entrepreneurship* (pp. 211–241). Hershey, PA: IGI Global. doi:10.4018/978-1-5225-2466-3.ch009

Briz-Ponce, L., Juanes-Méndez, J. A., & García-Peñalvo, F. J. (2016). The Role of Gender in Technology Acceptance for Medical Education. In M. Cruz-Cunha, I. Miranda, R. Martinho, & R. Rijo (Eds.), *Encyclopedia of E-Health and Telemedicine* (pp. 1013–1027). Hershey, PA: IGI Global. doi:10.4018/978-1-4666-9978-6.ch079

Briz-Ponce, L., Juanes-Méndez, J. A., & García-Peñalvo, F. J. (2016). A Research Contribution to the Analysis of Mobile Devices in Higher Education from Medical Students' Point of View. In L. Briz-Ponce, J. Juanes-Méndez, & F. García-Peñalvo (Eds.), *Handbook of Research on Mobile Devices and Applications in Higher Education Settings* (pp. 196–221). Hershey, PA: IGI Global. doi:10.4018/978-1-5225-0256-2.ch009

Brown-Jackson, K. L. (2018). Telemedicine and Telehealth: Academics Engaging the Community in a Call to Action. In S. Burton (Ed.), *Engaged Scholarship and Civic Responsibility in Higher Education* (pp. 166–193). Hershey, PA: IGI Global. doi:10.4018/978-1-5225-3649-9.ch008

Bwalya, K. J. (2017). Next Wave of Tele-Medicine: Virtual Presence of Medical Personnel. In K. Moahi, K. Bwalya, & P. Sebina (Eds.), *Health Information Systems and the Advancement of Medical Practice in Developing Countries* (pp. 168–180). Hershey, PA: IGI Global. doi:10.4018/978-1-5225-2262-1.ch010

Carlton, E. L., Holsinger, J. W. Jr, & Anunobi, N. (2016). Physician Engagement with Health Information Technology: Implications for Practice and Professionalism. *International Journal of Computers in Clinical Practice, 1*(2), 51–73. doi:10.4018/IJCCP.2016070103

Castillo-Page, L., Eliason, J., Conrad, S. S., & Nivet, M. A. (2016). Diversity in Undergraduate Medical Education: An Examination of Organizational Culture and Climate in Medical Schools. In C. Scott & J. Sims (Eds.), *Developing Workforce Diversity Programs, Curriculum, and Degrees in Higher Education* (pp. 304–326). Hershey, PA: IGI Global. doi:10.4018/978-1-5225-0209-8.ch016

Cebeci, H. I., & Hiziroglu, A. (2016). Review of Business Intelligence and Intelligent Systems in Healthcare Domain. In N. Celebi (Ed.), *Intelligent Techniques for Data Analysis in Diverse Settings* (pp. 192–206). Hershey, PA: IGI Global. doi:10.4018/978-1-5225-0075-9.ch009

Celik, G. (2018). Determining Headache Diseases With Genetic Algorithm. In U. Kose, G. Guraksin, & O. Deperlioglu (Eds.), *Nature-Inspired Intelligent Techniques for Solving Biomedical Engineering Problems* (pp. 249–262). Hershey, PA: IGI Global. doi:10.4018/978-1-5225-4769-3.ch012

Chakraborty, C., Gupta, B., & Ghosh, S. K. (2016). Mobile Telemedicine Systems for Remote Patient's Chronic Wound Monitoring. In A. Moumtzoglou (Ed.), *M-Health Innovations for Patient-Centered Care* (pp. 213–239). Hershey, PA: IGI Global. doi:10.4018/978-1-4666-9861-1.ch011

Chakraborty, S., Chatterjee, S., Ashour, A. S., Mali, K., & Dey, N. (2018). Intelligent Computing in Medical Imaging: A Study. In N. Dey (Ed.), *Advancements in Applied Metaheuristic Computing* (pp. 143–163). Hershey, PA: IGI Global. doi:10.4018/978-1-5225-4151-6.ch006

Chavez, A., & Kovarik, C. (2017). Open Source Technology for Medical Practice in Developing Countries. In K. Moahi, K. Bwalya, & P. Sebina (Eds.), *Health Information Systems and the Advancement of Medical Practice in Developing Countries* (pp. 33–59). Hershey, PA: IGI Global. doi:10.4018/978-1-5225-2262-1.ch003

Chen, E. T. (2016). Examining the Influence of Information Technology on Modern Health Care. In P. Manolitzas, E. Grigoroudis, N. Matsatsinis, & D. Yannacopoulos (Eds.), *Effective Methods for Modern Healthcare Service Quality and Evaluation* (pp. 110–136). Hershey, PA: IGI Global. doi:10.4018/978-1-4666-9961-8.ch006

Chin, S. (2016). Surviving Sandy: Recovering Collections after a Natural Disaster. In E. Decker & J. Townes (Eds.), *Handbook of Research on Disaster Management and Contingency Planning in Modern Libraries* (pp. 366–388). Hershey, PA: IGI Global. doi:10.4018/978-1-4666-8624-3.ch016

Chojnacki, M., & Wójcik, A. (2016). Security and the Role of New Technologies and Innovation in Medical Ethics. In A. Rosiek & K. Leksowski (Eds.), *Organizational Culture and Ethics in Modern Medicine* (pp. 52–77). Hershey, PA: IGI Global. doi:10.4018/978-1-4666-9658-7.ch003

Cılız, N., Yıldırım, H., & Temizel, Ş. (2016). Structure Development for Effective Medical Waste and Hazardous Waste Management System. In U. Akkucuk (Ed.), *Handbook of Research on Waste Management Techniques for Sustainability* (pp. 303–327). Hershey, PA: IGI Global. doi:10.4018/978-1-4666-9723-2.ch016

Ciufudean, C. (2018). Innovative Formalism for Biological Data Analysis. In M. Khosrow-Pour, D.B.A. (Ed.), Encyclopedia of Information Science and Technology, Fourth Edition (pp. 1814-1824). Hershey, PA: IGI Global. doi:10.4018/978-1-5225-2255-3.ch158

Ciufudean, C., & Ciufudean, O. (2016). Tele-Monitoring for Medical Diagnosis Availability. In M. Cruz-Cunha, I. Miranda, R. Martinho, & R. Rijo (Eds.), *Encyclopedia of E-Health and Telemedicine* (pp. 401–411). Hershey, PA: IGI Global. doi:10.4018/978-1-4666-9978-6.ch032

Colaguori, R., & Danesi, M. (2017). Medical Semiotics: A Revisitation and an Exhortation. *International Journal of Semiotics and Visual Rhetoric, 1*(1), 11–18. doi:10.4018/IJSVR.2017010102

Cole, A. W., & Salek, T. A. (2017). Adopting a Parasocial Connection to Overcome Professional Kakoethos in Online Health Information. In M. Folk & S. Apostel (Eds.), *Establishing and Evaluating Digital Ethos and Online Credibility* (pp. 104–120). Hershey, PA: IGI Global. doi:10.4018/978-1-5225-1072-7.ch006

Contreras, E. C., & Puente, G. J. (2016). How to Identify Rheumatic Diseases by General Physicians. In T. Gasmelseid (Ed.), *Advancing Pharmaceutical Processes and Tools for Improved Health Outcomes* (pp. 136–166). Hershey, PA: IGI Global. doi:10.4018/978-1-5225-0248-7.ch006

D'Andrea, A., Ferri, F., & Grifoni, P. (2016). RFID Technologies in Healthcare Setting: Applications and Future Perspectives. *International Journal of Computers in Clinical Practice, 1*(1), 15–27. doi:10.4018/IJCCP.2016010102

Damianakis, A., Kallonis, P., Loudos, G., Tsatsos, D., & Tsoukalis, A. (2016). Exploiting 3D Medical Equipment Simulations to Support Biomedical Engineering Academic Courses: Design Methodology and Implementation in a Small Scale National Project. In B. Khan (Ed.), *Revolutionizing Modern Education through Meaningful E-Learning Implementation* (pp. 277–295). Hershey, PA: IGI Global. doi:10.4018/978-1-5225-0466-5.ch015

Demiroz, E. (2016). Principles of Instructional Design for E-Learning and Online Learning Practices: Implications for Medical Education. In V. Wang (Ed.), *Handbook of Research on Advancing Health Education through Technology* (pp. 419–451). Hershey, PA: IGI Global. doi:10.4018/978-1-4666-9494-1.ch018

Deperlioglu, O. (2018). Intelligent Techniques Inspired by Nature and Used in Biomedical Engineering. In U. Kose, G. Guraksin, & O. Deperlioglu (Eds.), *Nature-Inspired Intelligent Techniques for Solving Biomedical Engineering Problems* (pp. 51–77). Hershey, PA: IGI Global. doi:10.4018/978-1-5225-4769-3.ch003

Dey, N., & Ashour, A. S. (2018). Meta-Heuristic Algorithms in Medical Image Segmentation: A Review. In N. Dey (Ed.), *Advancements in Applied Metaheuristic Computing* (pp. 185–203). Hershey, PA: IGI Global. doi:10.4018/978-1-5225-4151-6.ch008

Dey, N., Ashour, A. S., & Althoupety, A. S. (2017). Thermal Imaging in Medical Science. In V. Santhi (Ed.), *Recent Advances in Applied Thermal Imaging for Industrial Applications* (pp. 87–117). Hershey, PA: IGI Global. doi:10.4018/978-1-5225-2423-6.ch004

Di Virgilio, F., Camillo, A. A., & Camillo, I. C. (2017). The Impact of Social Network on Italian Users' Behavioural Intention for the Choice of a Medical Tourist Destination. *International Journal of Tourism and Hospitality Management in the Digital Age, 1*(1), 36–49. doi:10.4018/IJTHMDA.2017010103

Dias, C. M., Ribeiro, A. G., & Furtado, S. F. (2016). An Overview about the Use of Healthcare Applications on Mobile Devices. In M. Cruz-Cunha, I. Miranda, R. Martinho, & R. Rijo (Eds.), *Encyclopedia of E-Health and Telemedicine* (pp. 285–298). Hershey, PA: IGI Global. doi:10.4018/978-1-4666-9978-6.ch024

Dogra, A. K., & Dogra, P. (2017). The Medical Tourism Industry in the BRIC Nations: An Indian Analysis. In M. Dhiman (Ed.), *Opportunities and Challenges for Tourism and Hospitality in the BRIC Nations* (pp. 320–336). Hershey, PA: IGI Global. doi:10.4018/978-1-5225-0708-6.ch020

Drowos, J. L., & Wood, S. K. (2017). Preparing Future Physicians to Adapt to the Changing Health Care System: Promoting Humanism through Curricular Design. In V. Bryan & J. Bird (Eds.), *Healthcare Community Synergism between Patients, Practitioners, and Researchers* (pp. 106–125). Hershey, PA: IGI Global. doi:10.4018/978-1-5225-0640-9.ch006

Dulam, K. (2017). Medical Patents and Impact on Availability and Affordability of Essential Medicines in India. In R. Aggarwal & R. Kaur (Eds.), *Patent Law and Intellectual Property in the Medical Field* (pp. 41–57). Hershey, PA: IGI Global. doi:10.4018/978-1-5225-2414-4.ch003

Dutta, P. (2017). Decision Making in Medical Diagnosis via Distance Measures on Interval Valued Fuzzy Sets. *International Journal of System Dynamics Applications*, *6*(4), 63–83. doi:10.4018/IJSDA.2017100104

Edoh, T. O., Pawar, P. A., Brügge, B., & Teege, G. (2016). A Multidisciplinary Remote Healthcare Delivery System to Increase Health Care Access, Pathology Screening, and Treatment in Developing Countries: The Case of Benin. *International Journal of Healthcare Information Systems and Informatics*, *11*(4), 1–31. doi:10.4018/IJHISI.2016100101

El Guemhioui, K., & Demurjian, S. A. (2017). Semantic Reconciliation of Electronic Health Records Using Semantic Web Technologies. *International Journal of Information Technology and Web Engineering*, *12*(2), 26–48. doi:10.4018/IJITWE.2017040102

Ellouze, N., Rekhis, S., & Boudriga, N. (2016). Forensic Investigation of Digital Crimes in Healthcare Applications. In O. Isafiade & A. Bagula (Eds.), *Data Mining Trends and Applications in Criminal Science and Investigations* (pp. 169–210). Hershey, PA: IGI Global. doi:10.4018/978-1-5225-0463-4.ch007

Eneanya, A. N. (2016). Health Policy Implementation and Its Barriers: The Case Study of US Health System. In R. Gholipour & K. Rouzbehani (Eds.), *Social, Economic, and Political Perspectives on Public Health Policy-Making* (pp. 42–63). Hershey, PA: IGI Global. doi:10.4018/978-1-4666-9944-1.ch003

Entico, G. J. (2016). Knowledge Management and the Medical Health Librarians: A Perception Study. In J. Yap, M. Perez, M. Ayson, & G. Entico (Eds.), *Special Library Administration, Standardization and Technological Integration* (pp. 52–77). Hershey, PA: IGI Global. doi:10.4018/978-1-4666-9542-9.ch003

Ferradji, M. A., & Zidani, A. (2016). Collaborative Environment for Remote Clinical Reasoning Learning. *International Journal of E-Health and Medical Communications*, *7*(4), 62–81. doi:10.4018/IJEHMC.2016100104

Fisher, J. (2018). Sociological Perspectives on Improving Medical Diagnosis Emphasizing CAD. In M. Khosrow-Pour, D.B.A. (Ed.), Encyclopedia of Information Science and Technology, Fourth Edition (pp. 1017-1024). Hershey, PA: IGI Global. doi:10.4018/978-1-5225-2255-3.ch088

Flores, C. D., Respício, A., Coelho, H., Bez, M. R., & Fonseca, J. M. (2016). Simulation for Medical Training. In M. Cruz-Cunha, I. Miranda, R. Martinho, & R. Rijo (Eds.), *Encyclopedia of E-Health and Telemedicine* (pp. 827–842). Hershey, PA: IGI Global. doi:10.4018/978-1-4666-9978-6.ch064

Frank, E. M. (2018). Healthcare Education: Integrating Simulation Technologies. In V. Bryan, A. Musgrove, & J. Powers (Eds.), *Handbook of Research on Human Development in the Digital Age* (pp. 163–182). Hershey, PA: IGI Global. doi:10.4018/978-1-5225-2838-8.ch008

Garner, G. (2018). Foundations for Yoga Practice in Rehabilitation. In S. Telles & N. Singh (Eds.), *Research-Based Perspectives on the Psychophysiology of Yoga* (pp. 263–307). Hershey, PA: IGI Global. doi:10.4018/978-1-5225-2788-6.ch015

Gasmelseid, T. M. (2016). Improving Pharmaceutical Care through the Use of Intelligent Pharmacoinformatics. In T. Gasmelseid (Ed.), *Advancing Pharmaceutical Processes and Tools for Improved Health Outcomes* (pp. 167–188). Hershey, PA: IGI Global. doi:10.4018/978-1-5225-0248-7.ch007

Gavurová, B., Kováč, V., & Šoltés, M. (2018). Medical Equipment and Economic Determinants of Its Structure and Regulation in the Slovak Republic. In M. Khosrow-Pour, D.B.A. (Ed.), Encyclopedia of Information Science and Technology, Fourth Edition (pp. 5841-5852). Hershey, PA: IGI Global. doi:10.4018/978-1-5225-2255-3.ch508

Ge, X., Wang, Q., Huang, K., Law, V., & Thomas, D. C. (2017). Designing Simulated Learning Environments and Facilitating Authentic Learning Experiences in Medical Education. In J. Stefaniak (Ed.), *Advancing Medical Education Through Strategic Instructional Design* (pp. 77–100). Hershey, PA: IGI Global. doi:10.4018/978-1-5225-2098-6.ch004

Gewald, H., & Gewald, C. (2018). Inhibitors of Physicians' Use of Mandatory Hospital Information Systems (HIS). *International Journal of Healthcare Information Systems and Informatics, 13*(1), 29–44. doi:10.4018/IJHISI.2018010103

Ghosh, D., & Dinda, S. (2017). Health Infrastructure and Economic Development in India. In R. Das (Ed.), *Social, Health, and Environmental Infrastructures for Economic Growth* (pp. 99–119). Hershey, PA: IGI Global. doi:10.4018/978-1-5225-2364-2.ch006

Ghosh, K., & Sen, K. C. (2017). The Potential of Crowdsourcing in the Health Care Industry. In N. Wickramasinghe (Ed.), *Handbook of Research on Healthcare Administration and Management* (pp. 418–427). Hershey, PA: IGI Global. doi:10.4018/978-1-5225-0920-2.ch024

Ghrab, S., & Saad, I. (2016). Identifying Crucial Know-How and Knowing-That for Medical Decision Support. *International Journal of Decision Support System Technology*, *8*(4), 14–33. doi:10.4018/IJDSST.2016100102

Giokas, K., Tsirmpas, C., Anastasiou, A., Iliopoulou, D., Costarides, V., & Koutsouris, D. (2016). Contemporary Heart Failure Treatment Based on Improved Knowledge and Personalized Care of Comorbidities. In D. Fotiadis (Ed.), *Handbook of Research on Trends in the Diagnosis and Treatment of Chronic Conditions* (pp. 301–314). Hershey, PA: IGI Global. doi:10.4018/978-1-4666-8828-5.ch014

Gopalan, V., Chan, E., & Ho, D. T. (2018). Deliberate Self-Harm and Suicide Ideology in Medical Students. In C. Smith (Ed.), *Exploring the Pressures of Medical Education From a Mental Health and Wellness Perspective* (pp. 122–143). Hershey, PA: IGI Global. doi:10.4018/978-1-5225-2811-1.ch005

Goswami, S., Dey, U., Roy, P., Ashour, A., & Dey, N. (2017). Medical Video Processing: Concept and Applications. In N. Dey, A. Ashour, & P. Patra (Eds.), *Feature Detectors and Motion Detection in Video Processing* (pp. 1–17). Hershey, PA: IGI Global. doi:10.4018/978-1-5225-1025-3.ch001

Goswami, S., Mahanta, K., Goswami, S., Jigdung, T., & Devi, T. P. (2018). Ageing and Cancer: The Epigenetic Basis, Alternative Treatment, and Care. In B. Prasad & S. Akbar (Eds.), *Handbook of Research on Geriatric Health, Treatment, and Care* (pp. 206–235). Hershey, PA: IGI Global. doi:10.4018/978-1-5225-3480-8.ch012

Gouva, M. I. (2017). The Psychological Impact of Medical Error on Patients, Family Members, and Health Professionals. In M. Riga (Ed.), *Impact of Medical Errors and Malpractice on Health Economics, Quality, and Patient Safety* (pp. 171–196). Hershey, PA: IGI Global. doi:10.4018/978-1-5225-2337-6.ch007

Gürcü, M., & Tengilimoğlu, D. (2017). Health Tourism-Based Destination Marketing. In A. Bayraktar & C. Uslay (Eds.), *Strategic Place Branding Methodologies and Theory for Tourist Attraction* (pp. 308–331). Hershey, PA: IGI Global. doi:10.4018/978-1-5225-0579-2.ch015

Gürsel, G. (2016). Mobility in Healthcare: M-Health. In A. Panagopoulos (Ed.), *Handbook of Research on Next Generation Mobile Communication Systems* (pp. 485–511). Hershey, PA: IGI Global. doi:10.4018/978-1-4666-8732-5.ch019

Gürsel, G. (2017). For Better Healthcare Mining Health Data. In S. Bhattacharyya, S. De, I. Pan, & P. Dutta (Eds.), *Intelligent Multidimensional Data Clustering and Analysis* (pp. 135–158). Hershey, PA: IGI Global. doi:10.4018/978-1-5225-1776-4.ch006

Guzman-Lugo, G., Lopez-Martinez, M., Lopez-Ramirez, B., & Avila-Vazquez, D. (2016). City-Driven Approach to Determine Health Services Based on Current User Location and Collaborative Information. *International Journal of Knowledge Society Research, 7*(1), 53–62. doi:10.4018/IJKSR.2016010104

Gyaase, P. O., Darko-Lartey, R., William, H., & Borkloe, F. (2017). Towards an Integrated Electronic Medical Records System for Quality Healthcare in Ghana: An Exploratory Factor Analysis. *International Journal of Computers in Clinical Practice, 2*(2), 38–55. doi:10.4018/IJCCP.2017070103

Handayani, P. W., Sandhyaduhita, P. I., Hidayanto, A. N., Pinem, A. A., Fajrina, H. R., Junus, K. M., ... Ayuningtyas, D. (2016). Integrated Hospital Information System Architecture Design in Indonesia. In T. Iyamu & A. Tatnall (Eds.), *Maximizing Healthcare Delivery and Management through Technology Integration* (pp. 207–236). Hershey, PA: IGI Global. doi:10.4018/978-1-4666-9446-0.ch013

Hanel, P. (2017). Is China Catching Up?: Health-Related Applications of Biotechnology. In T. Bas & J. Zhao (Eds.), *Comparative Approaches to Biotechnology Development and Use in Developed and Emerging Nations* (pp. 465–520). Hershey, PA: IGI Global. doi:10.4018/978-1-5225-1040-6.ch016

Harmsen, C. A., & Royle, R. N. (2016). St. Stephen's Hospital Hervey Bay: Study of Developing a Digital Hospital. In J. Moon & M. Galea (Eds.), *Improving Health Management through Clinical Decision Support Systems* (pp. 127–153). Hershey, PA: IGI Global. doi:10.4018/978-1-4666-9432-3.ch006

Harp, D., Shim, R. S., Johnson, J., Harp, J. A., Wilcox, W. C., & Wilcox, J. K. (2016). Race and Gender Inequalities in Medicine and Biomedical Research. In U. Thomas & J. Drake (Eds.), *Critical Research on Sexism and Racism in STEM Fields* (pp. 115–134). Hershey, PA: IGI Global. doi:10.4018/978-1-5225-0174-9.ch006

Hartman, A., & Brown, S. (2017). Synergism through Therapeutic Visual Arts. In V. Bryan & J. Bird (Eds.), *Healthcare Community Synergism between Patients, Practitioners, and Researchers* (pp. 29–48). Hershey, PA: IGI Global. doi:10.4018/978-1-5225-0640-9.ch002

Hazra, J., Chowdhury, A. R., & Dutta, P. (2016). Cluster Based Medical Image Registration Using Optimized Neural Network. In S. Bhattacharyya, P. Banerjee, D. Majumdar, & P. Dutta (Eds.), *Handbook of Research on Advanced Hybrid Intelligent Techniques and Applications* (pp. 551–581). Hershey, PA: IGI Global. doi:10.4018/978-1-4666-9474-3.ch018

Hung, S., Huang, W., Yen, D. C., Chang, S., & Lu, C. (2016). Effect of Information Service Competence and Contextual Factors on the Effectiveness of Strategic Information Systems Planning in Hospitals. *Journal of Global Information Management*, *24*(1), 14–36. doi:10.4018/JGIM.2016010102

Iltchev, P., Śliwczyński, A., Szynkiewicz, P., & Marczak, M. (2016). Mobile Health Applications Assisting Patients with Chronic Diseases: Examples from Asthma Care. In A. Moumtzoglou (Ed.), *M-Health Innovations for Patient-Centered Care* (pp. 170–196). Hershey, PA: IGI Global. doi:10.4018/978-1-4666-9861-1.ch009

Iqbal, S., Ahmad, S., & Willis, I. (2017). Influencing Factors for Adopting Technology Enhanced Learning in the Medical Schools of Punjab, Pakistan. *International Journal of Information and Communication Technology Education*, *13*(3), 27–39. doi:10.4018/IJICTE.2017070103

Jagan, J., Dalkiliç, Y., & Samui, P. (2016). Utilization of SVM, LSSVM and GP for Predicting the Medical Waste Generation. In G. Hua (Ed.), *Smart Cities as a Solution for Reducing Urban Waste and Pollution* (pp. 224–251). Hershey, PA: IGI Global. doi:10.4018/978-1-5225-0302-6.ch008

Jagiello, K., Sosnowska, A., Mikolajczyk, A., & Puzyn, T. (2017). Nanomaterials in Medical Devices: Regulations' Review and Future Perspectives. *Journal of Nanotoxicology and Nanomedicine*, *2*(2), 1–11. doi:10.4018/JNN.2017070101

Jena, T. K. (2018). Skill Training Process in Medicine Through Distance Mode. In U. Pandey & V. Indrakanti (Eds.), *Optimizing Open and Distance Learning in Higher Education Institutions* (pp. 228–243). Hershey, PA: IGI Global. doi:10.4018/978-1-5225-2624-7.ch010

Jesus, Â., & Gomes, M. J. (2016). Web 2.0 Tools in Biomedical and Pharmaceutical Education: Updated Review and Commentary. In T. Gasmelseid (Ed.), *Advancing Pharmaceutical Processes and Tools for Improved Health Outcomes* (pp. 52–78). Hershey, PA: IGI Global. doi:10.4018/978-1-5225-0248-7.ch003

Joseph, V., & Miller, J. M. (2018). Medical Students' Perceived Stigma in Seeking Care: A Cultural Perspective. In C. Smith (Ed.), *Exploring the Pressures of Medical Education From a Mental Health and Wellness Perspective* (pp. 44–67). Hershey, PA: IGI Global. doi:10.4018/978-1-5225-2811-1.ch002

Joyce, B. L., & Swanberg, S. M. (2017). Using Backward Design for Competency-Based Undergraduate Medical Education. In J. Stefaniak (Ed.), *Advancing Medical Education Through Strategic Instructional Design* (pp. 53–76). Hershey, PA: IGI Global. doi:10.4018/978-1-5225-2098-6.ch003

Kaljo, K., & Jacques, L. (2018). Flipping the Medical School Classroom. In M. Khosrow-Pour, D.B.A. (Ed.), Encyclopedia of Information Science and Technology, Fourth Edition (pp. 5800-5809). Hershey, PA: IGI Global. doi:10.4018/978-1-5225-2255-3.ch504

Karon, R. (2016). Utilisation of Health Information Systems for Service Delivery in the Namibian Environment. In T. Iyamu & A. Tatnall (Eds.), *Maximizing Healthcare Delivery and Management through Technology Integration* (pp. 169–183). Hershey, PA: IGI Global. doi:10.4018/978-1-4666-9446-0.ch011

Kasina, H., Bahubalendruni, M. V., & Botcha, R. (2017). Robots in Medicine: Past, Present and Future. *International Journal of Manufacturing, Materials, and Mechanical Engineering*, *7*(4), 44–64. doi:10.4018/IJMMME.2017100104

Katehakis, D. G. (2018). Electronic Medical Record Implementation Challenges for the National Health System in Greece. *International Journal of Reliable and Quality E-Healthcare*, *7*(1), 16–30. doi:10.4018/IJRQEH.2018010102

Katz, A., & Shtub, A. (2016). Design and Build a Wizard of Oz (WOZ) Telemedicine Simulator Platform. In M. Cruz-Cunha, I. Miranda, R. Martinho, & R. Rijo (Eds.), *Encyclopedia of E-Health and Telemedicine* (pp. 128–141). Hershey, PA: IGI Global. doi:10.4018/978-1-4666-9978-6.ch011

Kaur, P. D., & Sharma, P. (2017). Success Dimensions of ICTs in Healthcare. In B. Singh (Ed.), *Computational Tools and Techniques for Biomedical Signal Processing* (pp. 149–173). Hershey, PA: IGI Global. doi:10.4018/978-1-5225-0660-7.ch007

Kaushik, P. (2018). Comorbidity of Medical and Psychiatric Disorders in Geriatric Population: Treatment and Care. In B. Prasad & S. Akbar (Eds.), *Handbook of Research on Geriatric Health, Treatment, and Care* (pp. 448–474). Hershey, PA: IGI Global. doi:10.4018/978-1-5225-3480-8.ch025

Khachane, M. Y. (2017). Organ-Based Medical Image Classification Using Support Vector Machine. *International Journal of Synthetic Emotions*, *8*(1), 18–30. doi:10.4018/IJSE.2017010102

Kirci, P. (2018). Intelligent Techniques for Analysis of Big Data About Healthcare and Medical Records. In N. Shah & M. Mittal (Eds.), *Handbook of Research on Promoting Business Process Improvement Through Inventory Control Techniques* (pp. 559–582). Hershey, PA: IGI Global. doi:10.4018/978-1-5225-3232-3.ch029

Kldiashvili, E. (2016). Cloud Computing as the Useful Resource for Application of the Medical Information System for Quality Assurance Purposes. *International Journal of Computers in Clinical Practice*, *1*(2), 1–23. doi:10.4018/IJCCP.2016070101

Kldiashvili, E. (2018). Cloud Approach for the Medical Information System: MIS on Cloud. In M. Khosrow-Pour (Ed.), *Incorporating Nature-Inspired Paradigms in Computational Applications* (pp. 238–261). Hershey, PA: IGI Global. doi:10.4018/978-1-5225-5020-4.ch008

Kldiashvili, E., Burduli, A., Ghortlishvili, G., & Sheklashvili, I. (2016). Georgian Experience in Telecytology. In M. Cruz-Cunha, I. Miranda, R. Martinho, & R. Rijo (Eds.), *Encyclopedia of E-Health and Telemedicine* (pp. 62–71). Hershey, PA: IGI Global. doi:10.4018/978-1-4666-9978-6.ch006

Ko, H., Mesicek, L., Choi, J., Choi, J., & Hwang, S. (2018). A Study on Secure Contents Strategies for Applications With DRM on Cloud Computing. *International Journal of Cloud Applications and Computing*, *8*(1), 143–153. doi:10.4018/IJCAC.2018010107

Komendziński, T., Dreszer-Drogorób, J., Mikołajewska, E., Mikołajewski, D., & Bałaj, B. (2016). Interdisciplinary Education for Research and Everyday Clinical Practice: Lessons Learned from InteRDoCTor Project. In A. Rosiek & K. Leksowski (Eds.), *Organizational Culture and Ethics in Modern Medicine* (pp. 78–110). Hershey, PA: IGI Global. doi:10.4018/978-1-4666-9658-7.ch004

Komendziński, T., Mikołajewska, E., & Mikołajewski, D. (2018). Cross-Cultural Decision-Making in Healthcare: Theory and Practical Application in Real Clinical Conditions. In A. Rosiek-Kryszewska & K. Leksowski (Eds.), *Healthcare Administration for Patient Safety and Engagement* (pp. 276–298). Hershey, PA: IGI Global. doi:10.4018/978-1-5225-3946-9.ch015

Konecny, L. T. (2018). Medical School Wellness Initiatives. In C. Smith (Ed.), *Exploring the Pressures of Medical Education From a Mental Health and Wellness Perspective* (pp. 209–228). Hershey, PA: IGI Global. doi:10.4018/978-1-5225-2811-1.ch009

Konieczna, A., & Słomkowski, P. (2016). Confrontation of Human Rights in Daily Clinical Situations. In A. Rosiek & K. Leksowski (Eds.), *Organizational Culture and Ethics in Modern Medicine* (pp. 255–281). Hershey, PA: IGI Global. doi:10.4018/978-1-4666-9658-7.ch011

Kromrei, H., Solomonson, W. L., & Juzych, M. S. (2017). Teaching Residents How to Teach. In J. Stefaniak (Ed.), *Advancing Medical Education Through Strategic Instructional Design* (pp. 164–185). Hershey, PA: IGI Global. doi:10.4018/978-1-5225-2098-6.ch008

Kulkarni, S., Savyanavar, A., Kulkarni, P., Stranieri, A., & Ghorpade, V. (2018). Framework for Integration of Medical Image and Text-Based Report Retrieval to Support Radiological Diagnosis. In M. Kolekar & V. Kumar (Eds.), *Biomedical Signal and Image Processing in Patient Care* (pp. 86–122). Hershey, PA: IGI Global. doi:10.4018/978-1-5225-2829-6.ch006

Kumar, A., & Sarkar, B. K. (2018). Performance Analysis of Nature-Inspired Algorithms-Based Bayesian Prediction Models for Medical Data Sets. In U. Singh, A. Tiwari, & R. Singh (Eds.), *Soft-Computing-Based Nonlinear Control Systems Design* (pp. 134–155). Hershey, PA: IGI Global. doi:10.4018/978-1-5225-3531-7.ch007

Kurtz, R. S. (2016). Fortitude: A Study of African Americans in Surgery in New York City. In U. Thomas & J. Drake (Eds.), *Critical Research on Sexism and Racism in STEM Fields* (pp. 153–169). Hershey, PA: IGI Global. doi:10.4018/978-1-5225-0174-9.ch009

Labbadi, W., & Akaichi, J. (2017). Efficient Algorithm for Answering Fuzzy Medical Requests in Pervasive Healthcare Information Systems. *International Journal of Healthcare Information Systems and Informatics*, *12*(2), 46–64. doi:10.4018/IJHISI.2017040103

Lagumdzija, A., & Swing, V. K. (2017). Health, Digitalization, and Individual Empowerment. In F. Topor (Ed.), *Handbook of Research on Individualism and Identity in the Globalized Digital Age* (pp. 380–402). Hershey, PA: IGI Global. doi:10.4018/978-1-5225-0522-8.ch017

Lamey, T. W., & Davidson-Shivers, G. V. (2017). Instructional Strategies and Sequencing. In J. Stefaniak (Ed.), *Advancing Medical Education Through Strategic Instructional Design* (pp. 30–52). Hershey, PA: IGI Global. doi:10.4018/978-1-5225-2098-6.ch002

Leon, G. (2017). The Role of Forensic Medicine in Medical Errors. In M. Riga (Ed.), *Impact of Medical Errors and Malpractice on Health Economics, Quality, and Patient Safety* (pp. 144–170). Hershey, PA: IGI Global. doi:10.4018/978-1-5225-2337-6.ch006

Lidia, B., Federica, G., & Maria, V. E. (2016). The Patient-Centered Medicine as the Theoretical Framework for Patient Engagement. In G. Graffigna (Ed.), *Promoting Patient Engagement and Participation for Effective Healthcare Reform* (pp. 25–39). Hershey, PA: IGI Global. doi:10.4018/978-1-4666-9992-2.ch002

Love, L., & McDowelle, D. (2018). Developing a Comprehensive Wellness Program for Medical Students. In C. Smith (Ed.), *Exploring the Pressures of Medical Education From a Mental Health and Wellness Perspective* (pp. 190–208). Hershey, PA: IGI Global. doi:10.4018/978-1-5225-2811-1.ch008

Lovell, K. L. (2017). Development and Evaluation of Neuroscience Computer-Based Modules for Medical Students: Instructional Design Principles and Effectiveness. In J. Stefaniak (Ed.), *Advancing Medical Education Through Strategic Instructional Design* (pp. 262–276). Hershey, PA: IGI Global. doi:10.4018/978-1-5225-2098-6.ch013

Lubin, R., & Hamlin, M. D. (2018). Medical Student Burnout: A Social Cognitive Learning Perspective on Medical Student Mental Health and Wellness. In C. Smith (Ed.), *Exploring the Pressures of Medical Education From a Mental Health and Wellness Perspective* (pp. 92–121). Hershey, PA: IGI Global. doi:10.4018/978-1-5225-2811-1.ch004

Luk, C. Y. (2018). Moving Towards Universal Health Coverage: Challenges for the Present and Future in China. In B. Fong, A. Ng, & P. Yuen (Eds.), *Sustainable Health and Long-Term Care Solutions for an Aging Population* (pp. 19–45). Hershey, PA: IGI Global. doi:10.4018/978-1-5225-2633-9.ch002

Mahat, M., & Pettigrew, A. (2017). The Regulatory Environment of Non-Profit Higher Education and Research Institutions and Its Implications for Managerial Strategy: The Case of Medical Education and Research. In L. West & A. Worthington (Eds.), *Handbook of Research on Emerging Business Models and Managerial Strategies in the Nonprofit Sector* (pp. 336–351). Hershey, PA: IGI Global. doi:10.4018/978-1-5225-2537-0.ch017

Maitra, I. K., & Bandhyopadhyaay, S. K. (2017). Adaptive Edge Detection Method towards Features Extraction from Diverse Medical Imaging Technologies. In S. Bhattacharyya, S. De, I. Pan, & P. Dutta (Eds.), *Intelligent Multidimensional Data Clustering and Analysis* (pp. 159–192). Hershey, PA: IGI Global. doi:10.4018/978-1-5225-1776-4.ch007

Mangu, V. P. (2017). Mobile Health Care: A Technology View. In C. Bhatt & S. Peddoju (Eds.), *Cloud Computing Systems and Applications in Healthcare* (pp. 1–18). Hershey, PA: IGI Global. doi:10.4018/978-1-5225-1002-4.ch001

Manirabona, A., Fourati, L. C., & Boudjit, S. (2017). Investigation on Healthcare Monitoring Systems: Innovative Services and Applications. *International Journal of E-Health and Medical Communications*, *8*(1), 1–18. doi:10.4018/IJEHMC.2017010101

Mannai, M. M., & Karâa, W. B. (2016). Biomedical Image Processing Overview. In W. Karâa & N. Dey (Eds.), *Biomedical Image Analysis and Mining Techniques for Improved Health Outcomes* (pp. 1–12). Hershey, PA: IGI Global. doi:10.4018/978-1-4666-8811-7.ch001

Manzoor, A. (2016). RFID in Health Care-Building Smart Hospitals for Quality Healthcare. *International Journal of User-Driven Healthcare*, *6*(2), 21–45. doi:10.4018/IJUDH.2016070102

Marwan, M., Kartit, A., & Ouahmane, H. (2018). A Framework to Secure Medical Image Storage in Cloud Computing Environment. *Journal of Electronic Commerce in Organizations*, *16*(1), 1–16. doi:10.4018/JECO.2018010101

Masoud, M. P., Nejad, M. K., Darebaghi, H., Chavoshi, M., & Farahani, M. (2018). The Decision Support System and Conventional Method of Telephone Triage by Nurses in Emergency Medical Services: A Comparative Investigation. *International Journal of E-Business Research*, *14*(1), 77–88. doi:10.4018/IJEBR.2018010105

McDonald, W. G., Martin, M., & Salzberg, L. D. (2018). From Medical Student to Medical Resident: Graduate Medical Education and Mental Health in the United States. In C. Smith (Ed.), *Exploring the Pressures of Medical Education From a Mental Health and Wellness Perspective* (pp. 145–169). Hershey, PA: IGI Global. doi:10.4018/978-1-5225-2811-1.ch006

Medhekar, A. (2017). The Role of Social Media for Knowledge Dissemination in Medical Tourism: A Case of India. In R. Chugh (Ed.), *Harnessing Social Media as a Knowledge Management Tool* (pp. 25–54). Hershey, PA: IGI Global. doi:10.4018/978-1-5225-0495-5.ch002

Medhekar, A., & Haq, F. (2018). Urbanization and New Jobs Creation in Healthcare Services in India: Challenges and Opportunities. In U. Benna & I. Benna (Eds.), *Urbanization and Its Impact on Socio-Economic Growth in Developing Regions* (pp. 198–218). Hershey, PA: IGI Global. doi:10.4018/978-1-5225-2659-9.ch010

Mehta, G., Dutta, M. K., & Kim, P. S. (2016). An Efficient and Lossless Cryptosystem for Security in Tele-Ophthalmology Applications Using Chaotic Theory. *International Journal of E-Health and Medical Communications*, *7*(4), 28–47. doi:10.4018/IJEHMC.2016100102

Mehta, P. (2017). Framework of Indian Healthcare System and its Challenges: An Insight. In V. Bryan & J. Bird (Eds.), *Healthcare Community Synergism between Patients, Practitioners, and Researchers* (pp. 247–271). Hershey, PA: IGI Global. doi:10.4018/978-1-5225-0640-9.ch011

Metelmann, B., & Metelmann, C. (2016). M-Health in Prehospital Emergency Medicine: Experiences from the EU funded Project LiveCity. In A. Moumtzoglou (Ed.), *M-Health Innovations for Patient-Centered Care* (pp. 197–212). Hershey, PA: IGI Global. doi:10.4018/978-1-4666-9861-1.ch010

Mi, M. (2017). Informal Learning in Medical Education. In J. Stefaniak (Ed.), *Advancing Medical Education Through Strategic Instructional Design* (pp. 225–244). Hershey, PA: IGI Global. doi:10.4018/978-1-5225-2098-6.ch011

Miglioretti, M., Mariani, F., & Vecchio, L. (2016). Could Patient Engagement Promote a Health System Free From Malpractice Litigation Risk? In G. Graffigna (Ed.), *Promoting Patient Engagement and Participation for Effective Healthcare Reform* (pp. 240–264). Hershey, PA: IGI Global. doi:10.4018/978-1-4666-9992-2.ch012

Misra, S. C., & Bisui, S. (2016). Feasibility of Large Scale Implementation of Personalized Medicine in the Current Scenario. *International Journal of E-Health and Medical Communications*, *7*(2), 30–49. doi:10.4018/IJEHMC.2016040103

Misra, S. C., Bisui, S., & Fantazy, K. (2016). Identifying Critical Changes in Adoption of Personalized Medicine (PM) in Healthcare Management. *International Journal of E-Health and Medical Communications*, *7*(3), 1–15. doi:10.4018/IJEHMC.2016070101

Mohammadian, M., Hatzinakos, D., Spachos, P., & Jentzsh, R. (2016). An Intelligent and Secure Framework for Wireless Information Technology in Healthcare for User and Data Classification in Hospitals. In V. Wang (Ed.), *Handbook of Research on Advancing Health Education through Technology* (pp. 452–479). Hershey, PA: IGI Global. doi:10.4018/978-1-4666-9494-1.ch019

Mokeddem, S., & Atmani, B. (2016). Assessment of Clinical Decision Support Systems for Predicting Coronary Heart Disease. *International Journal of Operations Research and Information Systems*, *7*(3), 57–73. doi:10.4018/IJORIS.2016070104

Mokrzycka, A., & Kowalska-Bobko, I. (2016). Public Health Legislation and Patient's Rights: Health2020 Strategy, European Perspective. In A. Rosiek & K. Leksowski (Eds.), *Organizational Culture and Ethics in Modern Medicine* (pp. 298–322). Hershey, PA: IGI Global. doi:10.4018/978-1-4666-9658-7.ch013

Moon, J. D., & Galea, M. P. (2016). Overview of Clinical Decision Support Systems in Healthcare. In J. Moon & M. Galea (Eds.), *Improving Health Management through Clinical Decision Support Systems* (pp. 1–27). Hershey, PA: IGI Global. doi:10.4018/978-1-4666-9432-3.ch001

Mosadeghrad, A. M., & Woldemichael, A. (2017). Application of Quality Management in Promoting Patient Safety and Preventing Medical Errors. In M. Riga (Ed.), *Impact of Medical Errors and Malpractice on Health Economics, Quality, and Patient Safety* (pp. 91–112). Hershey, PA: IGI Global. doi:10.4018/978-1-5225-2337-6.ch004

Moumtzoglou, A. (2017). Digital Medicine: The Quality Standpoint. In A. Moumtzoglou (Ed.), *Design, Development, and Integration of Reliable Electronic Healthcare Platforms* (pp. 179–195). Hershey, PA: IGI Global. doi:10.4018/978-1-5225-1724-5.ch011

Moumtzoglou, A., & Pouliakis, A. (2018). Population Health Management and the Science of Individuality. *International Journal of Reliable and Quality E-Healthcare, 7*(2), 1–26. doi:10.4018/IJRQEH.2018040101

Mpofu, C. (2016). International Medical Experiences Outbound New Zealand: An Economic and Medical Workforce Strategy. In D. Velliaris & D. Coleman-George (Eds.), *Handbook of Research on Study Abroad Programs and Outbound Mobility* (pp. 446–469). Hershey, PA: IGI Global. doi:10.4018/978-1-5225-0169-5.ch018

Mukhtar, W. F., & Abuelyaman, E. S. (2017). Opportunities and Challenges of Big Data in Healthcare. In N. Wickramasinghe (Ed.), *Handbook of Research on Healthcare Administration and Management* (pp. 47–58). Hershey, PA: IGI Global. doi:10.4018/978-1-5225-0920-2.ch004

Munugala, S., Brar, G. K., Syed, A., Mohammad, A., & Halgamuge, M. N. (2018). The Much Needed Security and Data Reforms of Cloud Computing in Medical Data Storage. In M. Lytras & P. Papadopoulou (Eds.), *Applying Big Data Analytics in Bioinformatics and Medicine* (pp. 99–113). Hershey, PA: IGI Global. doi:10.4018/978-1-5225-2607-0.ch005

Narasimhamurthy, A. (2016). An Overview of Machine Learning in Medical Image Analysis: Trends in Health Informatics. In N. Dey & A. Ashour (Eds.), *Classification and Clustering in Biomedical Signal Processing* (pp. 23–45). Hershey, PA: IGI Global. doi:10.4018/978-1-5225-0140-4.ch002

Ngara, R. (2017). Multiple Voices, Multiple Paths: Towards Dialogue between Western and Indigenous Medical Knowledge Systems. In P. Ngulube (Ed.), *Handbook of Research on Theoretical Perspectives on Indigenous Knowledge Systems in Developing Countries* (pp. 332–358). Hershey, PA: IGI Global. doi:10.4018/978-1-5225-0833-5.ch015

O'Connor, Y., & Heavin, C. (2018). Defining and Characterising the Landscape of eHealth. In M. Khosrow-Pour, D.B.A. (Ed.), Encyclopedia of Information Science and Technology, Fourth Edition (pp. 5864-5875). Hershey, PA: IGI Global. doi:10.4018/978-1-5225-2255-3.ch510

Ochonogor, W. C., & Okite-Amughoro, F. A. (2018). Building an Effective Digital Library in a University Teaching Hospital (UTH) in Nigeria. In A. Tella & T. Kwanya (Eds.), *Handbook of Research on Managing Intellectual Property in Digital Libraries* (pp. 184–204). Hershey, PA: IGI Global. doi:10.4018/978-1-5225-3093-0.ch010

Olaniran, B. A. (2016). ICTs, E-health, and Multidisciplinary Healthcare Teams: Promises and Challenges. *International Journal of Privacy and Health Information Management*, *4*(2), 62–75. doi:10.4018/IJPHIM.2016070105

Olaniran, B. A. (2016). ICT Use and Multidisciplinary Healthcare Teams in the Age of e-Health. *International Journal of Reliable and Quality E-Healthcare*, *5*(1), 18–31. doi:10.4018/IJRQEH.2016010102

Olivares, S. L., Cruz, A. G., Cabrera, M. V., Regalado, A. I., & García, J. E. (2017). An Assessment Study of Quality Model for Medical Schools in Mexico. In S. Mukerji & P. Tripathi (Eds.), *Handbook of Research on Administration, Policy, and Leadership in Higher Education* (pp. 404–439). Hershey, PA: IGI Global. doi:10.4018/978-1-5225-0672-0.ch016

Omidoyin, E. O., Opeke, R. O., & Osagbemi, G. K. (2016). Utilization Pattern and Privacy Issues in the use of Health Records for Research Practice by Doctors: Selected Nigerian Teaching Hospitals as Case Study. *International Journal of Privacy and Health Information Management*, *4*(1), 1–11. doi:10.4018/IJPHIM.2016010101

Omoruyi, E. A., & Omidele, F. (2018). Resident Physician and Medical Academic Faculty Burnout: A Review of Current Literature. In C. Smith (Ed.), *Exploring the Pressures of Medical Education From a Mental Health and Wellness Perspective* (pp. 171–189). Hershey, PA: IGI Global. doi:10.4018/978-1-5225-2811-1.ch007

Osop, H., & Sahama, T. (2016). Data-Driven and Practice-Based Evidence: Design and Development of Efficient and Effective Clinical Decision Support System. In J. Moon & M. Galea (Eds.), *Improving Health Management through Clinical Decision Support Systems* (pp. 295–328). Hershey, PA: IGI Global. doi:10.4018/978-1-4666-9432-3.ch014

Ossowski, R., & Izdebski, P. (2016). Ethical Aspects of Talking to a Patient. In A. Rosiek & K. Leksowski (Eds.), *Organizational Culture and Ethics in Modern Medicine* (pp. 203–235). Hershey, PA: IGI Global. doi:10.4018/978-1-4666-9658-7.ch009

Pandian, P. S. (2016). An Overview of Telemedicine Technologies for Healthcare Applications. *International Journal of Biomedical and Clinical Engineering*, *5*(2), 29–52. doi:10.4018/IJBCE.2016070103

Papadopoulou, P., Lytras, M., & Marouli, C. (2018). Bioinformatics as Applied to Medicine: Challenges Faced Moving from Big Data to Smart Data to Wise Data. In M. Lytras & P. Papadopoulou (Eds.), *Applying Big Data Analytics in Bioinformatics and Medicine* (pp. 1–25). Hershey, PA: IGI Global. doi:10.4018/978-1-5225-2607-0.ch001

Paraskou, A., & George, B. P. (2018). An Overview of Reproductive Tourism. In *Legal and Economic Considerations Surrounding Reproductive Tourism: Emerging Research and Opportunities* (pp. 1–17). Hershey, PA: IGI Global. doi:10.4018/978-1-5225-2694-0.ch001

Park, S., & Moon, J. (2016). Strategic Approach towards Clinical Information Security. In J. Moon & M. Galea (Eds.), *Improving Health Management through Clinical Decision Support Systems* (pp. 329–359). Hershey, PA: IGI Global. doi:10.4018/978-1-4666-9432-3.ch015

Pereira, D., Castro, A., Gomes, P., Areias, J. C., Reis, Z. S., Coimbra, M. T., & Cruz-Correia, R. (2016). Digital Auscultation: Challenges and Perspectives. In M. Cruz-Cunha, I. Miranda, R. Martinho, & R. Rijo (Eds.), *Encyclopedia of E-Health and Telemedicine* (pp. 910–927). Hershey, PA: IGI Global. doi:10.4018/978-1-4666-9978-6.ch070

Peters, R. A., & Cruz, M. (2016). The States as Generators of Incremental Change in American Health Care Policy: 1935 to 1965. In R. Gholipour & K. Rouzbehani (Eds.), *Social, Economic, and Political Perspectives on Public Health Policy-Making* (pp. 86–114). Hershey, PA: IGI Global. doi:10.4018/978-1-4666-9944-1.ch005

Phuritsabam, B., & Devi, A. B. (2017). Information Seeking Behavior of Medical Scientists at Jawaharlal Nehru Institute of Medical Science: A Study. In S. Ram (Ed.), *Library and Information Services for Bioinformatics Education and Research* (pp. 177–187). Hershey, PA: IGI Global. doi:10.4018/978-1-5225-1871-6.ch010

Pieczka, B. (2018). Management of Risk and Adverse Events in Medical Entities. In A. Rosiek-Kryszewska & K. Leksowski (Eds.), *Healthcare Administration for Patient Safety and Engagement* (pp. 31–46). Hershey, PA: IGI Global. doi:10.4018/978-1-5225-3946-9.ch003

Poduval, J. (2016). Curriculum Development. In *Optimizing Medicine Residency Training Programs* (pp. 45–102). Hershey, PA: IGI Global. doi:10.4018/978-1-4666-9527-6.ch003

Poduval, J. (2016). Ethics and Professionalism. In *Optimizing Medicine Residency Training Programs* (pp. 103–133). Hershey, PA: IGI Global. doi:10.4018/978-1-4666-9527-6.ch004

Poduval, J. (2016). Management Skills and Leadership. In *Optimizing Medicine Residency Training Programs* (pp. 182–205). Hershey, PA: IGI Global. doi:10.4018/978-1-4666-9527-6.ch008

Poduval, J. (2016). Medicine Residency Training. In *Optimizing Medicine Residency Training Programs* (pp. 1–27). Hershey, PA: IGI Global. doi:10.4018/978-1-4666-9527-6.ch001

Poduval, J. (2016). Personal Issues. In *Optimizing Medicine Residency Training Programs* (pp. 206–221). Hershey, PA: IGI Global. doi:10.4018/978-1-4666-9527-6.ch009

Poduval, J. (2017). Medical Errors: Impact on Health Care Quality. In M. Riga (Ed.), *Impact of Medical Errors and Malpractice on Health Economics, Quality, and Patient Safety* (pp. 33–60). Hershey, PA: IGI Global. doi:10.4018/978-1-5225-2337-6.ch002

Politis, D., Stagiopoulos, P., Aidona, S., Kyriafinis, G., & Constantinidis, I. (2018). Autonomous Learning and Skill Accreditation: A Paradigm for Medical Studies. In A. Kumar (Ed.), *Optimizing Student Engagement in Online Learning Environments* (pp. 266–296). Hershey, PA: IGI Global. doi:10.4018/978-1-5225-3634-5.ch012

Pomares-Quimbaya, A., Gonzalez, R. A., Quintero, S., Muñoz, O. M., Bohórquez, W. R., García, O. M., & Londoño, D. (2016). A Review of Existing Applications and Techniques for Narrative Text Analysis in Electronic Medical Records. In M. Cruz-Cunha, I. Miranda, R. Martinho, & R. Rijo (Eds.), *Encyclopedia of E-Health and Telemedicine* (pp. 796–811). Hershey, PA: IGI Global. doi:10.4018/978-1-4666-9978-6.ch062

Pomares-Quimbaya, A., González, R. A., Sierra, A., Daza, J. C., Muñoz, O., García, A., ... Bohórquez, W. R. (2017). ICT for Enabling the Quality Evaluation of Health Care Services: A Case Study in a General Hospital. In A. Moumtzoglou (Ed.), *Design, Development, and Integration of Reliable Electronic Healthcare Platforms* (pp. 196–210). Hershey, PA: IGI Global. doi:10.4018/978-1-5225-1724-5.ch012

Pouliakis, A., Margari, N., Karakitsou, E., Archondakis, S., & Karakitsos, P. (2018). Emerging Technologies Serving Cytopathology: Big Data, the Cloud, and Mobile Computing. In I. El Naqa (Ed.), *Emerging Developments and Practices in Oncology* (pp. 114–152). Hershey, PA: IGI Global. doi:10.4018/978-1-5225-3085-5.ch005

Queirós, A., Silva, A. G., Ferreira, A., Caravau, H., Cerqueira, M., & Rocha, N. P. (2016). Assessing Mobile Applications Considered Medical Devices. In M. Cruz-Cunha, I. Miranda, R. Martinho, & R. Rijo (Eds.), *Encyclopedia of E-Health and Telemedicine* (pp. 111–127). Hershey, PA: IGI Global. doi:10.4018/978-1-4666-9978-6.ch010

Raffaeli, L., Spinsante, S., & Gambi, E. (2016). Integrated Smart TV-Based Personal e-Health System. *International Journal of E-Health and Medical Communications*, *7*(1), 48–64. doi:10.4018/IJEHMC.2016010103

Rai, A., Kothari, R., & Singh, D. P. (2017). Assessment of Available Technologies for Hospital Waste Management: A Need for Society. In R. Singh, A. Singh, & V. Srivastava (Eds.), *Environmental Issues Surrounding Human Overpopulation* (pp. 172–188). Hershey, PA: IGI Global. doi:10.4018/978-1-5225-1683-5.ch010

Ramamoorthy, S., & Sivasubramaniam, R. (2018). Image Processing Including Medical Liver Imaging: Medical Image Processing from Big Data Perspective, Ultrasound Liver Images, Challenges. In M. Lytras & P. Papadopoulou (Eds.), *Applying Big Data Analytics in Bioinformatics and Medicine* (pp. 380–392). Hershey, PA: IGI Global. doi:10.4018/978-1-5225-2607-0.ch016

Rathor, G. P., & Gupta, S. K. (2017). Improving Multimodality Image Fusion through Integrate AFL and Wavelet Transform. In V. Tiwari, B. Tiwari, R. Thakur, & S. Gupta (Eds.), *Pattern and Data Analysis in Healthcare Settings* (pp. 143–157). Hershey, PA: IGI Global. doi:10.4018/978-1-5225-0536-5.ch008

Rawat, D. B., & Bhattacharya, S. (2016). Wireless Body Area Network for Healthcare Applications. In N. Meghanathan (Ed.), *Advanced Methods for Complex Network Analysis* (pp. 343–358). Hershey, PA: IGI Global. doi:10.4018/978-1-4666-9964-9.ch014

Rea, P. M. (2016). Advances in Anatomical and Medical Visualisation. In M. Pinheiro & D. Simões (Eds.), *Handbook of Research on Engaging Digital Natives in Higher Education Settings* (pp. 244–264). Hershey, PA: IGI Global. doi:10.4018/978-1-5225-0039-1.ch011

Rexhepi, H., & Persson, A. (2017). Challenges to Implementing IT Support for Evidence Based Practice Among Nurses and Assistant Nurses: A Qualitative Study. *Journal of Electronic Commerce in Organizations*, *15*(2), 61–76. doi:10.4018/JECO.2017040105

Reychav, I., & Azuri, J. (2016). Including Elderly Patients in Decision Making via Electronic Health Literacy. In M. Cruz-Cunha, I. Miranda, R. Martinho, & R. Rijo (Eds.), *Encyclopedia of E-Health and Telemedicine* (pp. 241–249). Hershey, PA: IGI Global. doi:10.4018/978-1-4666-9978-6.ch020

Richards, D., & Caldwell, P. H. (2016). Gamification to Improve Adherence to Clinical Treatment Advice: Improving Adherence to Clinical Treatment. In D. Novák, B. Tulu, & H. Brendryen (Eds.), *Handbook of Research on Holistic Perspectives in Gamification for Clinical Practice* (pp. 47–77). Hershey, PA: IGI Global. doi:10.4018/978-1-4666-9522-1.ch004

Rissman, B. (2016). Medical Conditions Associated with NLD. In B. Rissman (Ed.), *Medical and Educational Perspectives on Nonverbal Learning Disability in Children and Young Adults* (pp. 27–66). Hershey, PA: IGI Global. doi:10.4018/978-1-4666-9539-9.ch002

Rosiek, A. (2018). The Assessment of Actions of the Environment and the Impact of Preventive Medicine for Public Health in Poland. In A. Rosiek-Kryszewska & K. Leksowski (Eds.), *Healthcare Administration for Patient Safety and Engagement* (pp. 106–119). Hershey, PA: IGI Global. doi:10.4018/978-1-5225-3946-9.ch006

Rosiek, A., Leksowski, K., Goch, A., Rosiek-Kryszewska, A., & Leksowski, Ł. (2016). Medical Treatment and Difficult Ethical Decisions in Interdisciplinary Hospital Teams. In A. Rosiek & K. Leksowski (Eds.), *Organizational Culture and Ethics in Modern Medicine* (pp. 121–153). Hershey, PA: IGI Global. doi:10.4018/978-1-4666-9658-7.ch006

Rosiek, A., & Rosiek-Kryszewska, A. (2018). Managed Healthcare: Doctor Life Satisfaction and Its Impact on the Process of Communicating With the Patient. In A. Rosiek-Kryszewska & K. Leksowski (Eds.), *Healthcare Administration for Patient Safety and Engagement* (pp. 244–261). Hershey, PA: IGI Global. doi:10.4018/978-1-5225-3946-9.ch013

Rosiek-Kryszewska, A., Leksowski, Ł., Rosiek, A., Leksowski, K., & Goch, A. (2016). Clinical Communication in the Aspect of Development of New Technologies and E-Health in the Doctor-Patient Relationship. In A. Rosiek & K. Leksowski (Eds.), *Organizational Culture and Ethics in Modern Medicine* (pp. 18–51). Hershey, PA: IGI Global. doi:10.4018/978-1-4666-9658-7.ch002

Rosiek-Kryszewska, A., & Rosiek, A. (2018). The Involvement of the Patient and his Perspective Evaluation of the Quality of Healthcare. In A. Rosiek-Kryszewska & K. Leksowski (Eds.), *Healthcare Administration for Patient Safety and Engagement* (pp. 121–144). Hershey, PA: IGI Global. doi:10.4018/978-1-5225-3946-9.ch007

Rosiek-Kryszewska, A., & Rosiek, A. (2018). The Impact of Management and Leadership Roles in Building Competitive Healthcare Units. In A. Rosiek-Kryszewska & K. Leksowski (Eds.), *Healthcare Administration for Patient Safety and Engagement* (pp. 13–30). Hershey, PA: IGI Global. doi:10.4018/978-1-5225-3946-9.ch002

Roşu, S. M., Păvăloiu, I. B., Dragoi, G., Apostol, C. G., & Munteanu, D. (2016). Telemedicine Based on LMDS in the Urban/Metropolitan Area: A Romanian Case Study. In M. Cruz-Cunha, I. Miranda, R. Martinho, & R. Rijo (Eds.), *Encyclopedia of E-Health and Telemedicine* (pp. 96–109). Hershey, PA: IGI Global. doi:10.4018/978-1-4666-9978-6.ch009

Rouzbehani, K. (2017). Health Policy Implementation: Moving Beyond Its Barriers in United States. In N. Wickramasinghe (Ed.), *Handbook of Research on Healthcare Administration and Management* (pp. 541–552). Hershey, PA: IGI Global. doi:10.4018/978-1-5225-0920-2.ch032

Ruiz, I. M., Cohen, D. S., & Marco, Á. M. (2016). ISO/IEEE11073 Family of Standards: Trends and Applications on E-Health Monitoring. In M. Cruz-Cunha, I. Miranda, R. Martinho, & R. Rijo (Eds.), *Encyclopedia of E-Health and Telemedicine* (pp. 646–660). Hershey, PA: IGI Global. doi:10.4018/978-1-4666-9978-6.ch050

Sam, S. (2017). Mobile Phones and Expanding Human Capabilities in Plural Health Systems. In K. Moahi, K. Bwalya, & P. Sebina (Eds.), *Health Information Systems and the Advancement of Medical Practice in Developing Countries* (pp. 93–114). Hershey, PA: IGI Global. doi:10.4018/978-1-5225-2262-1.ch006

Sankaranarayanan, S., & Ganesan, S. (2016). Applications of Intelligent Agents in Health Sector-A Review. *International Journal of E-Health and Medical Communications*, *7*(1), 1–30. doi:10.4018/IJEHMC.2016010101

Santos-Trigo, M., Suaste, E., & Figuerola, P. (2018). Technology Design and Routes for Tool Appropriation in Medical Practices. In M. Khosrow-Pour, D.B.A. (Ed.), Encyclopedia of Information Science and Technology, Fourth Edition (pp. 3794-3804). Hershey, PA: IGI Global. doi:10.4018/978-1-5225-2255-3.ch329

Sarivougioukas, J., Vagelatos, A., Parsopoulos, K. E., & Lagaris, I. E. (2018). Home UbiHealth. In M. Khosrow-Pour, D.B.A. (Ed.), Encyclopedia of Information Science and Technology, Fourth Edition (pp. 7765-7774). Hershey, PA: IGI Global. doi:10.4018/978-1-5225-2255-3.ch675

Sarkar, B. K. (2017). Big Data and Healthcare Data: A Survey. *International Journal of Knowledge-Based Organizations*, *7*(4), 50–77. doi:10.4018/IJKBO.2017100104

Saxena, K., & Banodha, U. (2017). An Essence of the SOA on Healthcare. In R. Bhadoria, N. Chaudhari, G. Tomar, & S. Singh (Eds.), *Exploring Enterprise Service Bus in the Service-Oriented Architecture Paradigm* (pp. 283–304). Hershey, PA: IGI Global. doi:10.4018/978-1-5225-2157-0.ch018

Schmeida, M., & McNeal, R. (2016). Consulting Online Healthcare Information: E-Caregivers as Knowledgeable Decision Makers. *International Journal of Computers in Clinical Practice*, *1*(1), 42–52. doi:10.4018/IJCCP.2016010104

Sen, K., & Ghosh, K. (2018). Incorporating Global Medical Knowledge to Solve Healthcare Problems: A Framework for a Crowdsourcing System. *International Journal of Healthcare Information Systems and Informatics*, *13*(1), 1–14. doi:10.4018/IJHISI.2018010101

Shakdher, A., & Pandey, K. (2017). REDAlert+: Medical/Fire Emergency and Warning System using Android Devices. *International Journal of E-Health and Medical Communications*, *8*(1), 37–51. doi:10.4018/IJEHMC.2017010103

Shekarian, E., Abdul-Rashid, S. H., & Olugu, E. U. (2017). An Integrated Fuzzy VIKOR Method for Performance Management in Healthcare. In M. Tavana, K. Szabat, & K. Puranam (Eds.), *Organizational Productivity and Performance Measurements Using Predictive Modeling and Analytics* (pp. 40–61). Hershey, PA: IGI Global. doi:10.4018/978-1-5225-0654-6.ch003

Shi, J., Erdem, E., & Liu, H. (2016). Expanding Role of Telephone Systems in Healthcare: Developments and Opportunities. In A. Dwivedi (Ed.), *Reshaping Medical Practice and Care with Health Information Systems* (pp. 87–131). Hershey, PA: IGI Global. doi:10.4018/978-1-4666-9870-3.ch004

Shijina, V., & John, S. J. (2017). Multiple Relations and its Application in Medical Diagnosis. *International Journal of Fuzzy System Applications*, *6*(4), 47–62. doi:10.4018/IJFSA.2017100104

Shipley, N., & Chakraborty, J. (2018). Big Data and mHealth: Increasing the Usability of Healthcare Through the Customization of Pinterest – Literary Perspective. In J. Machado, A. Abelha, M. Santos, & F. Portela (Eds.), *Next-Generation Mobile and Pervasive Healthcare Solutions* (pp. 46–66). Hershey, PA: IGI Global. doi:10.4018/978-1-5225-2851-7.ch004

Singh, A., & Dutta, M. K. (2017). A Reversible Data Hiding Scheme for Efficient Management of Tele-Ophthalmological Data. *International Journal of E-Health and Medical Communications*, *8*(3), 38–54. doi:10.4018/IJEHMC.2017070103

Sivaji, A., Radjo, H. K., Amin, M., & Abu Hashim, M. A. (2016). Design of a Hospital Interactive Wayfinding System: Designing for Malaysian Users. In N. Mohamed, T. Mantoro, M. Ayu, & M. Mahmud (Eds.), *Critical Socio-Technical Issues Surrounding Mobile Computing* (pp. 88–123). Hershey, PA: IGI Global. doi:10.4018/978-1-4666-9438-5.ch005

Skourti, P. K., & Pavlakis, A. (2017). The Second Victim Phenomenon: The Way Out. In M. Riga (Ed.), *Impact of Medical Errors and Malpractice on Health Economics, Quality, and Patient Safety* (pp. 197–222). Hershey, PA: IGI Global. doi:10.4018/978-1-5225-2337-6.ch008

Smith, C. R. (2018). Medical Students' Quest Towards the Long White Coat: Impact on Mental Health and Well-Being. In C. Smith (Ed.), *Exploring the Pressures of Medical Education From a Mental Health and Wellness Perspective* (pp. 1–42). Hershey, PA: IGI Global. doi:10.4018/978-1-5225-2811-1.ch001

Smith, S. I., & Dandignac, M. (2018). Perfectionism: Addressing Lofty Expectations in Medical School. In C. Smith (Ed.), *Exploring the Pressures of Medical Education From a Mental Health and Wellness Perspective* (pp. 68–91). Hershey, PA: IGI Global. doi:10.4018/978-1-5225-2811-1.ch003

Sobrinho, Á. A., Dias da Silva, L., Perkusich, A., Cunha, P., Pinheiro, M. E., & Melo de Medeiros, L. (2016). Towards Medical Systems to Aid the Detection and Treatment of Chronic Diseases. In D. Fotiadis (Ed.), *Handbook of Research on Trends in the Diagnosis and Treatment of Chronic Conditions* (pp. 50–69). Hershey, PA: IGI Global. doi:10.4018/978-1-4666-8828-5.ch003

Soczywko, J., & Rutkowska, D. (2018). The Patient/Provider Relationship in Emergency Medicine: Organization, Communication, and Understanding. In A. Rosiek-Kryszewska & K. Leksowski (Eds.), *Healthcare Administration for Patient Safety and Engagement* (pp. 74–105). Hershey, PA: IGI Global. doi:10.4018/978-1-5225-3946-9.ch005

Sołtysik-Piorunkiewicz, A., Furmankiewicz, M., & Ziuziański, P. (2016). Web Healthcare Applications in Poland: Trends, Standards, Barriers and Possibilities of Implementation and Usage of E-Health Systems. In I. Deliyannis, P. Kostagiolas, & C. Banou (Eds.), *Experimental Multimedia Systems for Interactivity and Strategic Innovation* (pp. 258–283). Hershey, PA: IGI Global. doi:10.4018/978-1-4666-8659-5.ch013

Soni, P. (2018). Implications of HIPAA and Subsequent Regulations on Information Technology. In M. Gupta, R. Sharman, J. Walp, & P. Mulgund (Eds.), *Information Technology Risk Management and Compliance in Modern Organizations* (pp. 71–98). Hershey, PA: IGI Global. doi:10.4018/978-1-5225-2604-9.ch004

Spinelli, R., & Benevolo, C. (2016). From Healthcare Services to E-Health Applications: A Delivery System-Based Taxonomy. In A. Dwivedi (Ed.), *Reshaping Medical Practice and Care with Health Information Systems* (pp. 205–245). Hershey, PA: IGI Global. doi:10.4018/978-1-4666-9870-3.ch007

Srivastava, A., & Aggarwal, A. K. (2018). Medical Image Fusion in Spatial and Transform Domain: A Comparative Analysis. In M. Anwar, A. Khosla, & R. Kapoor (Eds.), *Handbook of Research on Advanced Concepts in Real-Time Image and Video Processing* (pp. 281–300). Hershey, PA: IGI Global. doi:10.4018/978-1-5225-2848-7.ch011

Srivastava, S. K., & Roy, S. N. (2018). Recommendation System: A Potential Tool for Achieving Pervasive Health Care. In J. Machado, A. Abelha, M. Santos, & F. Portela (Eds.), *Next-Generation Mobile and Pervasive Healthcare Solutions* (pp. 111–127). Hershey, PA: IGI Global. doi:10.4018/978-1-5225-2851-7.ch008

Stancu, A. (2016). Correlations and Patterns of Food and Health Consumer Expenditure. In A. Jean-Vasile (Ed.), *Food Science, Production, and Engineering in Contemporary Economies* (pp. 44–101). Hershey, PA: IGI Global. doi:10.4018/978-1-5225-0341-5.ch003

Stanimirovic, D. (2017). Digitalization of Death Certification Model: Transformation Issues and Implementation Concerns. In S. Saeed, Y. Bamarouf, T. Ramayah, & S. Iqbal (Eds.), *Design Solutions for User-Centric Information Systems* (pp. 22–43). Hershey, PA: IGI Global. doi:10.4018/978-1-5225-1944-7.ch002

Stavros, A., Vavoulidis, E., & Nasioutziki, M. (2016). The Use of Mobile Health Applications for Quality Control and Accreditational Purposes in a Cytopathology Laboratory. In A. Moumtzoglou (Ed.), *M-Health Innovations for Patient-Centered Care* (pp. 262–283). Hershey, PA: IGI Global. doi:10.4018/978-1-4666-9861-1.ch013

Sukkird, V., & Shirahada, K. (2018). E-Health Service Model for Asian Developing Countries: A Case of Emergency Medical Service for Elderly People in Thailand. In M. Khosrow-Pour (Ed.), *Optimizing Current Practices in E-Services and Mobile Applications* (pp. 214–232). Hershey, PA: IGI Global. doi:10.4018/978-1-5225-5026-6.ch011

Sygit, B., & Wąsik, D. (2016). Patients' Rights and Medical Personnel Duties in the Field of Hospital Care. In A. Rosiek & K. Leksowski (Eds.), *Organizational Culture and Ethics in Modern Medicine* (pp. 282–297). Hershey, PA: IGI Global. doi:10.4018/978-1-4666-9658-7.ch012

Sygit, B., & Wąsik, D. (2016). The Idea of Human Rights in Conditions of Hospital Treatment. In A. Rosiek & K. Leksowski (Eds.), *Organizational Culture and Ethics in Modern Medicine* (pp. 236–254). Hershey, PA: IGI Global. doi:10.4018/978-1-4666-9658-7.ch010

Talbot, T. B. (2017). Making Lifelike Medical Games in the Age of Virtual Reality: An Update on "Playing Games with Biology" from 2013. In B. Dubbels (Ed.), *Transforming Gaming and Computer Simulation Technologies across Industries* (pp. 103–119). Hershey, PA: IGI Global. doi:10.4018/978-1-5225-1817-4.ch006

Tamposis, I., Pouliakis, A., Fezoulidis, I., & Karakitsos, P. (2016). Mobile Platforms Supporting Health Professionals: Need, Technical Requirements, and Applications. In A. Moumtzoglou (Ed.), *M-Health Innovations for Patient-Centered Care* (pp. 91–114). Hershey, PA: IGI Global. doi:10.4018/978-1-4666-9861-1.ch005

Tiago, M. T., Tiago, F., Amaral, F. E., & Silva, S. (2016). Healthy 3.0: Healthcare Digital Dimensions. In A. Dwivedi (Ed.), *Reshaping Medical Practice and Care with Health Information Systems* (pp. 287–322). Hershey, PA: IGI Global. doi:10.4018/978-1-4666-9870-3.ch010

Tripathy, B. (2016). Application of Rough Set Based Models in Medical Diagnosis. In S. Dash & B. Subudhi (Eds.), *Handbook of Research on Computational Intelligence Applications in Bioinformatics* (pp. 144–168). Hershey, PA: IGI Global. doi:10.4018/978-1-5225-0427-6.ch008

Turcu, C. E., & Turcu, C. O. (2017). Social Internet of Things in Healthcare: From Things to Social Things in Internet of Things. In C. Reis & M. Maximiano (Eds.), *Internet of Things and Advanced Application in Healthcare* (pp. 266–295). Hershey, PA: IGI Global. doi:10.4018/978-1-5225-1820-4.ch010

Unwin, D. W., Sanzogni, L., & Sandhu, K. (2017). Developing and Measuring the Business Case for Health Information Technology. In K. Moahi, K. Bwalya, & P. Sebina (Eds.), *Health Information Systems and the Advancement of Medical Practice in Developing Countries* (pp. 262–290). Hershey, PA: IGI Global. doi:10.4018/978-1-5225-2262-1.ch015

Urooj, S., & Singh, S. P. (2016). Wavelet Transform-Based Soft Computational Techniques and Applications in Medical Imaging. In P. Saxena, D. Singh, & M. Pant (Eds.), *Problem Solving and Uncertainty Modeling through Optimization and Soft Computing Applications* (pp. 339–363). Hershey, PA: IGI Global. doi:10.4018/978-1-4666-9885-7.ch016

Vasant, P. (2018). A General Medical Diagnosis System Formed by Artificial Neural Networks and Swarm Intelligence Techniques. In U. Kose, G. Guraksin, & O. Deperlioglu (Eds.), *Nature-Inspired Intelligent Techniques for Solving Biomedical Engineering Problems* (pp. 130–145). Hershey, PA: IGI Global. doi:10.4018/978-1-5225-4769-3.ch006

Waegemann, C. P. (2016). mHealth: History, Analysis, and Implementation. In A. Moumtzoglou (Ed.), M-Health Innovations for Patient-Centered Care (pp. 1-19). Hershey, PA: IGI Global. doi:10.4018/978-1-4666-9861-1.ch001

Watfa, M. K., Majeed, H., & Salahuddin, T. (2016). Computer Based E-Healthcare Clinical Systems: A Comprehensive Survey. *International Journal of Privacy and Health Information Management*, *4*(1), 50–69. doi:10.4018/IJPHIM.2016010104

Wietholter, J. P., Coetzee, R., Nardella, B., Kincaid, S. E., & Slain, D. (2016). International Healthcare Experiences: Caring While Learning and Learning While Caring. In D. Velliaris & D. Coleman-George (Eds.), *Handbook of Research on Study Abroad Programs and Outbound Mobility* (pp. 470–496). Hershey, PA: IGI Global. doi:10.4018/978-1-5225-0169-5.ch019

Witzke, K., & Specht, O. (2017). M-Health Telemedicine and Telepresence in Oral and Maxillofacial Surgery: An Innovative Prehospital Healthcare Concept in Structurally Weak Areas. *International Journal of Reliable and Quality E-Healthcare*, *6*(4), 37–48. doi:10.4018/IJRQEH.2017100105

Wójcik, A., & Chojnacki, M. (2016). Behavior and Ethical Problems in the Functioning of the Operating Theater (Case Study). In A. Rosiek & K. Leksowski (Eds.), *Organizational Culture and Ethics in Modern Medicine* (pp. 154–179). Hershey, PA: IGI Global. doi:10.4018/978-1-4666-9658-7.ch007

Wolk, K., & Marasek, K. P. (2016). Translation of Medical Texts using Neural Networks. *International Journal of Reliable and Quality E-Healthcare*, *5*(4), 51–66. doi:10.4018/IJRQEH.2016100104

Wong, A. K., & Lo, M. F. (2018). Using Pervasive Computing for Sustainable Healthcare in an Aging Population. In B. Fong, A. Ng, & P. Yuen (Eds.), *Sustainable Health and Long-Term Care Solutions for an Aging Population* (pp. 187–202). Hershey, PA: IGI Global. doi:10.4018/978-1-5225-2633-9.ch010

Wu, W., Martin, B. C., & Ni, C. (2017). A Systematic Review of Competency-Based Education Effort in the Health Professions: Seeking Order Out of Chaos. In K. Rasmussen, P. Northrup, & R. Colson (Eds.), *Handbook of Research on Competency-Based Education in University Settings* (pp. 352–378). Hershey, PA: IGI Global. doi:10.4018/978-1-5225-0932-5.ch018

Yadav, N., Aliasgari, M., & Poellabauer, C. (2016). Mobile Healthcare in an Increasingly Connected Developing World. *International Journal of Privacy and Health Information Management*, *4*(2), 76–97. doi:10.4018/IJPHIM.2016070106

Yadav, S., Ekbal, A., Saha, S., Pathak, P. S., & Bhattacharyya, P. (2017). Patient Data De-Identification: A Conditional Random-Field-Based Supervised Approach. In S. Saha, A. Mandal, A. Narasimhamurthy, S. V, & S. Sangam (Eds.), Handbook of Research on Applied Cybernetics and Systems Science (pp. 234-253). Hershey, PA: IGI Global. doi:10.4018/978-1-5225-2498-4.ch011

Yu, B., Wijesekera, D., & Costa, P. C. (2017). Informed Consent in Healthcare: A Study Case of Genetic Services. In A. Moumtzoglou (Ed.), *Design, Development, and Integration of Reliable Electronic Healthcare Platforms* (pp. 211–242). Hershey, PA: IGI Global. doi:10.4018/978-1-5225-1724-5.ch013

Yu, B., Wijesekera, D., & Costa, P. C. (2017). Informed Consent in Electronic Medical Record Systems. In I. Management Association (Ed.), Healthcare Ethics and Training: Concepts, Methodologies, Tools, and Applications (pp. 1029-1049). Hershey, PA: IGI Global. doi:10.4018/978-1-5225-2237-9.ch049

Yu, M., Li, J., & Wang, W. (2017). Creative Life Experience among Students in Medical Education. In C. Zhou (Ed.), *Handbook of Research on Creative Problem-Solving Skill Development in Higher Education* (pp. 158–184). Hershey, PA: IGI Global. doi:10.4018/978-1-5225-0643-0.ch008

Zarour, K. (2017). Towards a Telehomecare in Algeria: Case of Diabetes Measurement and Remote Monitoring. *International Journal of E-Health and Medical Communications*, *8*(4), 61–80. doi:10.4018/IJEHMC.2017100104

Zavyalova, Y. V., Korzun, D. G., Meigal, A. Y., & Borodin, A. V. (2017). Towards the Development of Smart Spaces-Based Socio-Cyber-Medicine Systems. *International Journal of Embedded and Real-Time Communication Systems*, *8*(1), 45–63. doi:10.4018/IJERTCS.2017010104

Zeinali, A. A. (2018). Word Formation Study in Developing Naming Guidelines in the Translation of English Medical Terms Into Persian. In M. Khosrow-Pour, D.B.A. (Ed.), Encyclopedia of Information Science and Technology, Fourth Edition (pp. 5136-5147). Hershey, PA: IGI Global. doi:10.4018/978-1-5225-2255-3.ch446

Ziminski, T. B., Demurjian, S. A., Sanzi, E., & Agresta, T. (2016). Toward Integrating Healthcare Data and Systems: A Study of Architectural Alternatives. In T. Iyamu & A. Tatnall (Eds.), *Maximizing Healthcare Delivery and Management through Technology Integration* (pp. 270–304). Hershey, PA: IGI Global. doi:10.4018/978-1-4666-9446-0.ch016

Ziminski, T. B., Demurjian, S. A., Sanzi, E., Baihan, M., & Agresta, T. (2016). An Architectural Solution for Health Information Exchange. *International Journal of User-Driven Healthcare, 6*(1), 65–103. doi:10.4018/IJUDH.2016010104

Zineldin, M., & Vasicheva, V. (2018). Reducing Medical Errors and Increasing Patient Safety: TRM and 5 Q's Approaches for Better Quality of Life. In *Technological Tools for Value-Based Sustainable Relationships in Health: Emerging Research and Opportunities* (pp. 87–115). Hershey, PA: IGI Global. doi:10.4018/978-1-5225-4091-5.ch005

About the Contributors

Sandul Yasobant is a Junior Researcher at the Center for Development Research (ZEF), Bonn, Germany. With technical qualification in public health, he has worked in health system research for several years in South East Asia regions especially in India. The major focus of his work has been in the area of the health system, surveillance, infectious disease, non-communicable disease, maternal child health through various translational and operational research. Other research areas of his interest include health system and policy research, global health governance, infectious diseases & one health, health technology application in action research. Beyond his research tenure, he is actively serving as an editorial board member/reviewer for many national and international scientific research journals in the field of public health.

Deepak Saxena is a Professor of Epidemiology with Indian Institute of Public Health Gandhinagar, Gujarat, India. He is a Physician by training and holds Ph.D. in Epidemiology and a Post Doc from Karolinska University, Sweden. The major focus of his work has been Emerging Infectious diseases, Anti-Microbial Resistance (AMR) and Water Sanitation and Hygiene (WASH). Other research areas of his interest include health system, Community trials, Cohort studies, health technology assessments and integrating technology for early detection of Outbreaks. He is actively serving as an Editor, editorial board member/reviewer for many national and international scientific research journals in the field of public health.

* * *

Walter Bruchhausen studies of medicine, theology and health care ethics at the universities of Bonn, Würzburg and Glasgow; work as medical doctor and health coordinator in Germany, Rwanda and East Congo; since 2004 senior lecturer at the universities of Bonn, Aachen and Cologne; since 2016 senior fellow in the NRW Fortschrittskolleg One Health and Urban Transformation at the Centre for Development Research, University of Bonn.

Pallab Chaudhuri has gained 15 years of experience in genetic engineering work involving different microbial pathogens. Experience of cloning and expression of genes in prokaryotic system, handling of laboratory animals, use of recombinant proteins, as immunogen, in the experimental animals. 12 years of teaching experience for the discipline of animal biotechnology and veterinary microbiology, guided 6 MVSc and 3 PhD students of IVRI deemed university for their thesis work. Availed DBT overseas associateship in the University of Wisconsin, USA. Attended a ICTTD sponsored bioinformatics workshop at the institute of Parasitology, Univ. of South Bohemia, Czech Republic. Availed NFID travel grant to attend 13th Annual conference on vaccine research, at Bethesda, Maryland, USA.

Ana Cláudia Coelho is a DVM (University of Trás-os-Montes and Alto Douro, 1997), a MSc in Health Promotion and Health Education (University of Trás-os-Montes and Alto Douro, 2001) and a PhD in Veterinary Sciences (University of Trás-os-Montes and Alto Douro, 2006). She has spent the last 20 years teaching at the Department of Veterinary Sciences of the University of Trás-os-Montes and Alto Douro.

Catarina Coelho is a DVM (University of Trás-os-Montes e Alto Douro, 2011) and a PhD in Animal Science (University of Trás-os-Montes e Alto Douro, 2015) . She has spent the last 14 years teaching at the Agrarian Superior School of the Polythecnic Superior Institute of Viseu.

Rita Cruz is a DVM by the University of Lisbon in 2002, working in private practice since 2002. She has spent the last 11 years teaching at the Agrarian Superior School of the Polytechnic Superior Institute of Viseu. She also has spent the last 16 years working as a private veterinary surgeon in ANCOSE and in Clinica Veterinária do Dão.

Utpal Das is a Graduate in Veterinary Science. Dr. Utpal Das did his Masters in Veterinary Public Health from All India Institute of Hygiene & Public Health, Kolkata; Presently, working as Superintending Veterinary Officer, Health Department, Kolkata Municipal Corporation, India. He has around thirty five years of clinical, academic and administrative experience. Dr. Das focused on comparative pathology of CTVS and developed an unique and revolutionary chemotherapeutic drug regimen to cure the mostly prevalent cancer (CTVS) of dogs. He characterized Veterinary Public Health fundamentally and strongly advocated for One Health Approach. Dr. Das provided significant inputs for elucidation of a number of zoonotic infections including rabies in India. He is life member and Governing Body member of various professional organizations and honored as FELLOW of Indian Public Health Association and Association for Public Health Veterinarians. He published more than 80 scientific papers in reputed journals. Dr. Das has been bestowed with Debrani Dutta Memorial Silver Medal, Dr. R. Swaminathan Iyer memorial Gold Medal, ISACP Award, Dr. R.R. Shukla Gold Medal, Rashtriya Gaurab Award, Best Citizens of India Award and many plaques of Honors.

Fernando Esteves is a DVM by the University of Trás-os-Montes e Alto Douro, working in private practice for 20 years. He is a Professor at the Agrarian Superior School of the Polythecnic Institute of Viseu.

Ana Sofia Ferreira graduated in Biology in the University of Trás-os-Montes and Alto Douro (2007) and obtained her Ph.D. in Veterinary Sciences by the Institute of Biomedical Sciences Abel Salazar (2015). She is a Post-Doctoral researcher in the University of Porto.

Sophia Inbaraj has been working as Scientist in the Division of Bacteriology and Mycology, ICAR Indian Veterinary Research Institute, India. She is currently pursuing her doctoral research in antimicrobial resistance in *Salmonella* sps., of animal and environmental origin. Her research interests include antimicrobial resistance in animal pathogens, serosurveillance of leptospirosis in farm and wild animals.

Ike Valentine Iyioke has multidisciplinary backgrounds in philosophy, international relations, journalism and teaching. His career started as a lecturer at the College of Ecumenical Education, Enugu, Nigeria, where he taught social studies, general studies, and philosophy of education classes. During the first part of his graduate studies at the Michigan State University he assisted with teaching a class in the Environmental Journalism program in the School of Journalism. Subsequently, Iyioke has taught several courses in philosophy including, bioethics, business ethics, African philosophy and environmental ethics. Iyioke's doctorate degree is in philosophy (bioethics). He likes to explore questions pertaining to moral philosophy, particularly bioethics. He is also interested in environmental ethics, environmental science public policy, and the role these play in moral thinking. His research interests include issues about research subject/participant selection; human experimentation; biomedical research partnerships between Africa & the West; environmental ethics; environmental justice/racism; eugenics; science of life extension; morality in primitive cultures; and, consumer right to know.

Punit Jhandai is Veterinarian by profession and currently a master scholar in the field of Veterinary Public health and Epidemiology at LUVAS, India. His research focus is on extended Spectrum beta-lactamase E.coli in food of animal origin, which includes both milk and chicken meat. His research interests include phenotypic and molecular detection of ESBLs.

Stefanovska Jovana, University St. Kiril and Methodius, Macedonia, is a DVM (University of Zagreb, 1991), MSc in Veterinary science (University of Belgrade, 1998), and PhD of Veterinary Science (University St. Cyril and Methodius, 2011). She has spent all this year since 1998 in Faculty of veterinary medicine – Skopje, Department of parasitology. At the moment she is associated professor of parasitology and chief of Veterinary institute in frame of FVM-S.

Adnan Khan graduated as a veterinarian from the University of Agriculture, Peshawar with distinction in 2012. He is a veteran professional working on zoo and wild animals since 2013 with the Wildlife Department of Khyber Pakhtunkhwa (Pakistan) and has got proficiency in exotic medicine aimed at management and conservation of wildlife. Meanwhile, he got his masters in veterinary medicine from Arid Agriculture University, Rawalpindi. His areas of special interest include management and husbandry of zoo species, avian medicine, one health and zoonoses.

Cristina Mega is a DVM (University of Lisbon, 1992), a MSc in Vision Science (University of Coimbra, 2007) and a PhD in Health Science - Biomedical Sciences (University of Coimbra, 2017). She has spent the last 14 years teaching at the Agrarian Superior School of the Polytechnic Superior Institute of Viseu.

João R. Mesquita received his DVM from the University of Trás-os-Montes e Alto Douro in 2005 and in 2012 he obtained a PhD in Microbiology. He is a Professor at the Agrarian Superior School of Viseu for the past 12 years.

Carla Santos received her DVM from the University of Trás-os-Montes e Alto Douro in 1998 and in 2012 she was awarded a Master in Animal Science. She is Professor at the Agrarian School of the Polytechnic Institute of Viseu for the past 19 years.

Blagica Sekovska, University St. Kiril and Methodius, Macedonia, is bachelor of agriculture and food (University of Cyril and Methodius, Skopje, 1993), MSc and PhD of economics (UKIM, 2001 and 2006). She has spent the last 25 years working on Faculty of veterinary medicine, last 15 years in Department of veterinary economics and management. At the moment she is full time professor at the same department.

Said Sajjad Ali Shah received his DVM from The University of Agriculture, Peshawar in 2012 and M.Phil in Veterinary Pathology from the same University in 2015. Currently, he is enrolled as PhD scholar in Veterinary Pathology, Animal Health Dept, The University of Agriculture, Peshwar. He is a dynamic veterinarian, interested in issues related to One Health. Currently, he is working as Research Officer in Livestock and Dairy Development (Research), Khyber Pakhtunkhwa, Peshawar-Pakistan.

Vamshi Krishna Sriram did BVSc. & AH from College of Veterinary Science, Hyderabad, P.V. Narsimha Rao Telangana Veterinary University, Telangana in 2010 and M.V.Sc from Department of Veterinary Microbiology, College of Veterinary and Animal Sciences, Mannuthy, Thrissur, Kerala Veterinary and Animal Sciences University, Kerala and obtained PhD in Bacteriology from Division of Bacteriology and Mycology, ICAR- Indian Veterinary Research Institute, Bareilly, U. P, India. Research areas of interest include diagnosis of bacterial diseases and worked on canine leptospirosis in Masters program and antimicrobial resistance in Pasteurella multocida during PhD.

Prasad Thomas is working as a Scientist (Senior Scale) in National Salmonella Centre (Veterinary), Division of Bacteriology and Mycology, ICAR- Indian Veterinary Research Institute, India. He has specialization in molecular diagnosis, bioinformatics, molecular epidemiology of bacterial pathogens, salmonellosis, clostridial diseases and antimicrobial resistance. He has been working in bacterial diseases (9 years) in association with Division of Bacteriology and Mycology, ICAR-IVRI to understand genetic diversity, development of diagnostics and vaccines for pathogens like Pasteurella, Clostridium, Salmonella and Brucella sps.. Involved in teaching theory and practical courses such as Enterobacteriaceae, Bacterial Genetics, Advanced Bacteriology and Mycology, Techniques in Microbiology and Mycoplasmology for Masters (M.V.Sc) and Doctoral students.

Helena Vala is a DVM (University of Trás-os-Montes e Alto Douro, 1993) and a PhD in Veterinary Sciences (University of Trás-os-Montes e Alto Douro, 2002). She has spent the last 21 years teaching at the Agrarian Superior School of the Polythecnic Superior Institute of Viseu.

Carmen Vasconcelos-Nobrega is a DVM (University of Trás-os-Montes e Alto Douro, 2001), a MSc in Quality Control - Water and Food (University of Oporto, 2007) and a PhD in Veterinary Sciences (University of Trás-os-Montes e Alto Douro, 2012). She has spent the last 13 years teaching at the Agrarian Superior School of the Polythecnic Superior Institute of Viseu.

Abhishek Verma is working as a scientist (SS) in the Division of Bacteriology at IVRI, Izatnagar, India. Currently, he is serving as a collaborator in an All India Network Programme on Neonatal Mortality project under which he is actively involved in studying the phenotypic and genotypic resistance of E coli associated with neonatal calves. He has vast expertise in isolation and identification of fungal pathogens associated with livestock diseases, molecular characterization and studying its antifungal susceptibility. He has involved in teaching theory and practical classes on General and systematic mycology and mycoses to post-graduate and doctoral students.

Index

A

All-in-One (One-in-All) 55
Animal 2-14, 17-19, 21-23, 34-35, 49, 59-62, 65-67, 70-74, 82-86, 89-91, 99-100, 104-106, 108, 113-116, 119-120, 122-123, 125-127, 129-134, 142-143, 146-147, 149-151, 153, 165, 172, 175, 179, 181, 184, 197-198, 200-203, 205
Animal Health 7-9, 12-13, 17, 19, 21-23, 34, 59-62, 82-83, 85, 90, 108, 114-116, 126, 129-131, 172, 201-202
Antibiotic 36, 123, 125, 130, 142-144, 146, 149-153, 203
Arboviruses 86, 91
Avian Influenza 16-17, 24, 60, 67, 85, 91, 126, 130

B

Bacterial 36, 82, 86, 91, 100, 123, 142, 146, 175, 181, 196, 201, 203
Bacteriology 1-2, 7, 9-12, 174, 176
Bio-Eco-Communalism (BEC) 37

C

Clinical Veterinary Public Health 125-127, 130
Cluster sampling 68-72
Communalism 37, 50
Communicable Disease 19
Coxiella burnetii 174, 176-177, 179, 196, 198, 200, 205-206

E

Ecosystem 19, 22, 41, 43, 45, 55, 60, 63-64, 74, 83, 125
Environment 2, 19, 21-24, 33-35, 37, 40-44, 46-50, 55-56, 74, 83, 87-90, 106, 108, 114, 116, 119, 122-126, 129-131, 149-150, 153, 161, 165, 172, 177, 179, 181-182, 184, 196-197
Epidemiology 9, 15-16, 18, 44, 61, 66-70, 115, 121, 162, 164-165, 170, 174, 181, 197, 206

F

Food Chain 41, 142, 149-152

G

Global Health 1-2, 12, 16, 18-20, 130-131, 172
Global North 38, 56
Global South 38, 56
GMM 34-35, 38-42, 48-50, 55

H

Holism 33-35, 40, 44-45, 47-51, 56
Human 2-14, 16-23, 33-37, 39-50, 55-56, 59-68, 72-74, 82-86, 88-90, 92-93, 95-96, 98, 101-102, 108, 114-116, 118-119, 121-127, 129-133, 142-143, 146, 149-153, 160, 164-166, 170-172, 174, 179-182, 196-197, 200, 202-204, 206

I

Interdependence 33, 45-46, 48, 56, 129

O

One Health 1-5, 8-10, 13, 16-24, 33-35, 48-49, 51, 56, 59-63, 66, 68-69, 73-75, 82-85, 108, 113-114, 122, 124-127, 129-135, 142, 150, 152, 159, 162, 172, 174, 182, 195-196, 202

P

Population 5, 17, 24, 38, 43, 61-62, 64, 67-69, 73, 83-85, 87-89, 91, 97, 99, 114, 118-119, 121, 124-126, 128-129, 134, 142, 146, 163, 165-167, 172, 182, 201, 206
Prevalence 63, 67, 69, 71-72, 95, 129, 182, 201, 205-206
Public Health 1, 14, 17-19, 22, 34, 38-40, 42, 51, 60, 64, 66-67, 73, 82, 84-86, 90, 108, 113-114, 116-122, 124-125, 127-131, 134-135, 150, 159-170, 172, 174, 195-197, 199, 201, 204

Q

Q fever 14, 170, 174-176, 180-183, 195-206

R

Religion 1
Resistance 17, 19, 23, 41, 64-65, 106, 123, 142-144, 146-147, 149-153, 177
Risk Communication 40-41, 159, 164, 168-169, 171-172
Risk Governance 159-161
Risk Perception 164

S

Surveillance 15-16, 59-62, 64-66, 74-75, 85-86, 108, 122-123, 125-126, 132, 143, 151-152, 179

T

Tangwa 37, 47
Therapeutic Veterinary Public Health 118, 125, 127-129
Tick Borne Infections 86, 91

V

Vector-Borne Diseases (VBD) 159-160
Veterinarians 2, 11, 19, 21, 23, 35, 51, 62-63, 65, 73-74, 82-85, 113-115, 122, 124-125, 127, 132-133, 149, 151, 164, 172, 182, 197
Veterinary Public Health 14, 64, 113-114, 116-118, 120-122, 124-130, 135, 174, 195
Viral 12, 15, 82, 86, 91, 98, 133, 146

W

World Health Organization (WHO) 116

Z

Zoonoses 1, 4-5, 8-9, 11-16, 18, 20, 22-23, 35, 60-64, 66, 73, 75, 82, 84, 86, 88, 92, 108, 114, 123, 125-126, 132-133, 149
Zoonosis 4, 7, 9-11, 13, 16, 59, 83, 86, 88, 91-92, 102, 125, 132, 181, 198

www.ingramcontent.com/pod-product-compliance
Lightning Source LLC
LaVergne TN
LVHW061545290926
849162LV00004B/908